PAIN: MECHANISMS AND MANAGEMENT

From The Publisher

In keeping with the fine tradition of the **Cailliet Pain Series,** the newest and quite possibly most extraordinary contribution, *Pain: Mechanisms and Management,* strives to set new standards by providing the most up-to-date, efficient, and practical information in the eminent style of Dr. Rene Cailliet.

Although there are certainly other technical resources available, no other forum provides as concisely the most relevant information required for effective assessment, diagnosis, and treatment of patients suffering from the various aspects of pain and its implications.

On this 30th Anniversary of Dr. Cailliet's Pain Series he presents us with a new, comprehensive, cutting edge addition

PAIN: MECHANISMS AND MANAGEMENT
The Key to the Entire Pain Series

We would like to offer special thanks and gratitude to *Susan L. Michlovitz,* who helped conceptualize this book as an integral part of the Cailliet Pain Series.

PAIN: MECHANISMS AND MANAGEMENT

RENE CAILLIET, MD

Professor Emeritus and Chairman
Department of Physical Medicine and Rehabilitation
University of Southern California School of Medicine
Los Angeles, California

Illustrations by R. Cailliet, MD

 F.A. DAVIS COMPANY • Philadelphia

F.A. Davis Company
1915 Arch Street
Philadelphia, PA 19103

Printed in the United States of America

Last digit indicates print number: 10 9 8 7 6 5 4 3 2 1

Publisher, Nursing: Robert G. Martone
Production Editor: Crystal S. McNichol
Cover Design By: Donald B. Freggens

As new scientific information becomes available through basic and clinical research, recommended treatments and drug therapies undergo changes. The author(s) and publisher have done everything possible to make this book accurate, up to date, and in accord with accepted standards at the time of publication. The authors, editors, and publisher are not responsible for errors or omissions or for consequences from application of the book, and make no warranty, expressed or implied, in regard to the contents of the book. Any practice described in this book should be applied by the reader in accordance with professional standards of care used in regard to the unique circumstances that may apply in each situation. The reader is advised always to check product information (package inserts) for changes and new information regarding dose and contraindications before administering any drug. Caution is especially urged when using new or infrequently ordered drugs.

Library of Congress Cataloging-in-Publication Data

Cailliet, Rene.
    Pain : mechanisms and management / Rene Cailliet.
        p.   cm. -- (Pain series)
    Includes bibliographical references and index.
    ISBN 0-8036-1635-X (softback : alk. paper)
    1. Pain   I. Title   II. Series.
    [DNLM: 1. Pain--etiology. 2. Pain--therapy. WL 704 C134p 1993]
    RB 127,C336 1993
    616'.0472--dc20
    DNLM/DLC
    for Library of Congress   93-9422
                                                                    CIP

Preface

Pain was undefineable until the International Association for the Study of Pain[1] officially offered a classification and description. John Bonica[2] was the father of the approach of pain with his classic 1953 text, which he updated in 1990.[3] Bonica introduced the concept that pain is a specific disease entity rather than merely a symptom.

Albert Schweitzer, the Nobel Laureate physician who practiced in the African jungle for two decades, wrote "We must all die. But that I can save him from days of torture, that is what I feel as my great and ever new privilege. Pain is a more terrible lord of mankind than even death itself."[4] History is replete with instances of pain having influenced the lives of philosophers, generals, artists, musicians, scientists, and even biblical figures. In *Paradise Lost* Milton[5] writes

Pain is perfect miserie, the worst
Of evils, and excessive, overturns
All patience

The presence of pain and its significance has therefore been the scourge of mankind, and its cause and purpose has been the basis of speculation throughout antiquity. In ancient Egypt, India, and China, pain was believed to be caused by the gods, demons, and spirits of the dead. Hippocrates, the founder of medicine, postulated that there were four humors that controlled our bodies: blood, phlegm, yellow bile, and black bile,[6] and when these were unbalanced in proportion pain resulted.

Plato[7] (427 to 347 BC) believed that pain not only arose from peripheral stimulation but as an emotional experience in the soul, which resided in the heart. Pain and pleasure were opposite sensations that resided in the heart and were passions of the soul. In respect to current concepts it is remarkable how prophetic his thoughts were. Hippocrates stated "Divinum est opus sedare dolorum," which translates into "Divine is the work to subdue pain."

Harvey (1628), who discovered the concept of blood circulation, believed that the heart was the site of pain perception.[8] Pain and its theories have been described in the literature since humankind began writing, and apparently, suffering.

As the sensation of pain and its ravages have been described so have the theories of its causes, mechanisms, and treatments.

Pain originally was considered to be merely a sensation apart from those of touch, temperature, and position. Specific nerves were considered to carry the sensation of pain, and these fibers had specific nerve endings exclusively structured for this sensation.[9]

von Frey[10] originated the specificity of the end organs that he considered were responsible for initiating the nerve conduct of pain. These have been refuted but are of historical significance. The summation of intensity capable of causing pain via normal fibers carrying sensation of touch, pressure, and temperature was expounded by Erb[11] in 1874. In 1894 Goldscheider[12] fully expounded the theory that pain resulted from intensity of peripheral stimulation that caused a summation of sensory input at the dorsal horn within the cord.

In 1943 Livingston[13] postulated that the intensive peripheral stimulation of the nerves was the result of local tissue damage that activated the nerve fibers that projected to internuncial neuron pools in the spinal cord. These impulses bombarded the spinal cord transmission (T) cells with ultimate transmission to the brain for translation.

The dual transmission theory currently in vogue was initiated in 1959 by Noordenbos[14] who formulated the concept that sensations were transmitted centrally via two systems: myelinated ("slow system") and unmyelinated ("fast system") nerves. This lead to the current concept of gate by Melzack and Wall,[15] which has been further studied and modified. The reader is encouraged to read the excellent historical evolution of pain reviewed in Bonica.[3]

Besides the neuroanatomic and neurophysiologic concepts of pain in the last quarter century, numerous psychologic behavioral theories of pain have arisen.[16–18] The learned aspects of pain are now being investigated.

The following text attempts to discuss all the aspects of pain as currently understood: neuroanatomic, neurophysiologic, and psychosocial, as well as the basis for therapeutic programs. The evolution of acute pain, recurrent to chronicity, is explored. The recent involvement of the sympathetic nervous system and its neurohormonal aspect, which is most recently emerging, is also discussed.

References

1. Mersky, H (ed): Classification of chronic pain: Description of chronic pain syndromes and definition of pain terms. Pain (Suppl 3):S1, 1986.

2. Bonica, JJ: The Management of Pain (With Special Emphasis on the Use of Analgesic Block in Diagnosis, Prognosis, and Therapy). Lea & Febiger, Philadelphia, 1953.

3. Bonica, JJ (ed): The Management of Pain, ed 2, Vols 1 and 2. Lea & Febiger, Philadelphia, 1990.

4. Schweitzer, A: On the Edge of the Primeval Forest. New York, Macmillan, 1931, p 62.

5. Milton, J: Paradise Lost, Vol VI, line 462.

6. Keele, KD: Anatomies of Pain. Oxford, Blackwell, 1957.

7. Plato: Phaedo. (G.W. Geddes, ed). London, Macmillan, 1885.

8. Procacci, P and Maresca, M: The pain concept in western civilization: A historical review. In Benedetti, C, Chapman, CR, and Moricca, G (eds): Advances in the Management of Pain: Advances in Pain Research and Therapy, Vol 7. New York, Raven Press, 1984.

9. Dallenbach, KM: Pain: History and present status. Am J Physiol 52:331, 1939.

10. von Frey, M: Ber Verhandl konig sachs. Ges Wiss, Leopzig. Beitrage zur Physiologie des Shmerzsinnes 46:185–188, 1894.

11. Luckey, GWA: Some recent studies of pain. Am J Psychol 7:109, 1895.

12. Goldscheider, A: Ueber den Schmerz im Physiologischer und Klinischer Hinsicht. Berlin, Hirschwald, 1894.

13. Livingston, WK: Pain Mechanisms. New York, Macmillan, 1943.

14. Noordenbos, W: Pain. Amsterdam, Elsevier, 1959.

15. Melzack, R and Wall, PD: Pain mechanism: A new theory. Science 150:971, 1965.

16. Mersky, H and Spear, FG: Pain: Psychologic and Psychiatric Aspects. London, Balliere, Tindall and Cassell, 1967.

17. Sternbach, RA: Chronic pain as a disease entity. Triangle 20:27, 1981.

18. Fordyce, WE: Behavioral Methods for Chronic Pain and Illness. St. Louis, CV Mosby, 1976.

Toxonomy: Definition of Terms

Numerous terms have been applied in defining pain. The following terms include those published by the International Association for the Study of Pain: Subcommittee on Toxonomy,[1] but they have been modified by the author.

Acute pain: Unpleasant sensory perceptual or emotional response to an acute noxious stimulation of a tissue or an organ. "Acute" is defined as sharp, severe, coming speedily to a crisis.[2]

Afferent: Carrying impulses "toward" a center.

Algologist: A student investigator or practitioner of algology.

Algology: The science and study of pain phenomena.

Allodynia: Pain resulting from a stimulus that does not normally provoke pain.

Analgesia: Absence of pain in response to stimulus that would normally be painful.

Analgesic: An agent that produces analgesia.

Anesthesia: Absence of all sensory modalities.

Anesthesia dolorosa: An anesthetic area that develops pain.

Anesthetic: An agent that produces regional anesthesia.

Angina: Anterior thoracic pain related to cardiac disease.

Arthralgia: Pain in a joint.

Benign pain: A pain that persists with no known nociceptive input from the periphery.[4,5]

Causalgia: Pain described as "burning."

Central pain: Pain associated within the central nervous system, as opposed to peripheral pain.

Chronic pain: Pain that persists a month beyond the usual course of an acute injury or disease. This definition varies according to the clinician.

Chronic pain syndrome: Persistent, intractible pain inappropriate to existing physical problems or illness, with which the sufferer has excessive preoccupation.[3]

viii

Deafferentiation pain: Pain due to loss of sensation of an afferent fiber or fibers.

Dermatome: Segmental sensory area of a precise sensory nerve root.

Dysesthesia: An unpleasant abnormal sensation, usually not considered "pain."

Efferent: Carrying "away from" a central organ.

Hypalgesia: Lessened sensitivity to a painful stimulus.

Hyperalgesia: An increased painful sensation in response to a stimulus.

Hyperesthesia: Increased sensitivity to applied stimulation.

Hyperpathia: A painful syndrome in which there is increased overreaction to a stimulus.

Hypoalgesia: Diminished sensitivity to an otherwise noxious stimulus.

Hypoesthesia: Diminished sensitivity to a stimulus (not necessarily painful).

Neuralgia: Pain in the distribution of an afferent nerve.

Neuritis: Inflammation of a nerve or nerves.

Neuropathy: Impaired function of a nerve.

Nociceptor: A receptor sensitive to a specific stimulus that can be considered noxious.

Noxious: Harmful.

Noxious stimulus: A stimulus that is capable of potential or actual damage or injury to a body tissue.

Pain: An unpleasant sensory and emotional experience associated with actual or potential tissue damage or described in terms of such damage.

Pain threshold: The least intensity of stimulus at which a subject experiences pain.

Pain tolerance level: The greatest level of pain that a subject is capable (or willing) of tolerating.

Paresthesia: An abnormal sensation not specifically unpleasant.

Radiculalgia: Pain in the distribution of a sensory nerve root or roots.

Radiculitis: Inflammation of one or more nerve roots.

Radiculopathy: Disturbance of function in the distribution of one or more nerve root areas.

Somatic: Pertinent to structures of the body.

Suffering: A state of severe distress associated with threat to the body.

Temporal: Pertinent to or limited in time.

Threshold: Point at which a psychologic or physiologic effect begins to be produced. A measure of sensitivity.

Trigger point: A hypersensitive area (site) within a muscle or connective tissue.

References

1. Mersky, H (ed): Classification of chronic pain: Description of chronic pain syndromes and definition of pain terms. Pain (Suppl 3):S1, 1986.

2. Webster, N (ed): Webster's New Twentieth Century Dictionary of the English Language, ed 2. William Collins and World Publishers, 1978.
3. Black, RG: The chronic pain syndromes. Surg Clin North Am 55:4, 1975.
4. Pinsky, JJ: Chronic, intractible, benign pain: A syndrome and its treatment with intensive short term group psychotherapy. J Human Stress 4:17–21, 1978.
5. Boas, RA: Chronic benign pain. Pain 2:359, 1976.

Contents

Illustrations

CHAPTER 1

Neuroanatomy of Pain Mechanisms

Pain is a warning signal that helps to protect the body from tissue damage. Sherrington defined pain as a psychologic adjunct to a protective reflex, the purpose of which is to cause the affected tissue to be withdrawn from the potentially noxious (and injurious) stimuli.[1] Pain, unlike most other sensory modalities, has an essential function in survival.

The sensation of pain originates from the activation of nociceptive primary afferents by intense thermal, mechanical, or chemical stimuli. These nociceptor sites are small, free nerve endings in the numerous tissues of the body. There are numerous nociceptive stimuli.

Two decades ago it was thought that tissue damage and injury produced increased sensitization of the peripheral nociceptors and that this was the basis for hyperalgesia at the site of injury.[2] It was also thought that peripheral injury increased excitability in the spinal dorsal horn.[3] These concepts had clinical significance because if the excitability of the injured tissues of the periphery were diminished, it seemed apparent that the excitability of the central spinal horn—and thus pain—could also be diminished.[4] Today these initial concepts are being documented and verified.

The accepted neurophysiology of pain, a sensation transmitted through the peripheral and central nervous system until its final interpretation in the cortex, has undergone many changes in recent decades.

In the past, it was thought that pain depended solely on the intensity of stimulation and not on stimulation of a particular pathway with specific receptors. Pain can be evoked by a variety of different stimuli such as excessive cold or warmth, and it can be heightened by the concurrent presence of excessive noise or bright light. Frey postulated that separate anatomic endings could be stimulated to produce precise types of pain sensation.[5]

1

This concept has been refuted, but today specific nerve fiber types are considered to transmit sensation that ultimately will be considered "pain." For the most part, these are small myelinated A-alpha fibers and unmyelinated C fibers. This has been confirmed by recording action potentials when a painful stimulus (squeezing a muscle or injecting hypertonic saline) has been applied.[6] In a peripheral nerve block by procaine, the smallest-diameter nerve is initially affected, resulting in the cessation of pain before sensation to touch is lost. If nerve sensation is blocked by pressure, the function of myelinated nerve fibers is diminished or lost before that of the unmyelinated nerve, and touch sensation is lost before that of pain.[7]

Cutaneous A-alpha fibers respond to mechanical, chemical, and thermal stimuli. Among the chemicals currently identified as stimulating these receptors are potassium and hydrogen ions, histamine, bradykinin, and substance P. Hypoxia is also a noxious stimulus to muscle tissue. Interestingly, the neural tissues of the brain are insensitive to noxious stimuli.

In the recovery of function after injury, it is less well understood which fiber type carries specific sensation because awareness of pain sensation returns earlier than awareness of touch.[8]

The nature of pain as a specific entity remains obscure. Identification of specific fiber types transmitting pain sensation has been physiologically ascertained, and there is evidence that these painful sensations are carried within specific tracts in the spinal cord. However, there is no guarantee that interruption of these tracts will eliminate or modify pain sensation, as has been noted in causalgia, postherpetic neuralgia, phantom pain, and pain from cancer.

In evaluating the efficacy of cordotomy in relieving chronic pain, positron emission tomography (PET) studies have indicated that high cervical cordotomy apparently works by decreasing the blood flow at the thalamic level, particularly in the anterior quadrant of the thalamus contralateral to the side of nociception.[9] No changes were noted in the prefrontal or primary somatosensory cortex. Neuronal firing in the hypothalamus decreased. These findings indicate that a peripheral mechanism activates subcentral mechanisms, probably at the thalamic level.

Paresthesia, an unpleasant sensation but not necessarily pain, is a common symptom of diseases of the peripheral and central nervous system. Paresthesia can be produced by pressure on peripheral nerves. Ischemia may also elicit paresthesia.

Pain-producing substances have become prominent in pain research. Chemical mediators are released or synthesized from the damaged tissue. When these mediators, known as algogenic substances, accumulate in sufficient quantity, they activate the nociceptor sites.

Among these chemical mediators are phospholipids, which break down from arachidonic acid to form prostaglandin E (Fig. 1–1). Inflammatory mediators called leukotrienes are also liberated from trauma. These leuko-

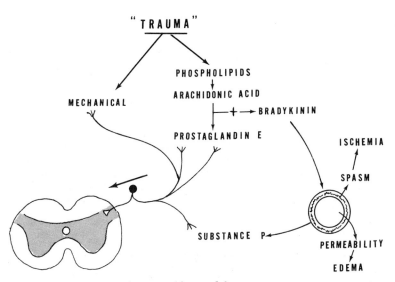

Figure 1–1. Nociceptive substances liberated from trauma.

Regardless of the type of trauma, the traumatized tissue liberates breakdown products from phospholipids into arachidonic acid and ultimately prostaglandins.

The trauma also affects the blood vessels causing spasm, edema, and liberation of platelets that break down to liberate serotonin and substance P. Other kinins and toxic substances are nociceptive products that irritate nerve endings and cause ultimate pain.

trienes do not undergo the same breakdown sequence as phospholipids and are not influenced by nonsteroidal anti-inflammatory drugs (NSAIDs). Trauma also causes a breakdown of blood platelets. This releases serotonin, which acts as a vasoconstrictor and causes local edema (Fig. 1–2). The resultant

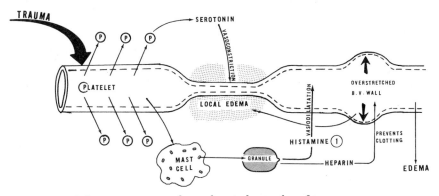

Figure 1–2. Schematic concept of vasochemical sequelae of trauma.

The microhemorrhage or macrohemorrhage releases serotonin, which causes vasoconstriction and releases mast cells. The granules of these mast cells release histamine, which causes vasodilation with resultant edema.

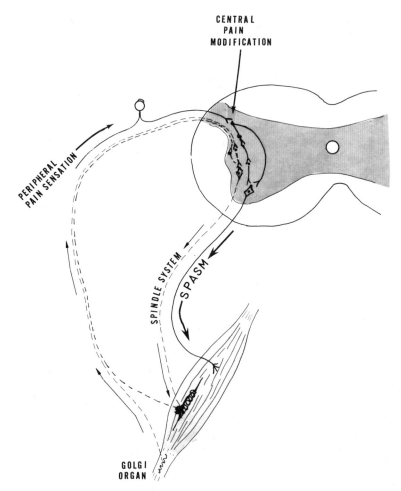

Figure 1–3. Neural pattern for production of spasm resulting from pain (postulated). The nociceptive impulses ascending to the dorsal horn become modified at the rexed layers. A mononeural reflex traverses to the ipsilateral anterior horn cell causing contraction of the extrafusal fibers of the muscle. The spindle system is also influenced and "reset."

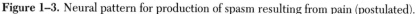

muscle spasm that locally accompanies trauma is possibly mediated through a neural pattern, wherein the nociceptor impulses emanating through the dorsal root ganglia (DRG) send impulses via neuronal connections to the anterior horn cell (AHC), with resultant muscular contraction (Fig. 1–3).[10] The nociceptor stimuli can emanate from the skin, blood vessels, joint capsules, ligaments, and muscles (Fig. 1–4). The muscle thus involved as recipient of the nociceptive reaction becomes an initiator of nociception, setting

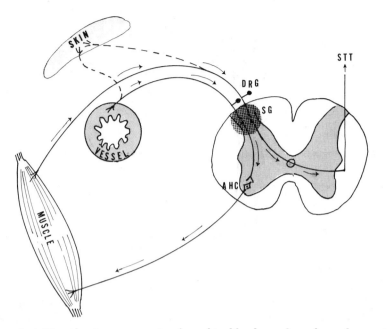

Figure 1–4. Neural patterns emanating from skin, blood vessels, and muscles causing "spasm." (A vicious cycle.)

The muscle held in sustained contraction (spasm) (Fig. 1–3) creates nociceptive substances that ascend through the dorsal root ganglia (DRG) into the substantia gelatinosum (SG) that traverses to the spinothalamic tracts (STTs) to the thalamus. A branch innervates the anterior horn cell (AHC), which causes further extrafusal muscle contraction. Muscle inflammation (ischemia, lactic acid, and so on) becomes the site of sustained nociception.

up a vicious cycle of painful muscle spasm which in turn becomes a nociceptor site of pain.

There are other chemical nociceptive mediators in addition to histamine, substance P, and the many leukotrienes which are being reported almost weekly in the research literature. Substance P, somatokinin, vasoactive polypeptides, and cholecystokinin are all present in small-diameter unmyelinated primary afferents that terminate in the superficial dorsal horn. Substance P is the most studied of these peptides, and its role of exciting transmission of the fibers that convey pain is well established.[11–12] Release of substance P from the peripheral terminals of these nerves produces a cutaneous wheal and flare so often noted in traumatic painful injury.[13] Inhibition of substance P transmission and peripheral emission could enhance the therapeutic armamentarium in controlling pain.[14]

The dorsal horn is divided into five laminas. The nociceptive fibers terminate in laminas I to IV (Fig. 1–5).[15–17] Areas of the dorsal horn of the

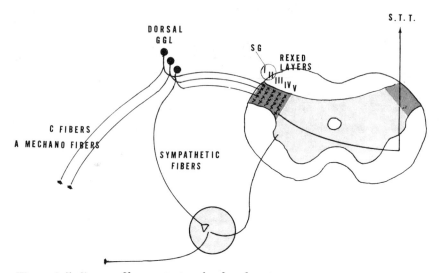

Figure 1–5. Sensory fibers entering the dorsal root.

The sensory C fibers, mechano A fibers, and sympathetic-sensory-afferent fibers enter the dorsal horn of the cord gray matter. The dorsal horn is divided into numerous (I–V or more) Rexed layers where the main sensory fibers enter Rexed layers I and II, which constitute the substantia gelatinosum (SG). Sensory impulses traverse the cord to ascend in the spinothalamic tracts (STTs).

One third of unmyelinated C fibers are considered to enter the dorsal column via the motor roots of the anterior horn (not shown).

spinal cord are innervated by both somatosensory and visceral autonomic fibers.

Lamina V responds to both cutaneous and visceral nerve stimulation.[18] Strong cutaneous stimulation can effect activity of preganglionic autonomic neurons in the lateral horns of the spinal cord.[19] These connections between somatic and sympathetic (autonomous) systems are of increasing clinical significance in determining the neurologic pathways of pain. Sympathetic discharges, fired over a long period of time, can initiate somatic muscle contractions, which become sites of nociception when their sustained contraction causes ischemia.

Two types of peripheral nociceptor fibers (fast and slow) have terminals in lamina V, although most terminate in laminas I to IV. Fully 80 percent of the afferent nerves which transmit the impulses that will ultimately evoke the sensation of pain are unmyelinated nerves (C fibers). These fibers conduct very slowly; they enter the dorsal column and immediately synapse with the neurons crossing through the anterior commissure to ascend to the thalamus via the spinothalamic tracts to the thalamus (Fig. 1–6). All of the remaining sensory nerves that can conduct noxious stimuli are myelinated nerves of small diameter. The larger-diameter myelinated sensory nerves respond to

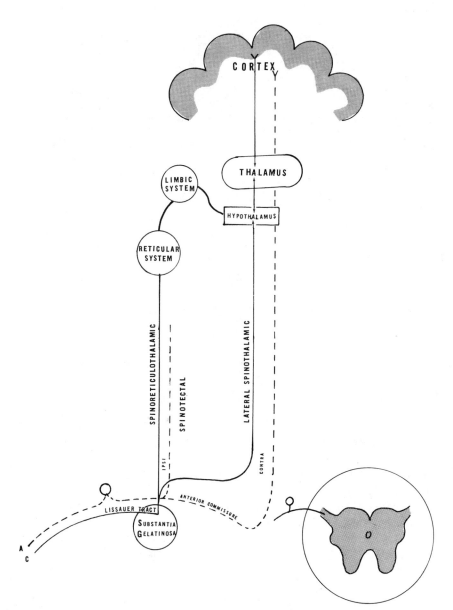

Figure 1–6. Major ascending sensory pathways of the spinal cord carrying pain mediating fibers.

The two major pathways for pain transmission are the spinothalamocortical system, which has spatiotemporal localization, and the spinoreticulothalamic system, which has no localization but is involved in emotional (limbic) and avoidance reaction. Both ascend through the substantia gelatinosum (SG) of Lissauer's tract (Rexed layers I and II). The reticular system associates with the hypothalamic-limbic system and relates emotions with sensation of pain.

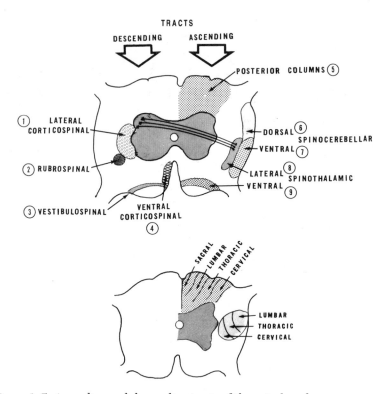

Figure 1–7. Ascending and descending tracts of the spinal cord.

In addition to the spinothalamic tracts[8,9] there are numerous tracts that carry motor, sensory, and coordinating functions. All are needed for function but not all transmit sensation nor all pain.

innocuous mechanical stimuli such as touch, temperature, and proprioceptive stimuli.

Anatomists have recently demonstrated that approximately one-third of all afferent small-diameter unmyelinated C fibers enter the cord through the anterior route.[20] The cell bodies of these fibers are also located in the DRG. This may well explain the mechanism of muscle pain, wherein descending motor fibers to the extrafusal fibers also carry ascending sensory fibers.

Pain sensation is also transmitted through the A-delta neurons that synapse in the dorsal horn of the cord and proceed superiorly through the lateral spinothalamic tracts (STTs) to the thalamus. Several sensations are transmitted via the STTs, of which an estimated 54 percent are pain sensations and 46 percent temperature sensations.

The unmyelinated C fibers are more numerous in the peripheral sensory fibers than the A-delta fibers and proceed cephalad in a different manner. The A-delta fibers have essentially one neuronal synapse, whereas the enter-

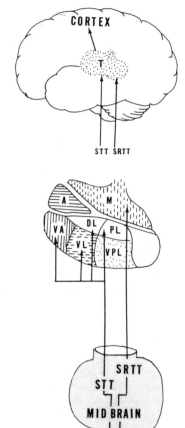

Figure 1–8. Thalamic pathways.

The thalamus (T) is a large ovoid gray mass located on either side of the third ventricle. The anterior tubercle (A) is thin and lies close to the midline. The posterior portion is known as pulvinar (P).

From the cord the ascending pathways that connect to the thalamus divide within the midbrain. They include the spinoreticulothalamic (SRTT) tract to the medial aspect of the thalamus and the spinothalamic tracts (STTs). They go directly to the lateral, ventral, and caudal regions. (A = anterior; VA = ventro anterior; DL = dorsolateral; VL = ventro lateral; PL = posterolateral; and VPL = ventropostero-lateral).

From the thalamus the pathways ascend to the cortex to as yet unknown areas of "representation."

ing C fibers synapse with numerous short intersegmental neurons that ascend cephalad through multiple ascending system (MAS) synaptic pathways. Some ascending paths are in the dorsal columns as well as in the anterolateral columns (Fig. 1–7). There are at least two major pathways in the spinal cord that are involved in rostral projection of the pain message: the STT and the spinoreticulothalamic tract (SRTT). Both ascend within the same tract in the cord, but the SRTT separates in the brainstem to synapse with neurons of the reticular system (Fig. 1–8). Activity of this latter pathway allegedly produces more diffuse and emotionally disturbing pain.[21]

Each of these tracts terminates at different sites in the thalamus: The SRTT is more medial and the STT projects into the lateral, ventral, and caudal lobes (Fig. 1–8). The two thalamic regions project to different cortical sites. At present, the action of these projections remains unclear.

The speed of impulse selectivity determines the type of pain transmitted. The A-delta fibers transmit faster and carry "sharp" pain, whereas the

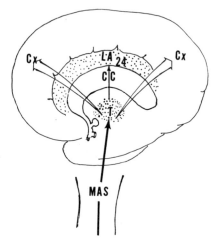

Figure 1–9. Thalamocortical projections. From the multiple ascending system (MAS) of the cord the tracts ascend to the thalamus (T) from which there are pathways to the limbic system (LA) thence to the cortical areas (Cx).

The limbic regions of the cingula above the corpus callosum (CC) are numbered according to the Brodmann designation.[24] (See Figure 51, page 178 in Gilman, S and Winans, SS (eds): Manter and Gatz's Essentials of Clinical Neuroanatomy and Neurophysiology, ed. 6. FA Davis, Philadelphia, 1982.)

C fibers are slower and carry a "dull," longer-lasting pain. In head and face pain, the trigeminal nerve consists of fibers that carry sharp pain and travel toward the thalamus within the lateral and trigeminal lemnisci, ending in the ventrobasal nucleus of the thalamus.

The ascending fibers of the MAS synapse with neurons of the thalamocortical aspects of the thalamus (Fig. 1–9) then proceed to the reticular system in the midbrain (Fig. 1–10), which processes diffuse fibers from all cranial nerves and upper motor-sensory brain systems including the cortex. The reticular system also relates to the hypothalamus and limbic systems, which interpose the emotions to the sensory system. The reticular system relates to another structure located at the floor of the fourth ventricle, the locus coeruleus, which appears to be directly related to the emotions of fear and anxiety as well as being involved in pain modulation. This area will be thoroughly evaluated in Chapter 4 of this text.

The thalamus divides into two major sytems: the MAS and the ventrobasal. The latter consists of the lateral and posterior nuclei, which receive the fast conducting impulses. This system is topographically organized, meaning that the sensations received relate to specific points of the face, head, and body. The neurons of the MAS are not specifically organized. These latter fibers radiate to the general cerebral cortex and the limbic system, which is concerned with memory and emotions.

Significant findings have emerged regarding the neural pathways to the thalamus as a result of percutaneous cordotomies and ultimate pathologic studies.[9] Anterolateral cordotomy in monkeys produced degeneration of the ipsilateral nucleus ventralis (ventral posterior lateral [VPL] nucleus) of the thalamus (Fig. 1–11). Studies with horseradish peroxidase demonstrated that 83 percent of the ventrothalamic tracts terminated in the ipsilateral thalamic nuclei. In 1937 Bowsher demonstrated that patients who underwent cor-

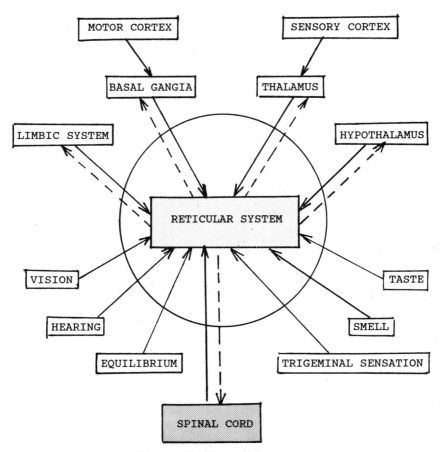

Figure 1–10. The reticular system.

dotomy for treatment of pain underwent massive bilateral degeneration of cells in the medial reticular formation (medulla) and some degeneration in the pons.[17] He reported that there was sparse degeneration in the thalamus, however.

These recent studies are significant, as pain results when the antero-lateral (contralateral) tracts of the cord are stimulated peripherally with noxious impulses. Because of the contralateral pathways of these ascending cord pathways, the finding that 17 percent of the ascending fibers are ipsilateral is significant. There are also direct or contralateral projections of STTs to the posterior thalamus and the periaqueductal gray area whose functional significance is unknown at present.

Stimulation of the VPI nucleus does not elicit pain, whereas stimulation of the more medial intralaminal nuclei does elicit pain. The relationship between these two thalamic projections remains unclear.

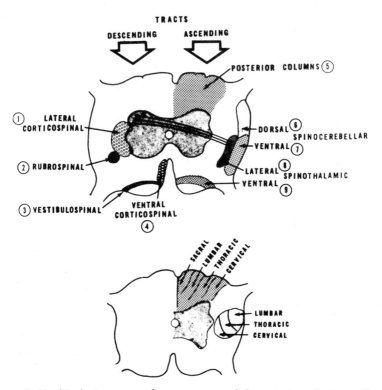

Figure 1–11. *(Top)*, Sensory and motor tracts of the spinal cord. Generally, the descending tracts (1,2,3,4) are motor, or for coordination, and the ascending tracts (5,6,7,8,9) carry sensation from the periphery to the higher centers. *(Bottom)*, The ascending tracts convey the sensations of pain, touch, proprioception, and discrimination for interpretation. Areas of the extremities are conveyed by the ascending *(dotted area)* and descending (lumbar, thoracic, and cervical) tracts.

Cordotomy, which causes a decrease of the cerebral blood flow (CBF) to the thalamus,[9] may alter the synaptic activity of the entering STT impulses. After successful cordotomy, the CBF increases. Glycerol injection into the trigeminal ganglion in the treatment of intractable trigeminal neuralgia has also been found to increase CBF.[22–23] This is further evidence that peripheral pain mechanisms perform with simultaneous associated central mechanisms.

The afferent fibers that enter the dorsal horn relay the information of the nociception (Fig. 1–9). These are termed projection, or transmission, fibers. This information is complex; it originates from both nociception and nonnociception, therefore carrying other innocuous sensations. In the dorsal root, besides unmyelinated sensory fibers carrying nociceptor impulses, there are afferent myelinated fibers, which enter the dorsal horn of the cord carrying inhibitory impulses (Fig. 1–12). The large myelinated fibers that enter the dorsal horn essentially moderate or inhibit the nociceptive impulses

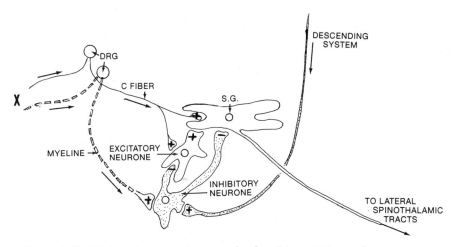

Figure 1–12. Nociceptive transmission to the dorsal horn of the cord.
A schematic version of nociceptive transmission to the dorsal horn is presented. X is the noxious stimulus that is transmitted through afferent C fibers and myelinated large diameter fibers. In the substantia gelatinosum (SG) of the dorsal horn the impulses go to and activate (+) the transmission cell of the SG. Impulses from the myelinated fibers activate the inhibitory neurons (−), which modulate the projection cell. Ultimately, the impulses are transmitted to the lateral spinothalamic tracts (LSTTs) where they ascend to the thalamus. The descending tracts also modulate the impulses arriving at the transmission cells.

transmitted via the unmyelinated C fibers. This explains the efficacy of transcutaneous electrical nerve stimulation (TENS), which is carried by the large myelinated fibers.

If the large myelinated fibers are interrupted, the nociceptive fiber impulses are uninhibited, causing the pain to be more severe. This indicates that a peripheral stimulus, either noxious or innocuous, reaches the dorsal horn and undergoes modulation at that site. As noxious stimuli are transmitted via all the sensory fibers—unmyelinated and myelinated—these sensations must be modulated at the cord level. This is known as the Wall-Melzack gate theory of pain modulation, as shown in Fig. 1–13. The modulation was thought to occur at the dorsal horn level, but is now known to occur at the dorsal root level and at more central levels in the midbrain area as well.

PAIN MODULATION

There are intrinsic factors in the system that modulate pain. This realization underlies much of our current understanding of how narcotic and

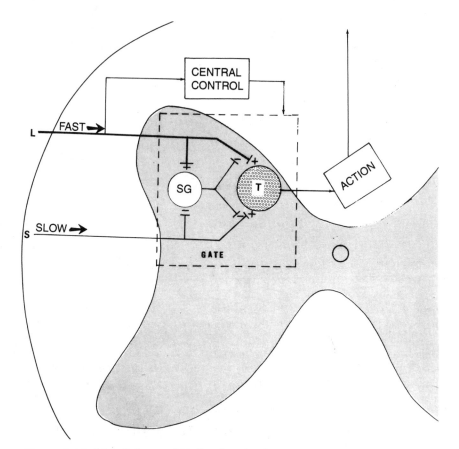

Figure 1–13. "Gate" theory of Wall and Melzack.
The gray area is the dorsal horn region of the cord. The Rexed layers I and II are the substantia gelatinosum (SG). The sensory afferent fibers carrying nociception are the "slow" C fiber neurons that activate (+) the SG. The impulses then proceed via the fibers ascending to the reticular formation via spinoreticulothalamic tracts and the spinothalamic tracts (STTs) to the thalamus and the reticular system. These impulses are ultimately interpreted at the cortex as pain.

Fast fibers (A-α) and mechano (A-Δ) (I) fibers are inhibitory (−) in that they modulate the intensity of the slower fiber activity.

analgesic drugs and various physical modalities work and indicates the direction for future studies.

Endogenous opioid substances are now considered to be synthesized by and within nerve cells. These substances, which mimic the action of narcotics and analgesics, are termed *endorphins (enkephalins)*.

As the neurologic sites became apparent, subsequent research elucidated the chemical and physiologic aspects of these pain-modulating processes in the hypothalamus, midbrain, periaqueductal gray area, and rostral medulla.

Fields and Levine[24] pose some interesting and as yet unanswered questions: Why does the brain need this pain-modulating system? When is it activated? And how are its actions manifested?

Enkephalins, which act at the peripheral neural sites, also occur at the DRG, spinal cord, midbrain, hypothalamus, periaqueductal gray area, and rostral medulla.[25] The first neuropeptides discovered were leucine and methionine enkephalin. Many more have been found since.

Currently identified are amino acids (glutaminic acid and aspartic acid), which act on N-methyl-D-aspartate (NMDA) receptors at the dorsal horn.[20] The hyperactivity of the central receptors can be initiated by electrical stimulation of C fibers, which apparently occurs via these NMDA receptors.[22] The hyperexcitability can be prevented by administration of D-CPP NMDA antagonists.[26] Ketamine, a noncompetitive NMDA antagonist, has been considered effective in reducing postoperative pain.[26] Similar drugs to ketamine are now being sought, and sites other than NMDA are also being researched.

Other neurochemical mediators from tissue damage have been found to initiate hyperexcitability of the central nervous system, and their antagonists afford promise in the future of pain management. Included among the numerous endorphins are norepinephrine and serotonin.

Serotonin (5-hydroxytryptamine) has been divided into three main types, each having a subtype of receptor. The dorsal raphe in the midbrain has the highest concentration of serotonin type $1a$ receptors in the brain.

The hypothalamus may be the activation site of migraine and cluster headaches. The posterior thalamus, which contains cells that regulate autonomic function, is closely related to the anterior hypothalamus, which contains the suprachiasmic nuclei. These nuclei control the principal circadian functions in mammals. This may explain the rhythmicity of many pains, including the time-related cluster headaches and other pains. This hypothalamic pacemaker is mediated by the serotonergic system.[27]

There is now evidence that NMDA plays a major role in several types of seizures, including epilepsy. The role of NMDA in migraine, migraine variants, and cluster headaches remains unclear.

The International Association for the Study of Pain (IASP) has characterized neural pain mechanisms along five axes: (1) site of pain, (2) physiologic system, (3) temporal pattern and recurrence, (4) intensity and duration, and (5) etiology.[28–29]

All the above neurologic mechanisms have been postulated on the mechanism introduced by Foster and Sherrington in 1897, implying that all messages transmitted within the central nervous system are transduced electrically.[30] There are numerous synapses (Fig. 1–14) along the course of the nerves where messages are converted into chemical (metabolic) impulses

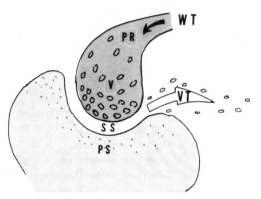

Figure 1–14. Synapse.
The wiring transmission (WT) functions by electrical stimulation of the preganglionic bulb (PR), which is charged with numerous vesicles (V) containing acetylcholine. When released across the synaptic space (SS) they cause depolarization of the postsynaptic membrane (PS) causing electrical-chemical direct neurotransmission.

The release of particles out of the synapse forms the vehicle that migrates (VT) in the interspaces to locate their receptors.

and then back to electrical impulses. These messages are considered to be diffusable molecules, termed *neurotransmitters*.

In this concept the postsynaptic neuron depolarizes thousands of signals at the synapse and thus generates an action potential. This constituted the neuron theory of Waldeyer and Cajal.[31] Golgi partially refuted this theory and offered instead a reticular network theory, terming his concept a "functional syncytium."[32] The term *syncytium* is defined as "a group of cells in which the protoplasm of one cell is continuous with that of adjoining cells."[31]

Agnati et al.[34] have recently proposed a provocative concept of neural transmission which questions the accuracy of the electrical continuity of presynaptic and postsynaptic transmission. This has been highlighted by electron microscopic studies. This hypothesis accepts transmission within the neural network (Waldeyer and Cajal), but it also postulates diffusion of electrochemical signals via the extracellular medium.

This supports Golgi's concept and does not refute the ultimate transmission of impulses through the central nervous system, the hypothalamus, the thalamus, and so forth. It merely questions the medium through which transmission occurs. The former system is termed *wiring transmission* (WT) and the latter *volume transmission* (VT) (Fig. 1–15).

Signals are conducted via electrical and chemical impulses through the extracellular fluid. Direct anatomic pathways cannot be identified, but the signal release site and the target can be identified (Fig. 1–16). The WT system fails to support morphologic coupling between neurotransmitter release sites and receptor sites (Fig. 1–17). The presynaptic nerve supposedly couples with numerous postsynaptic receptors, leading to the term *transmitter-receptor* mismatch.[35–36]

The VT concept requires that the specific target be present to accept the specific impulse being transmitted through an ill-defined transmission system. In this theory a "code" must exist.[37] The VT system theory seems

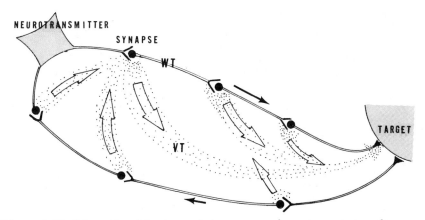

Figure 1–15. Schematic wiring transmission versus volume transmission of neurotransmission.

Direct neurotransmission resembling a direct wire transmission (WT) is depicted as going directly to its specific receptor *(dark arrows)* albeit via synapses.

At each synapse there allegedly leak chemical neurotransmitters that enter the interstitial spaces and chemically find their receptors. This transmission goes in afferent and efferent directions *(white arrows)*.

to have more validity than the WT system theory because it is more efficient. Although impulses are transmitted at low speed and with a high degree of divergence, only a limited number of transmission lines (axons) and switches (synapses) are required. Hence the VT system theoretically functions with

Figure 1–16. Transmission of wiring transmission versus volume transmission.

The wiring transmission (WT) indicates that a specific connection be made from the neurotransmitter to its specific receptors organ.

In the volume transmission (VT) concept the chemical neurotransmitters leave the synapse and are free to find their receptors wherever they are and as numerous as they may be.

One VT or WT does not replace the other but merely enhances each and explains chemical transmission (see text).

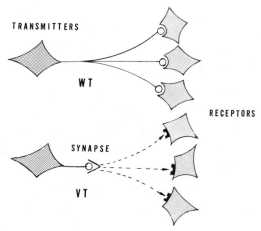

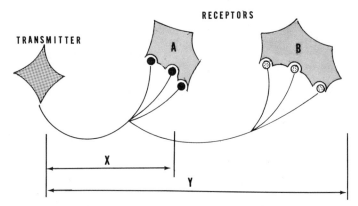

Figure 1–17. The concept of "mismatched" transmitter and receptors.
The mismatching between transmitters and receptors is schematically postulated in the above. The distance a neurotransmitter must go varies from distance X to distance Y causing B to receive the "message" later than receptor A.

Receptor A may have a higher affinity than receptor B and one may be in a higher density than the other. A different reaction results despite an initial similar transmitter release.

significantly less biologic costs. The type of energy used in the process of transmission has not been ascertained.

The results of certain experiments seem to confirm the presence of a VT transmission. For instance, a complex neuropeptide like neuropeptide-Y (NYP)[56] injected via microcannula into the striatum is able to reach distances over 1 mm in sufficient dosage to be an active neurotransmitter. Its ultimate presence initiates a sustained modulation of the central nervous system receptors creating a syndrome response. [38–39]

The ability to achieve analgesia resulting in insensitivity to pain without loss of consciousness is affected at all levels of the central nervous system by a "descending pain control system."[40]

Stress has been invoked as objectively and subjectively influencing pain perception. Two neuroendocrine systems are thought to be involved in the coping mechanism of stress: the hypothalamo-pituitary-adrenocortical system and the hypothalamo-sympatho-adrenocortical. The roles of these two systems are mediated by medullary-pontine catecholamine neurons and by corticotropin-releasing hormone (CRH) neurons. [41–42] The intricacy of these transport systems, which cause somatic visceral responses to stress, involve several neuronal systems of transportation that trigger "syndrome responses." The WT and VT systems are both involved.

The old concept of a single isolated system of afferent transmission relating to pain mechanisms is therefore no longer tenable. This concept was oversimplistic. More recent studies suggest another system, one that can explain the return of pain after a successful surgical lesion of ascending pathways has been performed for the relief of pain.

The concept of psychophysiologic pain may explain why chemical substances and hormones affect receptor sensitivity. Systemic opioids and epidural administration that are affective at the cord level now suggest that both VT and WT systems are operating.

CHRONIC PAIN MECHANISMS

Acute pain relates to recurrent pain and can ultimately become chronic pain. In the past, chronic pain was considered to be any pain that lasted longer than 3 months, but some pain states are considered chronic in shorter periods of time. The way in which acute or recurrent pain becomes chronic requires an understanding of the mechanisms of pain. The concept that pain is a specific sensation and that its intensity is proportional to the degree of tissue damage is no longer tenable. Pain is a sensory experience influenced by attention, expectancy, learning, anxiety, fear, and distraction.[28]

The selection and modification of the sensory component of noxious transmission is neurologically accepted (Fig. 1–6), but the receptive system of the dorsal horn and every higher level is directly influenced by attention, expectancy, learning, anxiety, and fear (among others) (Fig. 1–18).

Emotions affect the peripheral ventral mechanisms of pain transmission through the limbic system, which then affects the descending tracts to the dorsal horn of the cord and ascending tracts to the thalamus (lateral STTs and SRTTs), and finally the cortex (Fig. 1–19). These emotions are basically of three categories: (1) perceptual information locating the site of the noxious insult, (2) motivational tendency indicating the need for reaction by the patient, and (3) cognitive information which is based on previous information.[28] The perceptual information implies the significance of the tissue damaged and its sequelae. The motivational information causes fight or flight, and the cognitive information involves previous experiences and their sequelae. Anxiety, anger, depression, and so forth are all involved. Treatment of chronic pain must consider and attack all these sites.

Pain is modulated by chemical substances that are secreted by nerve cells (endorphins) that can be experimentally blocked by naloxone. The release of nociceptive substances that initiate ultimate pain and the resultant relief by endorphins can be blocked by naloxone. This has shed much light on causation of pain by trauma, stress, anxiety, and depression and clarifies the inhibition of pain within the central nervous system.

Chronic pain has too long been viewed by the medical profession as an organic-psychogenic dichotomy. We must now consider it to be a complex synthesis of biologic, psychologic, behavioral, and neurohormonal-chemical

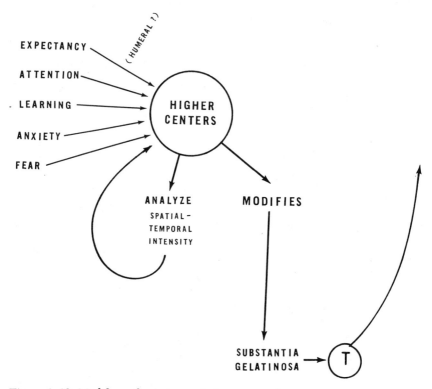

Figure 1–18. Modifiers of pain transmission.

The higher centers, which interpret pain as a sensation, are modified by humeral factors that involve expectation, attention, learning, anxiety, and fear. These factors modify and analyze sensation at the gray matter level (SG) of the cord (T) and at the thalamus-hypothalamus and the cervical cortex.

factors. The role of the autonomic nervous system in the realm of pain will be addressed in the next chapter.

In summary there are essentially three sensory centers (Fig. 1–20). The first center contains the peripheral receptors with fibers mediating impulses through the dorsal roots to the dorsal horn of the cord. The second center is at the midbrain level and involves the thalamus, reticular system, and so on. The third center contains the cerebral cortex, where the pain is localized and qualified.

ROLE OF THE CEREBRAL CORTEX IN PAIN PERCEPTION

A provocative theory has been offered by Melzack[43] in evaluating the role of the brain in perceiving pain. He questions the prevalent theory that

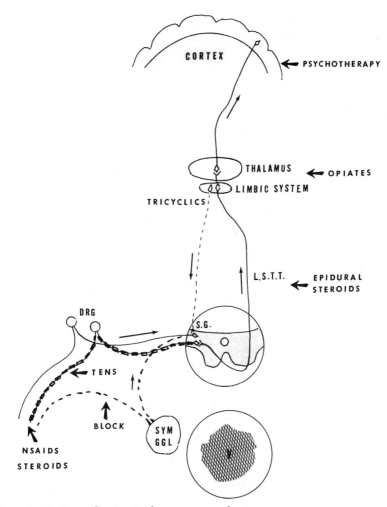

Figure 1–19. Sites of action in the treatment of pain.

The aspirin, steroid, and nonsteroidal sites of action are at the peripheral areas of noxious tissue injury. The myelinated nerves respond to TENS and the sympathetic nerves transmitting pain respond to sympathetic blocks. The lateral spinothalamic tracts (LSTTs) are the site of epidural steroids and anesthetic agents, and the thalamus is the site of opiates. Psychotherapy influences the interpretation of pain at the cortex level. Tricyclics and other antidepressants affect the descending tracts to the dorsal root (substantia ganglia [SG]). The dorsal root ganglion (DRG) also is affected by tricyclics.

the brain acts as a passive receptor of information from the outside world. He does not question the current concepts of transmission, and in fact accepts them. All current research verifies these concepts. How the pain is interpreted by the brain is his concern.

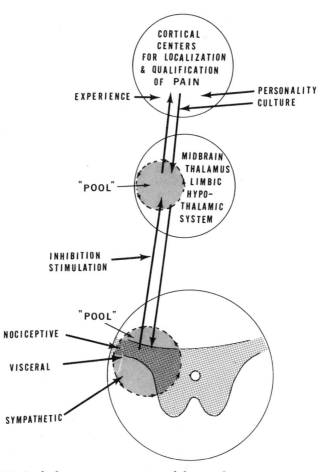

Figure 1–20. Pool of sensory centers in modulation of pain.
From the periphery the first pool is at the gray matter of the dorsal horn of the cord and ascends from there to the midbrain and ultimately the cortical centers. (See text for details.)

The direct ascent to the brain was postulated by Descartes in the 17th century. He held that the brain was the center of sensation and further postulated that pain was transmitted to the brain by means of small threads running from the skin to the brain (Fig. 1–21). The emphasis is on the periphery: receptors, fibers, nociceptive and other peripheral substances and pathways of the cord, thence to the midbrain, and finally the cortex. But this does not explain why paraplegics and quadriplegics can "feel" their bodies even though there is no nerve transmission. Melzack postulates that "the brain can generate every quality of experience which is normally triggered by sensory input."

Stimulus from the periphery can initiate sensory patterns, but it cannot

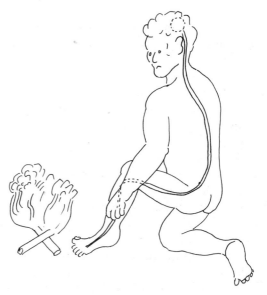

Figure 1–21. Kneeling man perceiving pain (Descartes). The Descartes kneeling figure (1596–1650) depicts a burning sensation irritating the filaments of a nerve in the foot ascending to the brain via the filaments of that nerve. (Rene Descartes' illustration from "De l'homme" was modified by the author).

produce them. According to Melzack, the patterns, in this case, pain, are present in the brain "substrate" with genetic specifications modified by experience. This substrate is a network of neurons, or loops, between the thalamus and the cortex which he terms the *neuromatrix*. The repeated cyclic processing and synthesis of the impulses through the neuromatrix form a *neurosignature*. A sentient neural hub converts the flow of these neurosignatures into a flow of "awareness," which in turn activates an action neuromatrix: a pattern of movements influenced by the awareness (in this case, pain).

The neuromatrix consists of a widespread network of neurons that form patterns felt and experienced as a "whole body." Melzack states: "We do not learn to feel qualities of experience: our brains are built to produce them." This concept is consistent with the molecular concept of neural activity postulated by Black,[44] in which environmental regulators effect changes in existing genetically encoded molecular structures. Black's molecular concept is consistent with Melzack's theory and gives insight into how the brain understands sensations from the periphery. Simplistically, both Black and Melzack postulate that our total body is encoded in the molecular structure of the central nervous system and is constantly being modified by external impulses. The concepts are made up of a chemical and electrical "neural language." These theories are now being documented in various laboratories.

Since the advent of PET, a test that ascertains the precise area of CBF, the brain region that is activated by peripheral stimulation can be determined.

There is evidence that there is frontal lobe involvement following noxious electrical skin stimulus. Painful peripheral heat application causes activation of both the anterior cingulate gyrus (a part of the limbic system) and the primary and secondary somatosensory cortices.[45] Nonnoxious stimulation activates only the primary somatosensory cortices. This suggests that the secondary cortices are involved in pain perception, whereas the primary cortices are involved in mechanoreception. Further radiation elicited by these noxious stimuli may reach and be modified by the parietal and frontal cortices after being modulated in the subcortical (hypothalamic and limbic) levels.

Studies also suggest that hormones may be involved in pain perception. Hormones are products created by endocrine glands that acted on distant organs. Recent studies now confirm that the brain is an endocrine organ. The study of psychoneuroendocrinology is evolving, but much remains to be clarified. It is feasible that in the future much of our understanding of pain will reside in this area (Fig. 1–22).

Neurotransmitters have been termed *paraneurons*, as they secrete substances significantly related to hormones. Structurally, hormones are proteins or polypeptides. Examples of these hormonal compounds include adrenocorticotropic hormone (ACTH), thryroxine, beta endorphine, and steroids. Most hormonal compounds exert their effect in a tonic rather than a phasic manner and act over a longer period of time than do neurotransmitters, which exert their neurotropic effect in milliseconds.

It is well known that corticotropin-releasing hormone (CRH), corticotropin, and cortisol are elevated in response to a variety of physical and psychic stresses.[46] The principal neuroanatomic site of action lies within the limbic midbrain and ascending reticular system. Although the release of glucocorticoids serves homeostatic needs (phasic), prolonged activity may result in structural neuropathology that is more lasting than an acute behavioral change.

The existence of endogenous opiate substances has been well documented, but their effect on appetite regulation, learning, memory, motor activity, and immune function are still under study.

Antidiuretic hormone (ADH; also called vasopressin) is released from the posterior pituitary gland but is triggered by pain and emotional stress. ADH is secreted by neurons that originate in the paraventricular nucleus and terminate in the median eminence of the hypothalamus. It is of interest that cerebrospinal fluid (CSF) ADH is lower in depressed patients than in normal patients.

Thyrotropin-releasing hormone is known to be involved in many systems, but its effect on neurotransmission remains sparce.

Not yet fully explored is the relationship of pain to *chronobiology*—the circadian rhythms. The identification of the central role of the hypothalamus in the regulation of circadian rhythms has raised the possibility that neural pathways pass temporal pathways to the hypothalamus. A pathway from the

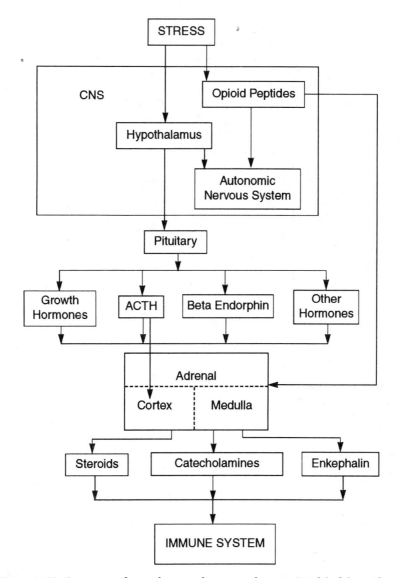

Figure 1–22. Sequence of neurohormonal aspects of stress. (Modified from Shavity, et al: J Immunol 135:836S, 1985.)

retina (retinohypothalamic tract [RHT]) has been identified projecting to the suprachiasmic nuclei (SCN).

The SCN are small, bilaterally symmetrical nuclei that lie above the optic chiasm of either side of the third ventricle in the ventral hypothalamus.

These nuclei receive fibers from the RHT. Two other afferent pathways to these nuclei are involved in the circadian system. One originates from the raphe nuclei of the midbrain and the other is a bilateral projection from the ventral lateral geniculate nuclei. The efferent pathways from the SCN are predominantly to the hypothalamus.[47]

Bilateral destruction of the SCN has eliminated the circadian secretion of corticosteroid in the rat. That and many other behavioral and physiologic functions are being discovered within the circuits of the SCN. Most biologic rhythms pass unnoticed unless they are disturbed by some disease states, work shifts, or meridional travel. Patients with major depressive disease have a disruption in their physiologic regulation of the sleep-wake cycle attributable to dysfunction of the circadian rhythm.[48]

Newer concepts will undoubtedly evolve that will implicate other neurophysiologic and psychoneuroendocrine pathways and related changes. The field of pain research is evolving rapidly.

REFERENCES

1. Sherrington, CS: The Integrative Action of the Nervous System. Yale University Press, New Haven, 1906/1947.
2. Woolf, CJ: Evidence for a central component of post-injury pain hypersensitivity. Nature 306:686–688, 1983.
3. Dunner, R: Neuronal plasticity and pain following peripheral tissue inflammation or nerve injury. In Bond, M, Charlton, E, and Woolf, CJ (eds): Proceedings of the VIth World Congress on Pain. Pain Research and Clinical Management, Vol 5. Elsevier, Amsterdam, 1991, pp 263–276.
4. Wall, PD: The prevention of postoperative pain. Pain 33:289–290, 1988.
5. Frey, M von: Beitrage zur Sinnesphysiologie des Schnerzsinns. Ber Sachs Ges Wiss Meth Phys Gl. 46:185, 196, 283–296, 1894.
6. Zotterman, Y: Touch, pain and tickling: An electrophysiological investigation on cutaneous sensory nerves. J Physiol 95:1–28, 1939.
7. Sinclair, DC and Hinshaw, JR: A comparison of the sensory dissociation produced by procaine and by limb compression. Brain 73:480–498, 1950.
8. Napier, JR: The return of sensibility in full thickness skin grafts. Brain 75:147–166, 1952.
9. Di Piero, V, Jones, AKP, Iannotti, F, Powell, M, Perani, D, Lenzi, GL, and Frackowiak, RSJ: Chronic pain: A PET study of the central effects of percutaneous high cervical cordotomy. Pain 46:9–12, 1991.
10. Dubner, R: Specialization in nociceptive pathways: Sensory discrimination, sensory modulation and neuronal connectivity. In Fields, HL, Dubner, R, and Cervero, F (eds): Advances in Pain Research and Therapy, Vol 9. Raven Press, New York, 1985, pp 111–133.
11. Hokfelt, T, Johannsson, O, Ljungdahl, A: Peptidergic neurones. Nature 284:515–521, 1980.
12. Hunt, SP, Kelly, JS, Emson, PC: An immunohistochemical study of neuronal populations containing neuropeptides or gamma-aminobutyrate within the superficial layers of the rat dorsal horn. Neuroscience 6:1883–1898, 1981.
13. Brimijoin S, Lundberg, JM, Brodin, E: Axonal transport of substance P in the vagus and sciatic nerves of the guinea pig. Brain Res 191:443–457, 1980.
14. Gamse, R, Holzer, P, and Lembeck, F: Decrease of substance P in primary afferent

neurones and impairment of neurogenic plasma extra-vasation by capsaicin. Br J Pharmacol 68:207–213, 1980.

15. Light, AR and Perl, ER: Reexamination of the dorsal root projection to the spinal dorsal horn including observations on the differential termination of coarse and fine fibers. J Comp Neurol 186:117–132, 1979.
16. Fields, HL and Basbaum, AI: Brainstem control of spinal pain-transmission neurons. Ann Rev Physiol 40:217–248, 1978.
17. Bowsher, D: Pain mechanisms in man. Res Staff Phys 29(12):26–34, 1983.
18. Selzer, M and Spencer, WA: Convergence of visceral and cutaneous afferent pathways in the lumbar spinal cord. Brain Res 14:331–348, 1969.
19. Aihara, Y, Nakamura, H, Sato, A, and Simpson, A: Neural control of gastric motility with special reference to cutaneo-gastric reflexes. In Brooks, C, (eds): Integrative Functions of the Autonomic Nervous System. Elsevier, New York, 1979, pp 38–49.
20. Davies, SN and Lodge, D: Evidence for involvement of N-methylaspartate receptors in "wind-up" of class 2 neurones in the dorsal horn of the rat. Brain Res 424:402–406, 1987.
21. Melzack, R and Casey, KL: Sensory motivational and central control determinants of pain. In Kenshalo, DR (ed): The Skin Senses. CC Thomas, Springfield, IL, 1968, pp 423–443.
22. Salt, TE and Hill, RG: Pharmacological differentiation between responses of rat medullary dorsal horn neurons to noxious mechanical and noxious thermal cutaneous stimuli. Brain Res 263:167–171, 1983.
23. Trans Dinh, YR, Thural, C, Serrie, A, Cunin, G, and Seylaz, J: Glycerol injection into the trigeminal ganglion provokes a selective increase in human cerebral blood flow. Pain 46:13–16, 1991.
24. Fields, HL and Levine, JD: Pain mechanisms and management. Western J Med 141(3):347–357, 1984.
25. Fields, HL and Basbaum, AI: Brainstem control of spinal pain-transmission neurons. Ann Rev Physiol 4:451–462, 1978.
26. Woolf, CJ and Thompson, SWN: The induction and maintenance of central sensitization is dependent on N-methyl-D-aspartic acid receptor activation: Implications for the treatment of post-injury pain hypersensitivity states. Pain 44:293–299, 1991.
27. Raskin, NH: Serotonin receptors and headache. New Engl J Med 325:353–354, 1991.
28. Mersky, H: Classification of chronic pain: Description of chronic pain syndromes and definitions. Pain (Suppl)3:S1–S225, 1986.
29. Melzack, R: Psychological concept and methods for the control of pain. In Advances in Neurology, Vol 4. Raven Press, New York, 1974, pp 275–280.
30. Fulton, JF: Physiology of the Nervous System. Oxford University Press, London, 1943, p 52.
31. Kandel, ER: Brain and behavior. In Kandel, ER and Swartz, JH (eds): Principles of Neural Science. Edward Arnold, London, 1983, p 4.
32. Luciani, L: Fisiolgia dell'Uomo. Societa' Editrice Libraria, Milano, 1912, p 239
33. Thomas, CL (ed): Taber's Cyclopedic Medical Dictionary, ed 15. FA Davis, Philadelphia, 1985.
34. Agnati, LF, Tiengo, M, Ferraguti, F, Biagini, G, Benfenati, F, Benedetti, C, Rigoli, M, and Fuxe, K: Pain, analgesia, and stress: An integrated view. Clinical J Pain 7(Suppl 1):S23–S37, 1991.
35. Kuhar, MJ: The mismatch problem in receptor mapping studies. Trends Neurosci 8:190–191, 1985.
36. Zoli, M, Agnati, LF, Fuxe, K, and Bjelke, B: Demonstration of NPY transmitter-receptor mismatches in the central nervous system of the male rat. Acta Physiol Scand 135:201–202, 1989.
37. Swartz, TW, Fuhlendorff, J, Langeland, N, Thogersen, H, Jorgensen, JC, and Sheikh, SP: Y1 and Y2 receptors for NPY. The evolution of PP-fold peptides and their receptors. In

Mutt, V, Fuxe, K, Hokfelt, T, and Lundberg, JM (eds): Neuropeptide Y. Raven Press, New York, 1989, pp 103–114.

38. Agnati, LF, Zoli, M, Merlo Pich, E, Benfenati, F, and Fuxe, K: Aspects of neural plasticity in the central nervous system, VIII. Theoretical aspects of brain communication and computation. Neurochem Int 16:479–500, 1990.

39. Agnati, LF, Zoli, M, Merlo Pich, E, Benfenati, F, Grimaldi, R, Zini, I, Toffanoo, G, and Fuxe, K: NPY receptors and their interactions with other transmitter systems. In Mutt, V, Fuxe, K, Hokfelt, T, and Lundberg, JM (eds): Neuropeptide Y. Raven Press, New York, 1989, pp 103–114.

40. Nieuwehuys, R (ed): Chemoarchitecture of the brain. Springer-Verlag, Berlin, 1985, p 36.

41. Kurosawa, M, Sato, A, Swensen, RS, and Takahashi, Y: Sympatho-adrenal medullary functions in response to intracerebroventricularly injected corticotropin-releasing factor in anaesthetized rats. Brain Res 367:250–257, 1986.

42. Ehlers, CL, Henrikson, SJ, Wang, M, Rivier, J, Vale, W, and Bloom, FE: Corticotropin releasing factor produces increases in brain excitability and convulsive seizures in rats. Brain Res 278:332–336, 1983.

43. Melzack, R: Central pain syndromes and theories of pain. In Casey, KL (ed): Pain and Central Nervous System Disease. Raven Press, NY, 1991, pp 59–75.

44. Black, RG: A laboratory model for trigeminal neuralgia. Adv Neurol 4:651–658, 1974.

45. Kalin, NH and Dawson, G: Neuroendocrine dysfunction in depression: Hypothalamic-anterior pituitary systems. Trends in Neurosci 9:261–266, 1986.

46. Ganong, W: The stress response: A dynamic overview. Hosp Prac 23(6):155–190, 1988.

47. Moore, RY: The suprachiasmic nucleus and the organization of a circadian system. Trends Neurosci 5:404, 1982.

48. Moore-Ede, MC, Sulzman, FM, and Fulle, CA: The Clocks That Time Us: Physiology of the Circadian Timing System. Harvard University Press, Cambridge, MA, 1982.

CHAPTER 2

Pain Mediated Through the Sympathetic Nervous System

The major part of the nervous system is under voluntary control and concerned with activation of the skeletal muscle system. It is also concerned with transmission of sensory impulses from the periphery for feedback information in neuromuscular activities and interpretation of noxious stimuli. Another division of the nervous system controls the activities of smooth muscles, cardiac musculature, and glandular secretion. This is the autonomic nervous system (ANS), which is not under voluntary control. The role of the ANS in the transmission of noxious sensory impulses currently remains unconfirmed.

The functional anatomy of the ANS is well documented (Fig. 2–1). The ANS includes the central portion at the cortical midbrain level, the spinal cord level, and the peripheral level. The peripheral portion consists of pre-ganglionic and postganglionic efferent and afferent fibers. Only the relationship of the ANS to the sensation of pain will be emphasized.

The ANS fibers transmit visceral sensations such as nociception, nausea, feelings of fullness, and so on.[1] The concept that the ANS is restricted merely to efferent function has been refuted. Function cannot be maintained merely by efferent nerve input because normal function, albeit reflex, requires feedback via afferent fiber function.

The peripheral efferent pathways of the ANS, unlike the single fiber of the somatic nervous system to the skeletal muscle fibers, consist of two neuron connections: a primary presynaptic (preganglionic) connection and a secondary postsynaptic (postganglionic) connection (Fig. 2–2). The cell bodies of the axons start as groups located in the brainstem and spinal cord. As they proceed toward their peripheral destinations, they pass through

29

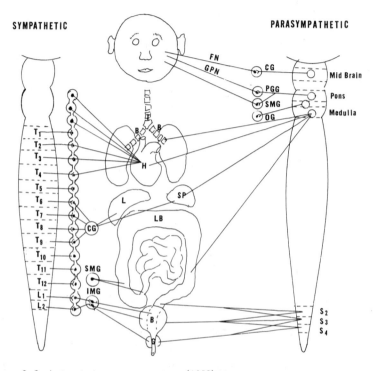

Figure 2–1. Autonomic nervous system (ANS).

A schematic description of the sympathetic and parasympathetic nervous system and its innervations. The ANS arises from the lateral horn cells of the thoracic vertebrae (T). The lateral horn cells in turn synapse with the celiac ganglia (CG), superior mandibular ganglia (SMG), and otic ganglion (OG).

These in turn innervate the organs depicted: The facial nerve (FN) and glossopharyngeal nerves (GPN) to the head and face, and the CG, SMG, and inferior mesenteric ganglia (IMG) to the large bowel and urinary tract.

The parasympathetic system derives from the midbrain, pons, and medulla, and the sacral system from S-2, S-3, and S-4 segments.

The sympathetic system innervates the heart (H), bronchi (B), spleen (SP), liver (L), and large bowel (LB). The bladder (B), genitalia (G), rectum and sigmoid are innervated by the sacral outflow.

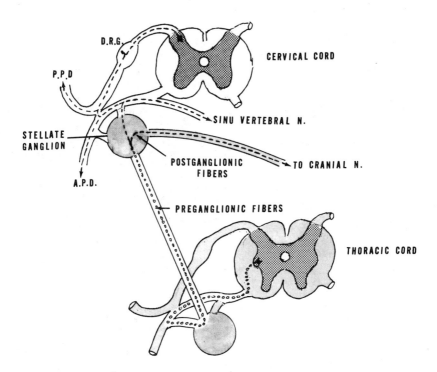

Figure 2–2. Sympathetic nervous system.

The preganglionic white fibers originate from the intermediolateral horn cells of the thoracic cord and ascend to the stellate ganglia where they synapse with the postganglionic gray fibers.

Sympathetic fibers accompany the somatic nerves within the anterior primary divisions (APD) and the posterior primary divisions (PPD) of nerve roots.

The sensory nerves enter the dorsal column via the dorsal root ganglia (DRG). The sympathetic nerves carry pain sensation (paresthesia) and are a motor to the blood vessels, sweat glands, and pilatory glands.

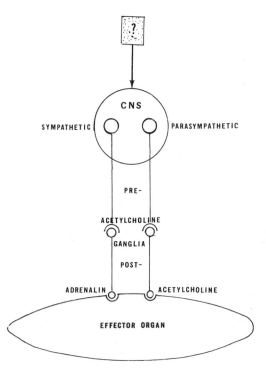

Figure 2–3. Transmitter sequence of autonomic nervous system.

The box represents the transmitter substance from numerous sources that initiate autonomic impulses in the sympathetic and parasympathetic central nervous systems (CNS).

At the termination of the preganglionic fibers acetylcholine is liberated at the ganglia. The postganglionic fibers release adrenaline at the effector organs, and the parasympathetic fibers liberate acetylcholine.

various ganglia, at which point they synapse to new fibers that eventually proceed to the effector organs (Fig. 2–3).

The preganglionic fibers leave the brainstem and spinal cord at three levels: the cranial outflow, the thoracolumbar outflow, and the sacral outflow.[2] The cranial and sacral portions form the parasympathetic nervous system, and the thoracolumbar portion forms the sympathetic nervous system.

The cranial outflow consists of the nucleus of Edinger-Westphal, the nucleus of Perlia, and the dorsal motor nucleus of the vagal system originating in the midbrain, the pons, and the medulla. The cranial outflow synapses in the celiac, oculomotor, pterygopalatine, submandibular, and otic ganglia. These, in turn, divide into the facial nerve and the glossopharyngeal nerve to innervate facial structure.[3] The sacral outflow (S-2, S-3, S-4) forms the pelvic nerve (N erigens). None of these segments contribute to the ANS.

The function of neurons is considered to be the axonal transport of protein, which is conveyed along the length of the nerve fiber (Fig. 2–4). This transported protein tissue is highly dependent on adequate blood supply. Pressure on the nerve axon causing blood vessel impairment impairs axonal transportation.

The terminals of the parasympathetic system liberate acetylcholine and are termed *cholinergic*. The postganglionic sympathetic fibers (except those

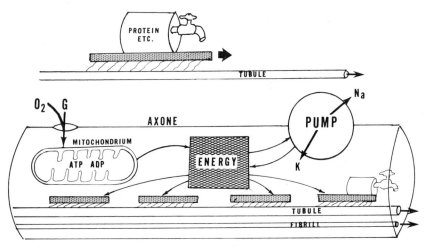

Figure 2–4. Axoplasmic neural transport: A theory.

The *flow* of protein and other derivatives begins with entry of glucose (G) into the fiber. Glycolysis and phosphorylation occur (O_2) in the mitochondria through metabolism of adenosine-triphosphate (ATP), which creates the energy to the sodium pump. This pump regulates balance of sodium (Na) and potassium (K) and determines nerve activity.

The transport *filaments* (F) move along the axon by oscillation and carry the nutritive protein elements along the nerve pathway. (Data from Ochs, S: Axoplasmic transport: A basis for neural pathology. In Dyck, PJ, Thomas, PK, Lambert, EN (eds): Peripheral Neuropathy. WB Saunders, Philadelphia, 1975, pp 213–230.)

to sweat glands) liberate epinephrine-like substances. Many systems are supplied by both systems where they have opposing action.

The preganglionic fibers of the sympathetic division leave the spinal cord along with other motor fibers of the ventral root, but they soon separate from the ventral roots to form the white rami communicants (Fig. 2–5). These fibers pass on to the paravertebral ganglia, which are long ganglionated chains of nerve fibers extending along either side of the entire vertebral column. Many of these white rami terminate in ganglia, but some do not synapse at these sites. Instead, they proceed on to synapse within the ganglia of the specific organ system (celiac or mesenteric). The postganglionic fibers, after synapse, form plexi that envelop the large blood vessels supplying the viscera. An example is the lower fibers forming the hypogastric plexus, which enters the pelvis and innervates the rectum, bladder, and reproductive organs.

The postganglionic fibers are unmyelinated and thus are termed gray rami communicants. Each spinal nerve receives a gray ramus fiber, which innervates specific blood vessels and sweat glands in their region. A major function of the sympathetic nervous system, one that causes a generalized

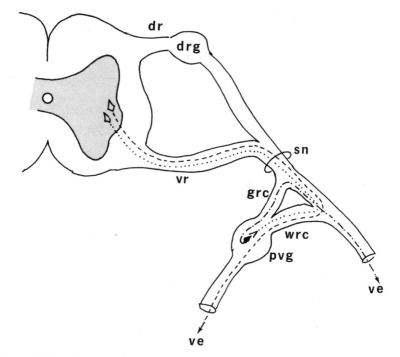

Figure 2–5. Autonomic fibers in a spinal nerve.

The lateral horn cells from which emerge the autonomic nerves are located in the gray matter of the cord. The dorsal root ganglia (DRG) is the site of emergence of the somatic nerves (DR).

The afferent autonomic nerves emerge via the ventral root on to the spinal nerve (SN), which then proceeds to the paravertebral ganglia (PVG). The preganglionic fibers enter the ganglia through the white ramus communicans (WRC) where some proceed without synapse and others synapse to reenter the spinal nerve through the gray ramus communicans (GRC). These proceed down the primary division of the nerve root. (VE = visceral efferent nerves.)

bodily reaction, is to supply the adrenal gland, which liberates adrenaline in addition to the adrenaline secreted at its terminals.

The medulla of the adrenal gland is innervated by preganglionic fibers that do not synapse in intervening ganglia. Because this nerve supply is involved in the glandular system of the body, it is associated with adrenaline secretion resulting from rage, fear, anger, and reaction to cold. It also explains the cardiac reaction relating to pulse rate and blood pressure, the dilation and constriction of the coronary blood vessels and pulmonary bronchioles, and even the spleen's release of red blood cells to the body.

In 1933, Cannon and Rosenbleuth postulated that there must be two sympathins: one excitatory and the other inhibitory.[4] This has now been ascertained: Noradrenaline is the principal postganglionic sympathetic trans-

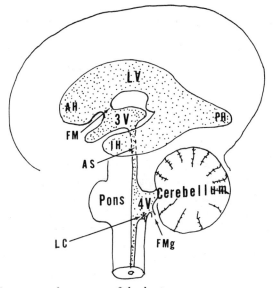

Figure 2–6. The ventricular system of the brain.

A schematic illustration of the ventricular system of the brain containing the spinal fluid. (LV = lateral ventricles; AH = anterior horn; PH = posterior horn; IH = inferior horn; FM = foramen of Monro; 3V = third ventricle; AS = aqueduct of Sylvius; 4V = fourth ventricle; FMg = foramen of Magendie; LC = site of locus coeruleus neurons.)

mitter, and adrenaline is liberated at the sympathetic nerve endings in smaller doses.

Adrenaline acts on two separate types of receptors, termed *alpha* and *beta*. Activation of alpha receptors produces effects that are blocked by ergotamine and causes vasoconstriction, uterine contraction, and pupil dilation. Beta activation causes vasodilation, cardiac acceleration, and relaxation of the bronchioles. Adrenaline acts equally on both receptors, whereas noradrenaline acts almost exclusively on alpha receptors.[5] How adrenaline and norepinephrine are deactivated after release remains unknown.[6] Adrenergic "blockade" implies blocking the catecholamine neurohumeral transmission system at any of the sites of action.[7] Originally, it was thought to be destroyed by the enzyme amine oxidase with reserpine as the blocking agent. These agents inhibit synthesis, storage, or release.

Control of the final common pathway of sympathetic release is currently believed to be the locus coeruleus (LC).[7,8] The LC is a small band of neurons located at the base of the fourth ventricle within the brain substance (Fig. 2–6).[9] The fourth ventricle is a cavity bound ventrally by the pons and dorsally by the cerebellum. It is connected to the third ventricle by the aqueduct of Sylvius and caudally to the central canal of the medulla. The floor, known as the rhomboid fossa, is formed by the dorsal surfaces of the medulla oblongata, and the lateral boundaries of the floor of the cerebellar peduncles. This is where the LC is located.

The LC consists of many neurons. The neurons have the highest density of norepinephrine (NE) of any neurons in the brain.[10] When stimulated the LC liberates NE to the cerebral cortex, limbic system, brainstem, and spinal cord.[11] This tends to create symptoms of anxiety and fear. When the stimulus abates, so do these emotions.[12] The LC may be the final pathway for the manifestation of psychologic stress, physical trauma, immune imbalance, and even viral infection causing a sympathetic-parasympathetic imbalance.[13]

During a state of anxiety the LC is maintained at a constant alert. This results in a depletion of the postganglionic presynaptic sympathetic endplates and may lead to a condition termed *sympathicotonia*, which is considered prevalent in many disease states, including chronic pain states.[13]

Stimulation of the LC in animals has raised questions as to whether the adjacent nonadrenogenic neurons in the region of the fourth ventricle are stimulated or ablated, causing the reaction attributed to the specific LC neurons. This site of action has also been questioned by noradrenaline blocking of the postsynaptic noradrenaline being released by propranolol, a beta blocker.[14]

Anxiety has been invoked in the mechanism of acute and chronic pain. In 1872, Darwin discussed fear merging into terror and described physiologic changes involving the sympathetic nervous system.[15] Adrenaline was thought to be the stimulating factor.[16] Failure of an infusion of adrenaline to induce emotional symptoms caused Cannon to postulate a central nervous system mechanism.[17] The limbic system was also thought to be involved.[18]

Areas of the parietal lobe of the brain have been implicated in anxiety. Area 24 of the cortical region has been related to the control of emotions as well as affective response to pain.[19,20] Area 24 receives ipsilateral projections from the ventral border of the thalamus, which has been implicated in the reception of nociceptive impulses. Neurosurgical resection of this cortical area in patients with intractable pain has caused the patient still to acknowledge pain but to "complain less."[21,21A]

Recent studies[22] have determined temporal and spatial features of pain to occur in the parietal area of the brain and an emotional reaction to pain to occur in the limbic region of the frontal lobes.

As mentioned in Chapter 1, there are two neuroendocrine systems that affect stress in the transmission of pain: the hypothalamo-pituitary-adrenocortical and the hypothalamo-sympatho-adrenomedullary. Corticotropin-releasing hormone (CRH) may be the main chemical that triggers the neuroendocrine response to stress, which is mediated via the wire transmission (WT) and volume transmission (VT) systems acting on its target.[23,24]

The delay in recognizing pain as emanating from the ANS was "Its lack of neurotomal distribution of symptomatology."[25] Review of the ANS and pain have clarified the problem.[26-28]

Fontaine and Leriche[29] electrically stimulated the cervical sympathetic trunk between the occiput and the middle ganglion and provoked painful anxiety but of no dermatomal distribution. This stimulation produced severe pain in the lower jaw teeth and behind the ipsilateral ear.

Patients whose spinal cords have been severed (quadriplegics) or who are under spinal anaesthesia feel pain when the arteries are constricted. Considering arteries to be "sensitive," Fontaine and Leriche felt that this phenomenon was a sympathalgia.[29] These topographic zones were considered to be the region of the vascular area supplied and were associated with vasomotor, sudomotor, and trophic changes.[30]

Three indications suggest the relevance of sympathetic nervous system involvement in pain.

1. Neuropathic pain is frequently exacerbated by stimuli, such as a startle reflex or other acute emotional activity, that evoke sympathetic discharges. It is unclear whether sympathetic discharge exacerbates or maintains the pain.[1] Hu and Zhu[31] demonstrated that nociceptors discharging after prolonged noxious stimulation, hence being algogenic, are further excited by sympathetic discharge and norepinephrine discharge. This merely explains that the sympathetic system may exacerbate and/or prolong the pain but not necessarily initiate or mediate it.

2. Neuropathic pain is frequently accompanied by signs and symptoms that indicate abnormal sympathetic activity such as excessive vasomotor or sweat reactions. In this respect, a causalgic hand that is pale, cold, and cyanotic—usually considered evidence of sympathetic vasoconstriction—may actually be due to circulating catecholamines "caused by" vasoconstriction. The opposite, a hot erythematous causalgic hand usually considered to be sympathetically caused by vasodilation, may be erythematous because of antidromic vasodilation from C fiber nociceptor sensitization.

3. Relief of pain has often been achieved by interrupting the sympathetic nervous system by chemical or surgical means. This is true in many, but not in all cases. It is thought that this interruption, whether surgical or chemical, may interrupt contiguous afferent nerve fibers running along the sympathetic fibers.

What indicates that there is a sympathetic influence in the provocation of pain is the finding that a regenerating axon from an injured or severed nerve forms "sprouts" (Fig. 2–7).[32] These sprouts develop sensitivity to NE, which has been created by the alpha-adrenergic receptors that release further discharges upon exposure to NE. Stimulation of the damaged nerves that have formed sprouts further liberate NE, which results in the firing of the nerve.[33] Injury to a nerve that severs axons creates NE receptors at the terminal endings of the nerve indicating that peripheral connections remain.[34]

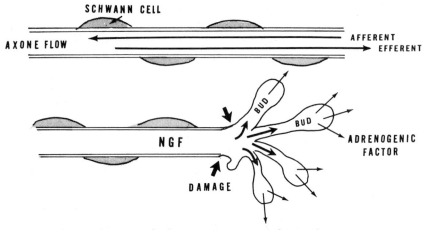

Figure 2–7. Axonal outgrowths forming a neuroma (schematic).

After a nerve injury with compression or partial to total severance, the nerve growth factor (NGF) stimulates the nerve to advance distally and form "buds," which create more endings than the normal nerve shown in the upper drawing.

By virtue of the greater secretion of adrenogenic factors, the nerve becomes more sensitive to adrenogenic agonists and transmits more potential pain fiber impulses to the spinal cord. (See also Fig. 2–10).

Trauma to a nerve can cause saccule formation of the membrane with the accumulation of catecholamines (Fig. 2–8). The normal transmission of impulses is modified. The catecholamines within the saccule now become "generators" as well as transmitters and veritable ectopic sites of causalgic pain. The adrenergic receptors that form on the surface of the saccule increase local sensitivity and may account for the resultant allodynia.

Nociceptors that are released in response to prolonged continuing noxious stimuli are further intensified by exposure to NE.[31] This implies that a connection exists between the afferent nociceptor reaction to noxious stimuli and sympathetic efferents.[35]

A local discharge of peptides in the area of tissue innervated by the injured nerve may send antidromic impulses that release further afferent peptides to the periphery: a domino concept.[1] All these findings, however, fail to clarify whether the resultant pain is caused by or is a sequela of abnormal sympathetic impulses.

The reason for performing a sympathectomy in an extremity that demonstrates hyposympathetic activity has been questioned.[36] Relief of pain from sympathetic intervention is also questioned as not all patients with identical conditions respond favorably from sympathetic interruption. The possibility has been raised that sympathectomies may also interrupt the primary afferent axons that are located in the region of the ganglion. When injected into the dorsal root ganglion (DRG), morphine alleviates the pain without any evi-

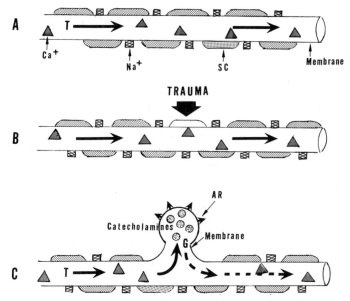

Figure 2–8. Ectopic generator evolving from nerve injury.
A, Normal nerve, which is a transmitter (T) of impulses within the membrane
(M). The Schwann cells (SC) of the membrane form the myelin sheath. The electrolytes sodium (Na⁺) and calcium (Ca⁺) generate the impulse. B, Trauma damages
the Schwann cells of the membrane. C, At the site of trauma there is a release of
catecholamines, and the membrane forms a saccule containing these catecholamines,
which become generators (G) of abnormal impulses *(broken line)*. Adrenergic receptors (AR) form on the membrane surface of the saccule explaining the hypersensitivity
of the nerve at that site. (Modified from Devor, M: Nerve pathophysiology and
mechanisms of pain in causalgia. J Autonom Nerv Sys 7:371–384, 1983.)

dence of sympathetic blockage.[37] Patients who have sympathectomies performed in the treatment of Raynaud's phenomenon often have causalgia after
the procedure.

A provocative research paper that questions clinical experiences[38] discussed the vasomotor changes resulting in peripheral nerve injuries resembling reflux sympathetic dystrophy (RSD). Reference was made to the article
by Wakisaka,[35] who created a laboratory model for RSD. Skin temperature
changes were described in the plantar skin following a mechanical constriction applied to the sciatic nerve (rat) that deviated from the expected sympathetic vasomotor reaction.[35]

Loose ligatures were applied to the sciatic nerve at midthigh causing
swelling and constriction of the nerve. Morphologic studies of the nerve at
this site revealed loss of large myelinated nerve fibers but sparing of the
unmyelinated nerves. Sprouting, indicating regeneration, occurred within
days at these injured nerve sites. This was considered to be an ideal model

of RSD, as the afflicted rats expressed behavioral reaction consistent with pain.

The commonly believed vasoconstriction activity occurring in painful neuropathies, cold or hot skin reaction attributed to sympathetic flow, was questioned.[39]

In Wakisaka's rats the skin in the region of the constricted nerve remained hotter than normal for 10 days and colder than normal for the remaining 3 to 4 weeks postconstriction. During the initial reaction the noradrenergic innervation of the plantar skin blood vessels appeared normal. When the skin became cold, noradrenaline, neuropeptides Y, and dopamine-b-hydroxylase were absent. These findings implied that skin temperature was not necessarily correlated to sympathetic activity.[39]

The unitary reaction of the sympathetic nervous system, described in the usual textbooks of physiology, are questioned as being different from severe stress in normal conditions and are dependent on the target organs regulated by the sympathetic central nervous system. There is no basis for the expectation of "generalized" sympathetic tone[40] from sympathetic intervention.

Human cutaneous blood vessels, as target organs, are complex. Blood vessels of the hands and feet have a noradrenergic supply in a normal ambient temperature. The blood flow through these vessels is directly related to sympathetic activity: cooling from adrenergic constriction, and warming from decreased sympathetic activity. Which of the arterial vessels—precapillary arterioles, postcapillary capacitance vessels, or arteriovenous anastamosis— receive significant specific sympathetic innervation is not known. Vasodilatory mechanism remains unclear.[40]

Environmental temperature changes affect the smooth muscles of the blood vessels and alter the reaction of sympathetic nerve control.[41] Whether cutaneous blood vessels are properly reinnervated after denervation is not clear;[42] the effect of "adaptive supersensitivity" following denervation[43] also is not clear.

Whether or not the dystrophic aspects of RSD are attributable to vasomotor activity remains controversial, or at least unproven. Clinically, the diagnosis of causalgia in everyday practice is rare, and the dystrophic aspects of RSD seen in clinical practice are not frequently recognized or appropriately evaluated and treated. The criteria for diagnosing RSD remain imprecise, the pathophysiology unclear, and the therapeutic approach ambiguous.[37] Tentative diagnostic criteria have been proposed.[44]

RSD is a descriptive term referring to a complex disorder or group of disorders that may develop as a consequence of trauma affecting the limbs, with or without obvious nerve lesion. RSD may also develop after visceral diseases and central nervous system lesions or, rarely, without an obvious antecedent event. It consists of pain and related sensory abnormalities, abnormal blood flow and sweating, abnormalities in the motor system, and

Figure 2–9. The principal nuclei of the hypothalamus. The various groups of the hypothalamus. The efferents passing to the thalamus are probably the major routes to the cortex. (NPV = nucleus paraventricularis; NPO = nucleus preopticus; NSO = nucleus supraopticus; NHP = nucleus hypothalamicus; NHD = nucleus hypothalamus dorsomedicalis; MMN = medial mamillary nucleus; NHR = nucleus hypothalamus retromedicalis; AC = anterior commissure; OC = optic chiasma; I = infundibulum.)

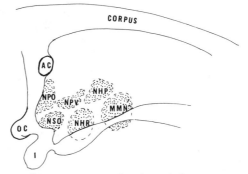

changes in structure of both superficial and deep tissues ("trophic" changes). It is not necessary that all components are present. The term RSD is used in a descriptive sense and does not imply specific underlying mechanisms.

A psychophysiologic model of RSD can be proposed merely based on a limited clinical experience, but more precise experimental and objective clinical study is needed to precisely explain the neurophysiology of RSD. The recent finding of an animal model will enhance the clarification of the central and peripheral components, the neuroeffector transmission, the neurovascular aspects of the affected blood vessels, and the mechanisms of the nociceptors and their identification and effect on the vascular smooth muscles. As clarification of neural mechanisms emerge, meaningful diagnostic criteria will ensue as will appropriate physiologic therapy.

The neuropsychologic-humoral aspect of pain merits discussion, especially since excessive NE released by anxiety, stress, and fear is considered important. Psychologic stress over a long period of time causes stimulation of the hypothalamus via the reticularis paragigantocellularis (RPG) in the medulla. From the medulla there are many projections to the hypothalamus, especially the paraventricular nuclei (PVN) (Fig. 2–9).[45] The PVN contains neurons that release vasopressin and oxytocin, which enter the posterior pituitary gland.

There is a chemical interplay between the posterior and anterior pituitary glands with a release of corticotropin (ACTH). This is termed "preponderance of sympathetic release." The resultant hypothalamic-pituitary-adrenal axis (HPA) is the neurologic and hormonal response to stress.[46-48]

In many painful states there is hypersensitivity of the involved tissues apparently mediated through mechanoreceptors in areas already hypersensitized. Clinically, pain can be elicited by mere touch. The theory explaining this concept is that repeated impulses from the nociceptor C fibers impinge on the substantia gelatinosum in the dorsal horn (layers of Rexed I and II), causing hypersensitivity of the wide dynamic range (WDR) neurons (see Fig.

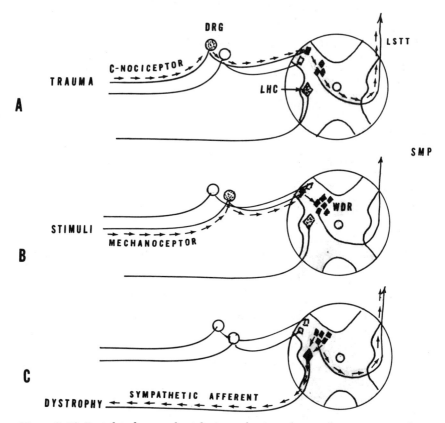

Figure 2–10. Postulated neurophysiologic mechanism of sympathetic maintained pain (SMP).

The transmission via C-nociceptor fibers *(A)* of impulses from the peripheral tissues that have been traumatized and created peripheral nociceptor chemicals (see details in text). These impulses pass through the dorsal root ganglion (DRG) to activate the gray matter of the cord in the Rexed layers. When sensitized, they are termed *wide dynamic range (WDR) neurons.* The WDR, becoming very irritated, receives impulses from the periphery via the A-mechanoreceptor fibers *(B)*, which normally transmit sensations of touch, vibration, temperature, and so on. When the periphery is stimulated (skin touch, pressure, or joint movement), these impulses enhance and maintain the irritability of the WDR. The impulses from the WDR continue cephalad through the lateral spinothalamic tracts (LSTTs) to the thalamic centers with resultant continued pain. The WDR impulses irritate the lateral horn cells (LHC), which generate sympathetic impulses that innervate the peripheral tissues, resulting in the symptoms and findings of dystrophy *(C)*.

1–5).[49] The WDR neurons become hypersensitive, accepting impulses from the myelinated mechanoreceptors (Fig. 2–10), which now become nociceptive. As a result, light touch now becomes painful.

There is also a neural connection in the cord where the WDR cells innervate the lateral horn cells of the ANS. This circuit, affecting the afferent autonomic fibers, explains in part the changes of RSD, discussed later in this chapter.

Because of these cord neuronal circuits there are also synapses with the anterior horn cells that initiate muscle contraction ("spasm") at the segmental level. This muscular contraction, when excessive and sustained, becomes an additional nociceptor. The vascular reaction of sustained muscular contraction becomes a sympathetic mediated nociceptor.

Cerebral mechanisms of pain reception also involve the ANS. As was noted in Chapter 1, PET studies show that pain perception affects the anterior cingulate gyrus and the primary and secondary somatosensory cortices. Painful peripheral heat application[50] causes activation of the contralateral anterior cingulate somatosensory cortices. Nonnoxious stimulation activates only the primary somatosensory cortices. This would imply that secondary cortices are involved in pain perception, whereas primary cortices are involved in mechanoreception.

The anterior cingulate gyrus, a part of the limbic system, includes the emotions and affective responses.

As well as the neurophysiologic aspects of pain there is also evidence of hormonal involvement. The ANS is obviously also involved.

Recent studies have related chronic fatigue syndrome to sympathetic mediated pain.[51] This concept envisions four phases of the syndrome:

1. An inciting event stimulates the posterior thalamus, which is responsible for sympathetic action (fight or flight). Such an event may be viral; an immune imbalance, either congenital or secondary to the viral invasion; prolonged psychologic stress; or physical trauma.

2. These inciting events (essentially nociceptors or algogens) initiate an inflammatory nociceptor process.[52] As stated in Chapter 1, lymphoid cells liberate histamine, serotonin, bradykinin, arachidonic acid, and prostaglandin.[53] These inflamed nociceptors result in hyperalgesia and myalgia.[54,55]

3. Progressive sympathetic flow results in a preponderance of sympathetic output. Whether the physiologic result of the output is organ-specific or generalized remains in question, but there is stimulation of the adrenals.

4. The sympathetic preponderance, considered up-regulation, reaches the postganglionic presynaptic nerves and then the terminal autonomic nerves to "leak" NE from the vesicles that store catecholamines. This continued leakage decreases the sensitivity of the alpha$_2$ receptors. The balance between alpha and beta receptors is upset.

Patients with endogenous depression have an up-regulated alpha$_2$ regulation. Because there is a relationship between chronic pain, depression, and chronic fatigue, tricyclic antidepressants may be beneficial to a number of patients.

The relationship of the ANS to chronic pain has many ramifications and relationships that are as yet not fully documented.

REFLEX SYMPATHETIC DYSTROPHY

RSD has emerged as a specific syndrome of sympathetic mediated pain. Frequently it is diagnosed and treated as if it were a prevalent entity. Any feature of RSD in a medical, orthopedic, neurologic, or rheumatologic entity immediately implies that the condition is a manifestation of RSD, and a treatment protocol is initiated. RSD has become a veritable "homogeneous" diagnosis with an equally homogeneous treatment protocol.[56]

Janig[57] addressed this quandary when he participated in an IASP committee developing a consensus definition of RSD. The resultant decision specified that RSD involved (1) pain (but not necessarily "burning" in quality) with (2) unspecified "abnormalities" of sensation, motor function, and blood flow, and (3) sweating and trophic changes in the skin and soft tissues of the involved extremity. This definition is as vague as is the term "syndrome."

The sensory abnormalities mentioned in the IASP definition, albeit not clarified, have been studied.[58] They include heat-induced hyperalgesia, low-threshold A-beta–mediated or high-threshold mechanical allodynia, and slow summation of mechanical allodynia.

Janig later proposed three types of RSD:

1. Algodystrophy, which includes pain and "all" the features of dystrophy. This was considered to be the full-blown syndrome.
2. RSD "without pain" but presenting all the other features of dystrophy.
3. Sympathetically maintained pain (SMP), not necessarily exhibiting dystrophic tissue changes.

Essentially, Janig's definitions of RSD, which included vasomotor sudomotor tissue changes, were unexplained by any other causes.

In previous definitions of RSD, confirmation of the diagnosis was dependent on relief of symptoms by sympathetic nerve block.[51] Given Janig's definition, could a diagnosis of RSD be entertained if a sympathetic nerve block was ineffectual?

Another problem surfaced regarding the efficacy of sympathetic nerve blocks: Did the analgesic agent injected for a sympathetic nerve block involve the somatic nerves within the area of the block and afford relief "not" mediated by sympathetic nerves? Also, could the benefit from the attempted sympathetic nerve block result from systemic absorption of the injected agent (usually lidocaine)?

There are RSD-like syndromes resulting from damaged nerve tissues that benefit from systemically administered lidocaine. There are conditions following nerve damage in which pain, allodynia, skin temperature changes, and atrophy result, but with no sympathetic involvement.[59,60] Lidocaine given intravenously has relieved neuropathic pains.[61]

True RSD must have the subjective and objective aspects of the syndrome to be diagnosed correctly. Numerous diagnostic terms are currently applied to RSD syndrome, which further confuse its classification. Among many terms the following are variously used:

Algoneurodystrophy
Chronic traumatic edema
Minicausalgia
Minor causalgia
Painful osteoporosis
Peripheral trophoneurosis
Posttraumatic pain syndrome
Reflex algodystrophy
Shoulder-hand syndrome
Sudeck's atrophy
Sympathalgia
Traumatic angiospasm

Clinically, since RSD is related to the dysfunctional pathomechanics of the ANS, a correct diagnosis of RSD will involve a description of the type of pain and other related physical findings.

Type of Pain

RSD pain has certain characteristics:

• Pain is out of proportion to the injury.
• Pain is described as neuralgic or dysesthetic. Patient uses such terms as "burning," "numbness," "tingling," "itching," and so forth.
• Pain may be confined to a neurologic dermatomal area, but it is often more diffuse, less precise, and of a vascular distribution.
• Pain is usually restricted to a distal peripheral limb, although the face, tongue, or other body part may be involved.
• Often there is no objective neural lesion.
• Superficial nonnoxious stimulus such as touch, air, or vibration accentuates the pain.
• Significant and often inappropriate behavioral responses occur; patient may become reclusive or withdrawn.

Physical Findings

RSD may be classified as stage 1, 2, or 3 according to its acuteness or chronicity.[55] The following physical findings may be present:

- Soft puffy edema of the extremity
- Skin color changes—either rubor or pallor—compared to the contralateral side
- Cold or warm sensation of the skin compared to the contralateral extremity
- Excessive moisture or dryness of the skin
- Increased hair or nail growth
- Edema progressing to induration
- Joint limitation, both passive and active
- Muscle atrophy
- X-ray changes indicating osteoporosis
- Gradual atrophic arthritic changes of the joints of the involved extremity
- Pain relieved or diminished by a sympathetic intervention[62,63]
- Increased uptake on radioisotope scan before osteoporosis is noted on routine x-rays.[64]

Hyperalgesia

Hyperalgesia has also been attributed to activation of peripheral adrenergic receptors (alpha$_1$ and alpha$_2$ fibers) in the involved area.[65] In a provocative paper, Campbell et al.[66] postulate that after trauma, norepinephrine is released from the sympathetic terminals in the peripheral tissues at the end organs of the nociceptors. This activates these nociceptors and causes the sensation of pain (Fig. 2–11).[67]

After sympathectomy, stimulation of the peripheral (not the central) cut end reproduces the pain.[68] Anesthetic blockage of the sympathetic ganglion abolishes the hyperalgesia, as does regional intravenous guanethidine, which depletes peripheral catecholamines. These factors all indicate that hyperalgesia is dependent on or markedly influenced by the sympathetic innervation of the painful peripheral part. Therefore, therapy should address this peripheral aspect of the pain.

Intradermal injection of norepinephrine restores the hyperalgesia in RSD, whereas intradermal epinephrine does not cause hyperalgesia in normal skin. A nonspecific alpha-adrenergic antagonist relieves hyperalgesia. Phenoxybenzamine hydrochloride (dibenzyline hydrochloride) work well. A suggested dosage is 10 mg/d increased by 10 mg/d until desired results are achieved.

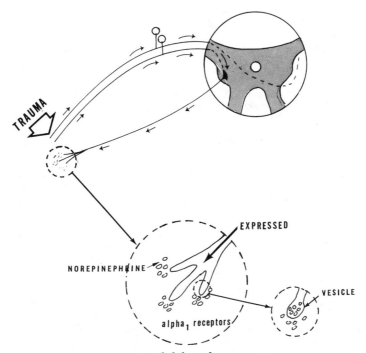

Figure 2–11. Nociceptor activation of alpha$_1$ adrenoreceptors.
Trauma causes the sympathetic nerves going to the area to express norepinephrine that is contained within the vesicles. The liberated norepinephrine reacts with the alpha$_1$ receptors to create causalgic symptoms.

Apparently hyperalgesia is directly related to activation of adrenergic receptors, especially alpha$_1$ and alpha$_2$ receptors. Addressing these receptors topically with antagonists should afford relief to the patient. Local application of clonidine hydrochloride (Antepres. Parke-Davis: Transdermal system) 2.5, 5.0, and 7.5 mg four times a day for 1 week is the suggested dosage. Clonidine is an alpha-adrenergic blocking agent that works by activating presynaptic adrenergic autoreceptors, resulting in reduction of epinephrine release.[69] No alpha-adrenergic antagonist is commercially available but clonidine is available as a transdermal patch and has been highly effective.

Apparently, peripheral alpha$_1$-adrenergic receptors are active in sympathetically maintained pain and are initiated after injuries.[70,71] Before intervention of the innervation to the allegedly injured part, local administration of appropriate medications should also be considered in conjunction with other modalities more centrally directed.

Hannington-Kiff raises the possibility of failed natural opioid modulation in regional sympathetic ganglia.[72] In this concept the plasticity of the DRG, the spinal horn cells, and the wide dynamic range (WDR) cells increase as a result of repeated or intensive nociception from the periphery.[73–75] The

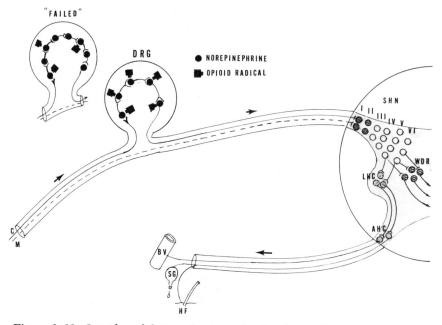

Figure 2–12. Opioid modulation of pain in the dorsal root ganglion after trauma: "failed modulation."

Opioid radicals in the normal dorsal root ganglia (DRG) modulate the norepinephrine contained within the small saccules in the ganglion.

Normally, afferent impulses from C fibers (C) transmitting nociceptive impulse to the spinal horn nuclei (SHN) impinge on Rexed layers I and II. These impulses react with wide dynamic range (WDR) cells in the cord (Rexed layer VII) with impulses going cephalad to the lateral spinothalamic tract (*small arrows*). Fibers connect the Rexed layer cells with lateral horn cells (LHC) that innervate the sympathetic fibers to blood vessels (BVC), sweat glands (SG), and hair follicles (HF).

Repeated or intense nociceptive impulses increase (plasticity) the number of norepinephrine cells within the DRG, increasing sensitivity to even mechanoreceptor (M) impulses. Hence allodynia.

In "failed" opioid modulation (upper left drawing) the epinephrine cells are increased and the opioid radicals are proportionately decreased. Hence, bombardment to SHN is increasing the number of WDR cells.

normal modulating opioid radicals contained within the DRG also increase to prevent excessive sympathetic activity. The increased activity affects the blood vessels, sweat glands, and hair follicles as well as other sympathetically controlled activities.

Normally, the opioid radicals modulate the NE activity. The theory here is that the increased NE within the gland is not balanced with commensurate opioid radical activity (Fig. 2–12). Excess bombardment of the spinal horn cells, WDR cells, and lateral horn cells results, causing RSD.

Treatment

Although the diagnosis of RSD is currently made exclusively on clinical grounds and is often confirmed by a favorable response to interruption of the sympathetic nervous system, diminution of the pain and other treatment modalities are justified.

Pain treatment involves treatment of the sympathetic mediated pain. The use of sympathetic blocks is valid and often effective, but other modalities of pain relief (discussed in Chapter 4) are also valid. The multidiscipline approach, involving physical, pharmacologic, and psychologic treatment is encouraged so that a treatment plan can meet the individual needs of the patient.

The dystrophic changes envisioned in RSD are specified and require attention. These should never be neglected. In fact, often the pain is abated, diminished, or even eliminated by appropriate attention to the dystrophic aspects of RSD.

Urgent comprehensive treatment is indicated independent of the intensity of the pain, the stage, the peripheral tissue involvement, and the functional impairment because the ultimate sequelae of RSD are potentially devastating and irreversible. The functional impairment imposed on the patient by the soft tissue changes often exceeds the impairment caused by pain alone.

The following treatment procedures, based on understanding the pathomechanics of the syndrome, have been advocated:

- Early recognition.
- Early active therapeutic involvement.
- Patient involvement, including a meaningful explanation, in understandable terms, of the symptoms and the physical findings and their significance.
- Local application of heat or ice as tolerated by the patient for vasodilation or vasoconstriction of the overlying skin. (The rationale for these modalities is discussed in Chapter 4.)
- Passive and active motion of the extremity.
- Elevation of the involved extremity as often and as long as feasible on a daily basis.
- Passive and active removal of the edema with compression dressing and vasoconstrictive equipment.
- Injection of local "trigger" areas with an anesthetic agent with or without steroids.
- Vasocoolant spray followed by stretch of the restricted myofascial tissues.
- Use of TENS if pain is significant.[76]

Various kinds of nerve blocks may be effective:

- Specific nerve blocks of the involved area with an anesthetic agent. Be aware that these blocks will intercept not only the A-mechanoreceptors, but also the A-delta and C fibers and the sympathetic nerve fibers.
- Sympathetic nerve blocks. For the upper extremities a cervicothoracic or stellate ganglion nerve block is effective. Paraspinous sympathetic nerve blocks are effective in the lower extremities. Epidural anesthetic blocks have effect.[77] Admittedly, the latter have been used most often in the lower extremity, but a cervical epidural injection of steroids has had recent advocacy.[78]
- Continuous epidural blockades have been effective in intractable pain.
- Epidural Demerol has recent endorsement.
- Bier blocks have been an alternative to perineural local anesthetic injections.[79] In this block a vasoactive drug is administered intravenously along with an anesthetic agent. With the veins of the afflicted extremity blocked by a tourniquet inflated 100 mm above systolic blood pressure, a solution of guanethidine (10 to 40 mg), reserpine (1 to 2 mg), and 0.5% lidocaine is administered through a venous cannula. This block, used in Europe, is currently not available in the United States, as parenteral reserpine is banned and parenteral guanethidine is still considered experimental.
- When a temporary chemical sympathetic block is effective but the symptoms return, permanent interruption of the sympathetic nerve supply may be considered. A solution of 6 to 7% phenol may be applied to the sympathetic ganglia.[80] More recently, radiofrequency thermal applications have been used. Surgical resection of the sympathetic nerve remains the standard approach.

This protocol is treatment of the acute and subacute phase and, hopefully, prevention of chronicity of the neurogenic pain and the soft tissue dystrophy, which itself can be a basis for continued pain.

Treatment of RSD pain also relies on medication, albeit empirically.

- Nonsteroidal anti-inflammatory medications (NSAIDs) are generally considered early in the treatment and may have some value, but long-term results have been disappointing. Their main value appears to be as an adjunct to intensive physical therapy.
- A short (2-week) course of oral steroids (60 to 80 mg prednisone) followed by a 2-week tapering program has its advocates. The reason for many failures is that the pathogenesis of the pain from nociception and the dystrophy are not in the realm of steroid response.
- Heterocyclic antidepressants,[81] such as amitriptyline (10 to 50 mg HS) or trazadone (50 to 150 mg HS) have some value, although their precise pharmacologic mechanism remains conjectural.

• Carbamazepine (initially 200 mg), essentially an anticonvulsant, is effective in trigeminal neuralgia and has some benefit in RSD.[82]
• Assuming a vasomotor component in dystrophic changes, beta blockers (propranolol) and alpha-adrenergic blockers (prazosin and phenoxybenzamine) have been reported of value.[83]
• Topical application of capsaicin relieves the hypersensitivity of the affected region in many patients.[84]

REFERENCES

1. Bennett, GJ: The role of the sympathetic nervous system in painful peripheral neuropathy. Pain 45:221–223, 1991.
2. Goldman, S and Newman, SW: Manter and Gatz's Essentials of Clinical Neuroanatomy and Neurophysiology, ed. 7. FA Davis, Philadelphia, 1987.
3. Cailliet, R: Head and Face Pain Syndromes. FA Davis, Philadelphia, 1992.
4. Cannon, WB and Rosenbleuth, A: Studies on conditions of activity in endocrine organs, XXIX. Sympathin E and Sympathin I. Am J Physiol 184:557–574, 1933.
5. Ahlquist, RP: A study of adrenotrophic receptors. Am J Physiol 153:586–600, 1948.
6. Lenman, JAR: Clinical Neurophysiology. Blackwell Scientific Publications, Oxford, 1975, p 250.
7. Gennaro, AR (ed): Remington's Pharmaceutical Sciences, Mack Publishing Company, Easton, PA, 1990, p 898.
8. Redmond, DE and Huang, YH: II. New evidence of the locus coeruleus norepinephrine connection with anxiety. Life Sciences 25:2149–2162, 1979.
9. Swanson, LW: Brain Res 110:338–356, 1976.
10. Nashold, BS, Wilson, WP, Slau, B, Nashold, BS, Wilson, WP, Slaughter, G: Adv Neurol 4, 1974.
11. Kerr, FWC: Pain 1:325–356, 1975.
12. Sladek, JR and Walker, P: Brain Res 134:359–366, 1977.
13. Korr, IM: Sustained sympathicotonia as a factor in disease. In The Collected Papers of Irvin M. Korr. American Academy of Osteopathy, 1979.
14. Nobin, A and Bjorkland, A: Acta Physiol Scand (Suppl) 388: 1–40, 1973.
15. Darwin, C: The Expression of Emotion in Man and Animals. Philosophical Library, New York, 1975, p 134.
16. Eliot, TR: J Physiol 32:401–467, 1905.
17. Cannon, WB: Am J Psychol 39:196, 1927.
18. Papez, JW: Proposed mechanisms of emotion. Arch Neurol Psychiat 38:725–744, 1937.
19. MacLean, PD: Psychosomatic Med 11:338, 1949.
20. Vogt, BA, Reosene, DL, Pandya, DN: Science 204–205, 1979.
21. Foltz, EL and Lowell, EW: J Neurosurg 19:89, 1962.
21a. Hurt, RW and Ballantine, Jr, HT: Clin Neurosurg 21:334, 1973.
22. Talbot, JD, Marrett, S, Evans, AC, Meyer, E, Bushnell, MC, and Duncan, GH: Multiple representations of pain in human cerebral cortex. Science 251:1355–1358, 1991.
23. Goldstein, S and Halbreich, U: Hormones and stress. In Nemeroff, C and Loosen, P (eds): Handbook of Clinical Psychoneuroendocrinology. Wiley, New York, 1987, pp 460–469.
24. Dunn, A and Berriodge, C: Is corticotropin-releasing factor a mediator of stress response? In Koob, G, Sandman, C, and Strand, F (eds): A Decade of Neuropeptides. New York Academy of Sciences, New York, 1990, pp 183–191.

25. Palkovits, M: Organization of the stress response at the anatomical level. Neuropeptides and brain function. Prog Brain Res 72:47–55, 1987.
26. Bonica, JJ: Anesthesiology 29:793, 1968.
27. Laux, W: Akt Fragen Psychiat Neurol 3:138, 1966.
28. Head, H: Sensibilitatsstorungen der Haut bei visceralen Erkrankungen. Hirschwald-Verlag, Berlin, 1898.
29. Leriche, R: Schmerzchirurgie. Joh Ambrosius Barh Verlag, Leipzig, 1958. (Translation of La chirurgie de la douleur, ed 3. Verlag Masson, Paris, 1959.)
30. Gross, D: Pain and the autonomic nervous system. Adv Neurol 4:93–103, 1974.
31. Hu, S and Zhu, J: Sympathetic facilitation of sustained discharges of polymodal nociceptors. Pain 38:85–90, 1989.
32. Devor, M and Janig, W: Activation of myelinated afferents ending in a neuroma by stimulation of the sympathetic supply in the rat. Neurosci Lett 24:43–47, 1981.
33. Sato, J and Perl, FR: Peripheral nerve injury causes cutaneous nociceptor to be excited by activation of catecholamine receptors. Soc Neurosci Abst 16:1072, 1990.
34. Levine, JD, Coderre, TJ, and Basbaum, AI: The peripheral nervous system and the inflammatory process. In Dubner, R, Gebhart, GF and Bond, MR (eds): Pain Research and Clinical Management, Vol. 3. Proceedings of the 5th World Congress on Pain. Elsevier, Amsterdam, 1988, pp 33–43.
35. Wakisaka, S, Kajander, KC and Bennett, GJ: Abnormal skin temperature and abnormal sympathetic vasomotor innervation in experimental painful peripheral neuropathy. Pain 46:299–313, 1991.
36. Schott, GD: Mechanisms of causalgia and related clinical conditions. Brain 109:717–738, 1980.
37. Shir, Y and Seltzer, Z: Effects of sympathectomy in a model of causalgiform pain produced by partial sciatic nerve injury in rats. Pain 45:309–320, 1991.
38. Janig, W: Experimental approach to reflex sympathetic dystrophy and related syndrome (guest editorial). Pain 46:241–245, 1991.
39. Janig, W: The sympathetic nervous system in pain: Physiology and pathophysiology. In Stanton-Hicks, M (ed): Pain and the Sympathetic Nervous System. Kluwer, Dordrecht, 1990, pp 17–89.
40. Cassell, JF, McLachlan, EM, Sittiracha, T: The effect of temperature on neuromuscular transmission in the main caudal artery of the rat. J Physiol 397:31–44, 1988.
41. Janig, W, Koltzenburg, M: Sympathetic activity and neuroeffector transmission changes after chronic nerve lesions. In Bond, MR, Charlton, JE and Woolf, CJ (eds): Pain Research and Clinical Management. Elsevier, Amsterdam, 1991, pp 365–371.
42. Fleming, WW, Westfall, DP: Adaptive supersensitivity. In Trendelenburg, U and Weiner, N (eds): Catecholamines I. Handbook of Experimental Pharmacology, vol. 90/I. Springer-Verlag, Berlin, 1988, pp 509–559.
43. Janig, W, Blumberg, HG, Boas, RA, and Campbell, JN: The reflex sympathetic dystrophy syndrome. Consensus statement and general recommendations for diagnosis and clinical research. In Bond, MR, Charlton, JE and Woolf, CJ (eds): Pain Research and Clinical Management. Proceedings of the 6th World Congress on Pain, Elsevier, Amsterdam, 1991, pp 373–376.
44. Price, DD, Bennett, GJ, Raffii, A: Psychophysical observations on patients with neuropathic pain relieved by sympathetic block. Pain 36:273–288, 1989.
45. Sawehenko, PE and Swanson, LW: The organization of noradrenergic pathways from the brain stem to the paraventricular and supraoptic nuclei in the rat. Brain Res Rev 4:275–325, 1982.
46. Kalin, NH and Dawson, G: Neuroendocrine dysfunction in depression: Hypothalamic-anterior pituitary systems. Trends Neurosci 9:261–266, 1986.
47. Ganong, W: The stress response: A dynamic overview. Hosp Pract 23(6):155–190, 1988.

48. Stokes, PE and Sikes, CR: The hypothalamic-pituitary-adrenocortical axis in major depression. Endocrinol Metab Clin North Am 17:1–19, 1988.
49. Roberts, WJ: A hypothesis on the physiological basis for causalgia and related pains. Pain 24:297, 1986.
50. Devor, M: Nerve pathophysiological and mechanisms of pain in causalgia. J Auton Nerv Syst 7:371, 1983.
51. Cheu, J and Findley, T: Pathophysiology of he Chronic Fatigue Syndrome (CFS). UMDNJ Kessler Institute: Personal correspondence, 1990.
52. Rubin, E and Farber, JL: The gastrointestinal tract. In Rubin, E and Farber, JL (eds): Pathology. JB Lippincott, Philadelphia, 1988, pp 628–721.
53. Chahl, LA: Pain induced by inflammatory mediators. In Beers, RF and Bassett, EG (eds): Mechanisms of Pain and Analgesic Compounds. Raven Press, New York, 1979, p 273.
54. Perl, ER: Pain and nociception. In Darian-Smith, I (ed): Handbook of Physiology, Sect I, the Nervous System. Vol 3. The Sensory Processes. American Physiological Society, Bethesda, MD, 1984, pp 915–975.
55. Schaible, HG and Schmidt, RF: Effects of an experimental arthritis on the sensory properties of fine articular afferent units. J Neurophysiol 54:1109–1122, 1985.
56. Fields, HL: Editorial comment. Pain 49:161–162, 1992.
57. Janig, W: Pathobiology of reflex sympathetic dystrophy: some general considerations. In Stanton-Hicks, M, Janig, W and Boas, RA (eds): Reflex Sympathetic Dystrophy. Kluwer, Boston, 1990, pp 42–54.
58. Evans, JA: Reflex sympathetic dystrophy. Surg Gynecol Obstet 82:36–43, 1946.
59. Wall, PD and Gutnick, M: Ongoing activity in peripheral nrves: The physiology and pharmacology of impulses originating from a neuroma. Exp Neurol 43:580–593, 1974.
60. Tanelian, DL and MacIver, MB: Analgesic concentrations of lidocaine suppress tonic A-delta and C fiber discharges produced by acute injury. Anesthesiology 74:934–936, 1991.
61. Rowbotham, MC, Reisner-Keller, MB and Fields, HL: Both intravenous lidocaine and morphine reduce the pain of postherpetic neuralgia. Neurology 41:1024–1028, 1991.
62. Cailliet, R: Reflex sympathetic dystrophy. In Shoulder Pain, ed 3. FA Davis, Philadelphia, 1991, pp 227–252.
63. Wang, JK, Johnspon, KA and Ilstrup, DM: Sympathetic blocks for reflex sympathetic dystrophy. Pain 23:13–17, 1985.
64. Kosin, F, McCarthy, DJ, Sims, J, Genant, H: The reflex sympathetic dystrophy syndrome. Am J Med 60:321–331, 1976.
65. Davis, KD, Treede, RD, Raja, SN, Meyer, RA and Campbell, JN: Topical application of clonidine relieves hyperalgesia in patients with sympathetically maintained pain. Pain 47:309–317, 1991.
66. Campbell, JN, Meyer, RA and Raja, SN: Is nociceptor activation by alpha-1 adrenoreceptors the culprit in sympathetically maintained pain? APS J 1(1):3–11, 1992.
67. Janig, W: Can reflex sympathetic dystrophy be reduced to an alpha-adrenoreceptor disease? APS J 1(1):16–22, 1992.
68. Walker, AE and Nulsen, F: Electrical stimulation of the upper thoracic portion of the sympathetic chain in man. Arch Neurol Psychiat 59:559–560, 1948.
69. Starke, K: Alpha-adrenoreceptor subclassification. Rev Physiol Biochem Pharmacol 88:199–236, 1981.
70. Roberts, W and Elardo, SM: Sympathetic activation of A-delta nociceptors. Somatosens Mot Res 3:33–44, 1985.
71. Sanjue, H and Jun, Z: Sympathetic facilitation of sustained discharges of polymodal nociceptors. Pain 38:85–90, 1989.
72. Hannington-Kiff, JG: Does failed natural opioid modulation in regional sympathetic ganglia cause reflex sympathetic dystrophy? Lancet 338:1125–1127, 1991.

73. Cook, AJ, Woolf, CJ, Wall, PD and McMahon, SB: Dynamic receptive field plasticity in rat spinal cord dorsal horn following C-primary afferent input. Nature 325:151–153, 1987.
74. Dubusisson, D, Fitzgerald, M and Wall, PD: Ameboid receptive fields of cells in laminae 1, 2 and 3. Brain Res 177:376–378, 1979.
75. Woolf, CJ and Fitzgerald, M: The properties of neurones recorded in the superficial dorsal horn in rat spinal cord. J Comp Neurol 221:313–328, 1983.
76. Richlin, DM, Carron, H, Rowlingson, JC: Reflex sympathetic dystrophy: Successful treatment by transcutaneous nerve stimulation. J Pediatr 93:84, 1978.
77. Ladd AL, DeHaven, KE, Thanik, J, Patt, RB and Feuerstein, M: Reflex sympathetic imbalance: Response to epidural blockade. Am J Sports Med 17:660–667, 1989.
78. Dirksen, R, Rutgers, MJ and Coolen, JMW: Cervical epidural steroids in reflex sympathetic dystrophy. Anesthesiology 66:71–73, 1987.
79. Fink, BR: History of local anesthesia. In Cousins, MJ and Bridenbaugh, PO (eds): Neural Blockade. JB Lippincott, Philadelphia, 1980, pp 3–18.
80. Payne, R: Neuropathic pain syndromes, with special reference to causalgia and reflex sympathetic dystrophy. Clin J Pain 2:59–73, 1986.
81. Max, MB, Culnane, M, Scafer, SC, Sussman, MD, Baugher, H, and Goldner, ED: Amitriptyline relieves diabetic neuropathy in patients with normal or depressed mood. Neurology 37:589–596, 1987.
82. Talor, JC, Brauer, S and Espir, MLE: Long-term treatment of trigeminal neuralgia with carbamazepine. Postgrad Med J 57:816, 1981.
83. Abram, SE and Lightfoot, RW: Treatment of long-standing causalgia with prazosin. Reg Anaeth 6:79–81, 1981.
84. Simone, DA and Ochoa, J: Early and late effects of prolonged topical capsaicin on cutaneous sensibility in neurogenic vasodilatation in humans. Pain 47:285–294, 1991.

CHAPTER 3
Psychologic Testing in Patients with Chronic Pain

Pain has traditionally been considered a stimulus-evoked response with the response equivalent to the stimulus. Relief of pain should therefore follow the removal of the noxious stimulus. Repeated stimuli over a course of time, however, modifies, diminishes, or eliminates the relationship of time to stimulus, and the response becomes dependent on other factors.[1]

Through generalized stimuli, sensations similar to the original noxious stimulus acquire the ability to elicit a pain response. These stimuli are then considered to be "conditioned" and "learned." The pain response loses its correspondence with the original stimulus and becomes a response to a variety of stimuli not necessarily similar to the original.[2]

The phenomenon of pain can be conceptualized as a behavior controlled by the initial unconditioned (pathologic) stimulus and conditioned (ecologic) stimuli that follow.[3] Initially, tissue pathology initiates the noxious stimulus, which is transmitted throughout all the neural mechanisms (Chapter 1). A pain "behavior" evolves.

Pain measurement is needed to achieve objective documentation, verification, and quantification of the emotional and psychologic aspects influencing the complaints of pain, especially chronic complaints. The usual index of pain is the patient's verbal report, which, at best, is a poor correlation of the pathology with the subjective complaint.

In a patient with minimal objective findings, measurement remains a significant concern to practitioners treating the patient with pain. A confirmable and reproducible pain indicator, or "dolorimeter," is needed.[4] A physiologic indicator that equates verbal reporting is the quest of algologists.

Psychologic testing has several potential uses.[5] It provides

1. Routine screening of patients whose pain complaints are considered to have a large psychologic component.
2. A means of affirming and confirming a precise psychiatric diagnosis.
3. A basis for an appropriate treatment protocol.
4. A basis for research.
5. A baseline measure for outcome assessment of treatment modalities and protocols. (Long-term follow-up has been lacking in most recommended procedures.)

STANDARD PSYCHOLOGIC TESTS

Numerous tests substantiating and quantifying pain have been reported in the literature. Only some of these tests will be discussed, but all have some validity, acceptance, and outcome assessments. It must be stated that any test must be carefully used to diagnose a patient with pain. The initial assumption that there is a psychologic basis for the pain, which may then be therapeutically pursued, must be validated. The treatment, as well as the diagnosis, must not be based solely on the outcome of the test.

Interpretation of any test must also take into account the patient's age, sex, cultural background, and educational level as well as any potential secondary gains to the patient, including economic (litigation). Treatment assessment must include acceptance by the patient and the competence of the therapist.

A test that has had acceptance for years is the Minnesota Multiphasic Personality Inventory (MMPI) (Fig. 3–1).[6] This is a self-administered true-false test. The long version has 550 questions, and the abbreviated version has 399 questions. The test is scored and interpreted by computer. It is a checklist of present and past physical and emotional symptoms.

Scores vary in patients with acute versus chronic pain. In the latter, patients score higher in hypochondriasis, depression, and hysteria, whereas patients in acute pain score lower in hypochondriasis and hysteria but higher in agitation.

Critics of the MMPI point out that the group used to define the norm or average was not a good representation of the general public. The original group included 700 men and women, all white and residents of Minnesota. The average members of the group interviewed were semiskilled workers or farmers with an eighth-grade education. The phrasing of the statements was also considered awkward and not clear. Many topics such as drug abuse, alcoholism, and suicidal tendencies were not addressed. The revised version, MMPI-2, corrected these flaws; it now consists of 567 items and includes a posttraumatic stress scale and a gender role scale. Its efficacy is being reevaluated.[7]

In evaluating an MMPI score one cannot determine whether the scales

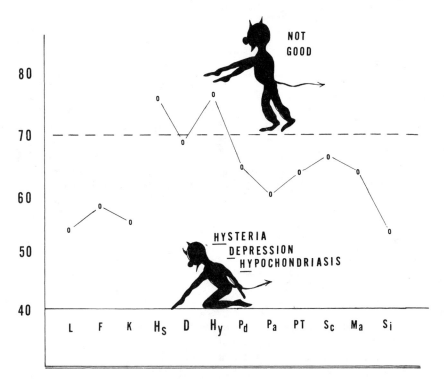

Figure 3–1. Minnesota Multiphasic Personality Inventory (MMPI).

were elevated prior to or as a result of the chronic pain.[8] Another disadvantage to the MMPI is the time needed for the patient to perform the test and the different interpretations placed on it by psychologists.

The Eysenck Personality Test (EPI) measures stability versus neuroticism and introversion versus extroversion.[9] This test basically indicates the stability of the patient's reaction to stress and the tendency of the patient to breakdown. A high N does not indicate neuroticism but does indicate susceptibility and introversion. Extroverts allegedly complain more freely than do introverts but have a higher threshold to pain. The EPI test is not as much help in therapy as it is in evaluating the patient's susceptibility to decompensate under stress.

The Beck Depression Inventory consists of 21 items.[10] It is self-administered and can be executed in 5 minutes. Each item relates to a factor regarding depression but not to other psychologic factors aggravating pain.

Hendler[11] has propounded an excellent test validating the complaint of chronic pain but it has been used essentially for low back pain. Its validity

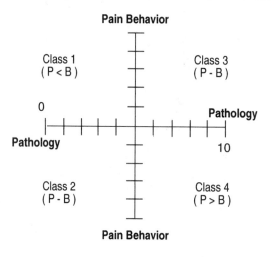

Figure 3–2. Emory University Pain Clinic "Pain Estimate Chart." (From Brena, SF and Koch, DL: A "pain estimate" model for quantification and classification of chronic pain states. Anesthesiology Review 2:8, 1975.

in substantiating other types of chronicity pending successful outcome from surgical intervention remains untested.

An approach to pain estimation has been advocated by Hendler et al.[12] in which the pain stimulus is held constant with the type of pathology categorized and the pain response recorded from which the relative pain behavior is calibrated. In this model the "objective" pain is based on physical examination and radiologic and laboratory studies, which, in themselves, cannot be fully accepted as objective. The pain assessment is in turn based on (1) a semantic inventory, (2) an activities checklist, (3) a drug use rating scale and (4) the MMPI. On the basis of these findings a rating is derived that relates objective damage to the degree of pain expression.

Just as the objective evaluation of significant pathology is questionable, so are the factors of pain assessment: The semantic inventory is verbalization by the patient, and interpretation of the MMPI has its variables. What is pertinent and valuable in this model is the activities checklist—what activities remain possible "in spite of pain"—and the use of drugs. The scale that documents this model is depicted in Fig. 3–2. All the numeric components in the model have a derivation that can be acquired in the proposal. Each component, such as the semantic inventory, is numbered, as are the activity checklist, the drug use rating scale, and the MMPI. Obviously, all are variable and mostly subjective.

The physician's assessment of pathology is also subjective. It is listed in classes and subdivisions and is based on 100 pain estimates. This model has potential, but only outcome assessment and time trial will verify its consistency, objectivity, and accuracy.

CAVEATS IN THE USE OF TESTS

It is apparent that there is a strong emotional component to any significant pain, and the proportion frequently remains obscure—often to the detriment of the patients and to the frustration of the therapist. Cultural and educational factors in today's society imply potential ominous sequelae of any pain in that region.

Because psychologic factors are prevalent in patients complaining of orofacial pain, this relationship is included in the psychiatric-psychologic medical literature. The International Association for the Study of Pain and the American Psychiatric Association both have classified orofacial pain of psychogenic origin, with the former claiming that orofacial pain is psychogenic only if no known physical cause or pathofunction can account for the pain and if contributing factors are undeniably present.[13] The American Psychiatric Association originally classified orofacial pain as a "psychogenic pain disorder" and later defined it as a "somatoform pain disorder."[14,15]

With these claims and implications it is evident that many facial and head pains, being subjective complaints with little if any confirmatory objective findings, tend to be labeled psychogenic. Failure of the patient to respond to what is considered "appropriate" treatment lends further support to a psychogenic basis rather than to an organic etiology. Accusation rather than diagnosis results, and pain becomes chronic, resilient, and intractable. Inappropriate exotic treatments ensue, and failures further frustrate the patient.

Patient-physician rapport and communication are the crux of appropriate examination, diagnosis, and treatment. Listening to the complaint and interpreting it properly is the initial basis of diagnosis and the beginning of effective treatment. The examiner should have knowledge of the presence of an underlying psychologic aspect of any, if not all, pain complaints, especially in evaluating orofacial and head pain.

The use of understandable language in explaining the cause and effects of a patient's pain is mandatory. It can never be denied that a patient's cooperation begins with a clear understanding of the problem. The presence of a psychologic component to the acceptance of pain—either as a cause or as an aggravation—can and must be portrayed to the patient. Its acceptance is the beginning of relief and even cure.

This is not to demean the validity of psychologic testing, but its value in determining pain etiology needs clarification before a treatment protocol is initiated and evaluated. In too many chronic pain centers the psychologic aspect is overstressed, if not even used to the exclusion of other modalities. There is no one exact psychologic test, and follow-up assessment of treatment is essential. The use of a standard test and conventional treatment protocol, regardless of the specific diagnosis for the individual, leads to failure.

The need for accurate measurement of pain was well documented when

Wiltse[16] performed a double-blind study and confirmed that patients who had minimal psychologic findings did better postoperatively, albeit in the presence of objective finding of lumbar discogenic disease, than those with severe hypochondriacal and conversional findings.

THE UNDESIRABLE PATIENT

Many patients with pain complaints presenting with significant or suggested psychopathology become "undesirable patients."[17] A patient so regarded by his or her physician can create a catastrophic situation. This patient is apt to have less than adequate study and care.

Undesirable patients are:

1. Socially undesirable. They are alcoholic, aged, dirty, uneducated, or very poor. Often their perceived undesirability may be based on religion, race, neighborhood, or country of origin.
2. Attitudinally undesirable. They are ungrateful patients, too inquisitive, "know too much," or arrogant.
3. Physically undesirable. They exhibit no positive findings and fail to respond to treatment. Often the presence of another serious illness, for example, a malignancy, may make the physician feel incompetent or helpless and add to the patient's undesirability.
4. Circumstantially undesirable. They arrive late, or the chart or laboratory studies are not available, or the physician is tired or ill, and so on.
5. Distractionally undesirable. The patient presents a medical problem not within the expertise or interest of the physician.

These and other forms of undesirability may interfere with adequate patient study, care, or concern, and both patient and physician suffer. Labeling the patient rather than the problem may result in an incorrect diagnosis.

PAIN BEHAVIOR

Behavioral psychologists base pain management on an evaluation of pain behavior to indicate the presence and severity of pain.[18] These behaviors may be verbal or nonverbal and include willingness to take pain medication, attitudes, postures, and facial expressions.[19] In an effort to objectively document behavior, some assessors are using electromechanical devices to record activity and gait patterns.[20]

Most frequently, pain behaviors are directly observed and recorded. Observations can be based on performance in either a natural or a standardized situation. The latter is intended to stimulate the natural occasion of pain production and may be videotaped for further evaluation.[21]

Objectivity depends on how well trained the observer is. Most criteria are considered too simplistic; they focus on behavior that denies the presence of pain and question whether the behavior is an expression of pain or merely a "coping mechanism."[22] Albeit a valid method of documenting pain, evaluation of behavior may be grossly misapplied and its value questioned.[23]

FACIAL EXPRESSION OF PAIN

After onset of pain a physical effort to withdraw from the source of trauma, called a "nociceptive reflex," occurs. This reflex is accompanied by guarded movements, postures, and characteristic "facial grimaces." Vocalization, including crying, moaning, anger, and so on, may be elicited, but the facial expression has often remained overlooked.[24]

Nonverbal signs of physical distress have been noted for centuries—Shakespeare concluded in *Macbeth*, act 1, scene 4: "There's no art to find the mind's construction in the face"—but are only now receiving scientific studies.[25] Physicians have actually claimed to be able to determine the location of pain more accurately through nonverbal pain expression than through verbal information.[26]

The quantification of pain has eluded the clinician. Most qualifications of severity have been based on verbal statements of the patient,[27] which imply that much information may be missed.[28]

Nonverbal expression of pain may provide collateral and confirming information, and it may contradict the credibility of the verbal complaint. Dispassionate display of agony may accompany severe verbal information, yet verbal expression of pain is influenced by experience, interpretation of significance, and psychosocial loss.

A Facial Action Coding System (FACS) is emerging in pain research.[29] This testing requires videotaping or filming of patients. The videotapes and films are then compared to standards.[30] The conclusion so far reached is that nonverbal communication, of which facial expression is a major factor, has its greatest validity when accompanying the verbal expression. The latter is more subject to self-interpretation, whereas the former is more probably an accurate experience of the pain.

For children, whose verbal expression is limited if even possible, facial expression is very important in evaluating pain (Chapter 12).

REFERENCES

1. Melzack, R: The Puzzle of Pain. Basic Books, New York, 1974.
2. Fordyce, WE, Fowler, RS, Lehman, JF, and Delateur, BJ: Some implications of learning in problems of chronic pain. J Chronic Dis 21:179, 1968.

3. Brena, SF and Koch, DL: A "pain estimate" model for quantification and classification of chronic pain states. Anesthesiology Rev 2:8–13, 1975.
4. Hardy, JD, Wolff, HG, and Goodell, H: A new method for measuring pain threshold: Observations on spatial summation of pain. J Clin Invest 19:649, 1940.
5. Rome, HP, Harness, DM, and Kaplan, HJ: Psychological and behavioral aspects of chronic facial pain. In Jacobson, AL and Donlon, WC (eds): Headache and Facial Pain. Raven Press, New York, 1990.
6. Dahlstrom, WG, Welsh, GS, and Dahlstrom, LE: An MMPI Handbook, Vol 1. University of Minnesota Press, Minneapolis, 1960.
7. Kingsbury, SJ: Why has the MMPI been revised? Harvard Medical School, Mental Health Letter 1991.
8. Naliboff, BD, Cohen, MJ, and Yellen, AN: Does the MMPI differentiate chronic illness from chronic pain? Pain 13:333–341, 1982.
9. Bond, MR: Pain: Its nature, analysis and treatment. In Personality and Pain. Churchill Livingstone, London, 1984, pp 45–50.
10. Beck, AT, Ward, CH, Mendelson, M, Mock, J, and Erbaugh, J: An inventory for measuring depression. Arch Gen Psychiatry 4:561–571, 1961.
11. Hendler, NH: The four stages of pain. In Hendler, NH, Long, DM, and Wise, TN (eds): Diagnosis and Treatment of Chronic Pain. Wright-PSG, Boston, 1982, pp 1–8.
12. Hendler, N, Viernstein, M, Gucer, P, and Long, D: The Hendler Ten-Minute Screen Test for Chronic Back Pain Patients, rev ed. Johns Hopkins Hospital, Chronic Pain Treatment Center, Baltimore, MD.
13. Mersky, H: Classification of chronic pain, descriptions of chronic pain syndromes, and definitions of pain terms. Pain (Suppl)3:S1–S225, 1986.
14. American Psychiatric Association: Diagnostic and Statistical Manual of Mental Disorders, ed. 3. Washington, DC, 1980.
15. American Psychiatric Association: Diagnostic and Statistical Manual of Mental Disorders, ed 3 rev. Washington, DC, 1987.
16. Wiltse, LL and Rocchio, PD: Predicting success of low back surgery by the use of preoperative psychological tests. Paper presented at the annual meeting of the American Orthopedic Association, Hot Springs, VA, June 1973.
17. Papper, S: The undesirable patient. J Chron Dis 22:777–779, 1970.
18. Keefe, FJ and Dunsmore, J: Pain behavior: Concepts and controversies. APS Journal 1(2):92–100, 1992.
19. Fordyce, WE: Behavioral Methods for Chronic Pain and Illness. CV Mosby, St Louis, 1976.
20. Keefe, FJ and Hill, RW: An objective approach to quantifying pain behavior and gait patterns in low back pain patients. Pain 21:153–161, 1985.
21. Follick, MJ, Ahern, DK, and Aberger, EW: Development of an audio-visual taxonomy of pain behavior: Reliability discriminate validity. Health Psych 4:555–568, 1985.
22. Turk, DC, Wack, JT, and Kerns, RD: An empirical examination of the "pain behavior" construct. J Behav Med 8:119–130, 1985.
23. Keefe, FJ: Behavioral measurements in pain. In Chapman, CR and Loeser, JD (eds): Advances in pain research and therapy. Raven Press, New York, 1989.
24. Craig, KD: The facial expression of pain: Better than a thousand words? Focus. 1(3):153–162, 1992.
25. Johnson, M: Assessment of clinical pain. In Jacox, AK (ed): Pain: A source book for nurses and other health professionals. Little, Brown, Boston, 1977, pp 130–166.
26. Rosenthal, R: Skill in nonverbal communication: Individual differences. Oelgeschlager, Cambridge, 1979.
27. Max, MB, Portenoy, RK, and Laska, EM (eds): The Design of Clinical Trials: Advances in Pain Research and Therapy, vol 18. Raven Press, New York, 1991.

28. Gracely, RH: Pain psychophysics. In Chapman, CR and Loeser, JD (eds): Issues in Pain Measurement. Raven Press, New York, 1989, pp 211–230.
29. Ekman, P and Friesen, W: Facial Action Coding System: A technique for the measurement of facial movement. Consulting Psychologists Press, Palo Alto, 1978.
30. LeResche, L and Dworkin, SF: Facial expression of pain and emotions in chronic TMD patients. Pain 35:71–78, 1988.

CHAPTER 4
Physical Intervention in Pain

Discussion and evaluation of the mechanisms of pain is intended to influence and instruct the clinician in treating the appropriate sites of pain and its associated symptomatology. The neuromusculoskeletal and psychologic basis for any treatment modality must be ascertained to make that treatment plausible.

However, addressing all aspects of tissue pain in every organ system of the body in one volume is not possible, nor is it intended here. All the author intends to discuss in this volume is the intervention of pain based on the physiologic, pharmacologic, psychologic, hormonal, and even dietary aspects of the mechanisms of pain resulting from various pathologies. The neuromusculoskeletal system, of which the author claims some expertise, will be highlighted, but every other organ system experiencing pain as a symptom will also be considered.

Once the symptom of pain has been evaluated and its significance determined, pain is initially treated by eliminating the nociceptor input and allaying the patient's apprehension and impairment. Acute or recurrent pain should be interrupted to prevent the ultimate occurrence of chronic pain, which in itself may become a disease rather than merely a symptom.

Interruption of the acute pathways of pain in every region of the body has been clearly discussed by Bonica[1] in his classic two-volume text. Here we will merely highlight the major concepts. Every organ system that elicits pain when injured has a precise mechanism that, once understood, makes interruption of pain sensation more meaningful. Tissue sites in every organ system are responsible for the production of pain; these can be identified and the mechanism by which they are inflamed can also be understood. Acute treatment addressing these changes therefore becomes sound and effective.

Acute pain consists of a complex constellation of unpleasant sensory, perceptual, and emotional experiences with certain associated autonomic, psychologic, emotional, and behavioral responses to a noxious stimulus produced by injury and/or disease.[1] These tissues relate to superficial cutaneous, deep somatic, and visceral sites, either direct or referred.

Pain, considered a warning sign to the patient, is the basis for clinical consultation. Injuries constitute the vast majority of these painful occurrences. Loss of function and work interruption is the dreaded result. Injuries can vary from fractures, dislocations, strains, and sprains to the residual of burns. In addition, pain can occur as a symptom of menstrual, gastric, cardiovascular, dental, and malignancy etiology. With the thrust of medical science being the eradication of the causative and life-threatening aspect of these disease syndromes, their resultant pains must also be addressed.

The quality of pain varies as to the tissue responsible for the pain. Various terms such as "sharp," "pricking," "burning," and "stabbing" are applied to the more superficial tissue sites such as skin and subcutaneous tissues. Pain is described as "aching" or "tightening" for deeper tissues. Quality of pain is also described in various terms such as "excruciating," "frightening," "unbearable," and so on, implying the significance of the pain to the patient. Pain can be localized and localizing, but it may be generalized and nonspecific as to the site or the organ involved. Differentiations and interpretation of these symptoms depend on the expertise and experience of the examiner.

When pain is associated with a precise incidence and is precisely localized with appropriate symptoms, the causative agent and organ site are easily discernible. Treatment aimed at the etiology is simplified, but management of the ensuing pain may remain a therapeutic challenge.

Benign pain—that is, pain that is not recurrent, progressive, or malignant[2]—poses a therapeutic challenge, as the cause is considered innocuous by the examiner but not so acknowledged or accepted by the patient. Pain for which no etiology or organic component can be determined understandably poses diagnostic and therapeutic problems.

Acute pain, from whatever etiology, poses a challenge as to its control. Sherrington[3] defined pain as "a psychological adjunct to an imperative protective reflex." Bonica[4] reconciled the varying opinions regarding the significance of pain by asserting that "pain and associated reflexes have an important biological function that prevents further tissue damage." To this statement can be added "and psychologic impairment."

Pain related to injury or disease, as well as being a warning, is deleterious to the organism. The production of nociceptors initiating the ultimate sensation of pain has been discussed (Chapter 1), as have the local biochemical changes—including capillary, smooth muscle, and hormonal changes—that alter the microenvironment. Pain, allegedly a chemical reaction of algogens, causes neurophysiologic changes that alter normal tissue physiology. These chemical changes must be altered not only to minimize pain but also to prevent the undesired tissue changes that are involved in the proposed mechanisms.

As well as interrupting the mechanisms of acute pain, there is the need to prevent ultimate chronic pain, which may be caused by persistent pathologic somatic tissue changes, prolonged dysfunction of the central nervous system, and inadvertent psychologic and environmental changes. All must be addressed.

The peripheral mechanisms responsible for chronic pain may be attributed to persistence of nociceptors released by chronic disease states such as rheumatoid arthritis, malignancies, chronic peptic ulcers, or peripheral vascular disease. They may occur from persistent benign conditions such as are considered to exist in vascular and nonvascular headache,[5] myofascial syndromes, and other similar conditions.

The thesis has been presented in Chapter 1 that tissue damage from injury or disease liberates endogenous chemical substances such as serotonin, histamine, bradykinin, phospholipids, substance P, and prostaglandins. These chemicals all have a neuroactive and vasoactive effect on the membrane structures of their receptor tissues. These tissue reactions impair local microcirculation with resultant tissue impairment. To manage this and modulate pain, the resultant tissue damage from the trauma must be addressed. Numerous modalities and medications can be used to intervene in the specific pain mechanisms.[6-8]

The local tissue damage to the microenvironment, albeit chemical, has mechanical effects, such as edema or ischemia, which cause pain transmission. Algogens such as substance P alter the threshold level to mechanical stimuli of A-delta and C fiber nociceptor afferents.[9] The dorsal horn neurons of lamina I and the neurons of the ventrobasal complex of the thalamus, all involved in pain transmission, undergo increased sensitivity from prolonged peripheral nociception.[10,11] Persistent local nociceptive agents at the peripheral site not only cause local damage but enhance pain transmission at various levels of the central nervous system.

The sensitization of the peripheral nociceptors by various types of trauma can also be enhanced by the application of certain modalities such as heat or ice.[12] This phenomenon causes pain from otherwise innocuous mechanical or thermal stimuli. There are many examples of this phenomenon, of which sympathetic mediated pain is a prime example.

Painful peripheral neuropathies with no demonstrable pathology add to the confusion of ascertaining the true mechanism of pain. This pain may be due to activation of unmyelinated fibers in the nervi nervorum, a neurochemical reaction, as is evident from its beneficial response to corticosteroids.

Persistent nociceptive impulses on the central nervous system being a factor in causation of chronic pain mandates effective therapy on the peripheral mechanisms. Central mechanisms, once involved, cause chronic pain and compound the problem of intervention.

The pathomechanics of pain dictate the precise modality to address that pain, yet many modalities have crossover effects in that they can be applied to any similar pain entity and thus are not necessarily specific. What is pertinent is that their use is effective regardless of the specific mechanism of the pain.

The noxious agents that accumulate at the peripheral trauma site, including histamine, kinins, and neuropeptides, have a vasomotor effect: either vasodilation or vasoconstriction. These nociceptive agents lower the threshold of the receptors of the A-delta and C fibers of the peripheral nervous system sending impulses cephalad.

The local area becomes hypersensitive, creating pain known as primary hyperalgesia. A secondary hyperalgesia occurs in the surrounding tissues from antidromic activation of the primary afferent C fibers. This releases substance P in the region.[13] This hypersensitivity may also be an aftereffect of the discharge from small primary afferents that release substance P. Electrical stimulation of the primary afferents has been shown to release substance P at their receptor ends.[14] Reactive local skeletal muscle spasm occurs, initiating a pain-spasm-pain cycle.

Chemical and mechanical substances produced at the peripheral tissue site following injury are a mechanism of pain production that must be addressed.

CRYOTHERAPY

Cryotherapy, the application of cold in the acute treatment of pain, has been an accepted modality for centuries. Three possible mechanisms for the effectiveness of local cold include (1) receptor adaptation,[15] (2) a counterirritant effect,[16] and (3) a neurogenic effect.[17] To date there is no evidence that cold thermal agents activate the endorphin system, as has been postulated.

Essentially, cold lowers the temperature of the skin and underlying tissues by removing heat from these tissues. Its local application as a treatment modality for a traumatized area is that (1) being a vasoconstrictor, it decreases or inhibits bleeding, (2) it decreases local tissue metabolism, which produces algogens, (3) it neutralizes the local histamine liberated by trauma, (4) it decreases local muscle spasm by decreasing the sensitivity of the muscle spindle system, and (5) it elevates the threshold of pain-transmitting nerves.

A local tissue reaction to trauma is the formation of local edema (Fig. 4–1). Edema occurs because of a change of hydrodynamics as the vasoconstriction is followed by reflex vasodilation. The afflicted vessels—the arterioles, capillaries, venules, and lymphatics—become distended. The endothelial cells separate, creating gaps between the cells so that greater filtration

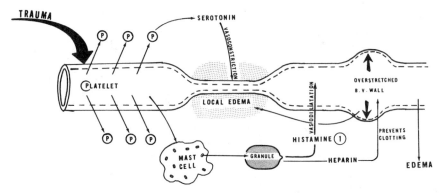

Figure 4–1. The effect of trauma, a vasochemical reaction.

of the serum with its contained constituents can enter the perivascular tissues.

At first, this edematous fluid is merely a transudate containing water and dissolved electrolytes. It has a specific gravity of 1.012, maintaining osmotic balance. As permeability increases, the transudate becomes an exudate containing cells and protein, with a specific gravity of more than 1.012; this causes an imbalance of osmotic pressure and further outflow to the perivascular tissues.

Both the transudate and the exudate cause a mechanical impedance to further blood flow, resulting in ischemia. The protein contained in the exudate gradually causes chemical "thickening" of the fluid, which impairs physiologic movement between fascial planes.

Ice or cold applied to the inflamed tissues intervenes in this transudate-exudate cycle by decreasing fluid transudate and metabolic rate.[18] Cold also decreases tissue sensitivity; this makes possible active and passive exercises that mechanically express the exudate and transudate from the tissues.

Nerves differ in their reaction to cold, depending on their degree of myelination.[19] The unmyelinated small-diameter fibers are less responsive to cold than are the A fibers; the large A-alpha motor fibers are the least affected.[20]

Exercise performed after the application of cold generates more muscular tension.[21] The combined effect of ice and exercise therefore decreases pain, alters the hydrodynamics, and permits greater strength of muscle contraction while decreasing edema and removing the accumulation of the nociceptive metabolites.

THERAPEUTIC HEAT

The effect of heat on tissues depends on the extent of temperature rise, the rate of application of heat energy, and the volume of tissue exposed to the heat.[22] Elevation between 40 and 50°C increases blood flow; this is the therapeutic objective.

Temperature elevation increases blood flow, which causes cooler blood to reach the site and remove the warm blood. The rate of temperature rise influences its efficacy. A slow rise of tissue temperature may defeat the objective of heat application as it brings "cooler" blood into the inflamed tissue site. Too rapid a temperature rise may also be deleterious, as the heat generated in the local tissues may stimulate pain receptors with adverse effect.

The effects of heat are an alteration in metabolic activity, hemodynamic function, neural response, skeletal muscle activity, and collagen tissue.[23] All these effects can be directly or indirectly related to the management of pain resulting from tissue trauma. The neural response more directly intervenes in transmission, but the other effects of heat relate to the tissue dysfunction, and this also enhances pain.

The neural effect of how heat provides analgesia and reduces muscle spasm—both involved in pain production—is not fully understood.[24,25] Reduction of muscle spasm is conceivably induced via the spindle system.[26] Heating the area over a peripheral nerve by high-intensity infrared radiation has induced analgesia distal to the application.[27] Much research remains to be done on the precise neurophysiologic basis for relief from pain.

Surface heating agents do not elevate muscle temperature needed to alter Ib or II afferent nerve activity, whereas skin temperature heating has decreased gamma efferent activity, which may relate to diminished muscle spasm and pain.[27]

Metabolic rate increases two- to threefold with every 10°C rise in temperature. Increasing the tissue temperature above 50°C burns the tissues, as their repair potential cannot cope with the protein denaturation of excessive heat. Chemical and metabolic activities are beneficially increased below that temperature.

The hemodynamic effect of increasing blood flow occurs as superficial heat causes reflex postganglionic sympathetic nerve activity to the smooth muscles of the blood vessels, supplying more blood flow to deeper organs such as muscle.[28]

The most effective heat modality proposed for therapeutic intervention is covered extensively in the literature and will not be thoroughly evaluated here.[29]

Moist heat transmitted via hot moist packs has many advocates.[30] Hot paraffin wax is effective in treating extremities, as are hydrotherapy,[31] ultrasound,[31] diathermy, pulsed electromagnetic fields, laser, and ultrasound. Whimsically, Licht[32] has commented that "the choice of source of heat will depend upon the training and experience of the physician, or empirically: the latter, a matter of local routine often based, regrettably, on such considerations as cost, availability, convenience, hand-me-down habits, custom or publicity."

Soft Tissue Modalities for Elongation

Connective tissue, which is so often impaired after injury or disease, benefits from heat application. Connective tissue—be it collagen, elastin, or fibrous—tends to shorten after injury.[33] The viscoelastic properties of connective tissues that permit elongation from physical stretch is known as plastic deformation.[34] Recoverable deformation is possible if the modalities of heat and passive-active stretch are applied to the deformed (shortened) tissues.[35]

The need to regain tissue flexibility in treating pain is apparent in that sensory nerves enclosed within the soft tissues have often become impaired after injury or prolonged tension from anxiety, anger, and emotional tension.

For damaged tissues to regain their normal length, the appropriate temperature intensity, site, and duration must be used. Consideration must also be given as to the extent of physical strength, including its intensity, duration, and velocity.[23] The techniques of stretch have been propounded; they vary from (1) constant load to overcome impaired elasticity, to (2) rapid stretch followed by holding the gained elongation, to (3) a slow progressive stretch.[36]

In the arthritides, where the synovial tissue components and their somatic and sympathetic nerve supply are involved, the approach to regaining flexibility presents a major aspect of treatment protocols.

ANALGESIC NERVE BLOCK

The subtitle of Bonica's *Management of Pain* placed special emphasis on the use of analgesic block in diagnosis, prognosis, and therapy. This laid the groundwork for interrupting all peripheral tissue sites of nociception by analgesic nerve blocks. This concept is still valid in acute and recurrent pain for its diagnostic localization, treatment, and even prognosis, as will be substantiated in subsequent discussions of varied musculoskeletal and other painful states. Its application in treating chronic pain is being questioned in view of later concepts of central pain and its modulation.

The purpose of analgesic nerve blocks is to interrupt the transmission of nociceptive impulses of the afferents to the cord from the damaged tissues. Diagnostically, the affected organ or tissue is identified by interruption of the somatic nerve to and from that tissue. Acute pain is interrupted, and therapeutic procedures on that organ or tissue are permitted during the period of anesthesia.

In acute pain, interruption of the afferent impulses allows a more normal healing process or at least some comfort to the patient during the healing process.

Knowing that repeated or continuous impulses from the end organs (terminals) increase the sensitivity of those fibers, the dorsal root ganglia, the dorsal column neurons, and even the thalamic pathways, interruption of the initial barrage of impulses diminishes the subsequent sensitivity enhancement.

In chronic pain continuing nociception from the periphery can be moderated by appropriate nerve blocks. Chronic pain does occur from pathology that persists and differs from chronic benign pain, where nerve blocks are less effective, if even indicated at all.

Techniques of performing nerve blocks have been extensively described in textbooks of anesthesia and acute pain. The precise nerve supply of every tissue and organ of the body is well known. Repetition of these numerous techniques and their tissue sites is beyond the scope of this text.

It is well documented that the analgesic value occurs not only during the presence of the injected drug but also after the chemical duration of the drug. The basis for this prolongation remains obscure.

A recent controversy has been raised as to the psychophysiologic benefits involved in nerve blocking for chronic pain.[37] This may be an oxymoron, because any modality that is beneficial in treating chronic pain remains in use regardless of its mechanism.[38] The numerous medications injected are well documented in the literature, but even this raises questions because there is benefit from insertion of a needle without the use of medication. The "dry needle" has proven effective.[39]

Use of operant conditioning has been a major component of standard chronic pain management. Chronic pain treatment involving operant conditioning and sympathetic nerve blocks was proposed using Minnesota Multiphasic Personality Inventory (MMPI) testing to determine susceptibility.[40] Patients demonstrating a "conversion valley" in the MMPI were considered acceptable.[41] This valley is an elevation of hypochondriasis (Hs) and hysteria (Hy) over depression (D). Hence: Hs > Hy > D. Controls were patients demonstrating a profile of Hs > D > Hy. This profile reflected patients having "purposeful operants."[42] In operant conditioning terms, the patient was experiencing a secondary gain, a "reward" from the chronic pain.

The outcome assessments in this study were termed "up time" and included time walking, performing daily chores, exercising, playing sports, and so on. Pain perception was ignored as is mandated in operant conditioning.[43]

The injections here were sympathetic nerve blocks performed weekly for 6 weeks using 0.25% butylpipecoloxylidide (Marcaine R) with epinephrine. Evaluation of up-time activities was performed weekly for 4 weeks, and then monthly for 6 months. Most patients (65 percent) who completed this program improved in their activities. Any further injections were given on the basis of improvement and were considered "reward."

The needle used here, admittedly to block the sympathetic nervous system, may contain a placebo or a medicative substance. The absence of pain relief here is also inconclusive. Several points need mention here. Current chronic pain management still relies on ambiguous criteria. The MMPI determination of "susceptibility" is vague. The benefit of a needle versus the benefit of sympathetic blockage is also unclear. The placebo effect looms prominent in these suggestions as in many extolled modalities used in chronic pain.

Nerve blocks—somatic and/or sympathetic—will be discussed in relation to specific tissues, organs, and syndromes in subsequent chapters.

EXERCISE

Despite the statement that "exercise therapy is the cornerstone treatment for subacute and chronic pain,"[43] Lee et al[44] note that "During acute pain, exercise generally is contraindicated except for maintaining self-administered passive range of motion (ROM) of all extremities and the trunk." Subacute pain, however, "is less intense . . . therefore therapeutic exercise is highly desirable and realistic 'for restoration of function to the affected area.' " This statement implies that exercise is mainly directed to the functional impairment of trauma or illness and only indirectly applies to relief from pain.

In treating chronic pain, exercise is directed to the effects of decreased activity leading to atrophy, weakness, and contracted joints, with pain only indirectly addressed. In Basmajian's[45] treatise on therapeutic exercise, the use of exercise in treating painful syndromes is directed at specific organ systems such as low back, arthritis, and so forth without mention of exercise as a modality treating pain per se. DeVries[46] does not mention pain at all in his discussion of the physiology of exercise.

Fordyce,[47] whose operant conditioning has become an accepted procedure in the treatment of chronic pain, uses exercise only to increase activity level. He states that "exercise is, with few exceptions, also a behavior that is incompatible with pain behavior."[47]

There is no doubt that muscular weakness prevalent in many musculoskeletal pain syndromes, as well as the fatigue and debility that accompanies depression from chronic pain, can be altered in part by exercise.[48] In that respect exercise to regain strength and endurance as well as flexibility and mobility is a powerful adjunct in the treatment of pain.

Exercise appears to increase the endorphin level.[49] Endorphins are accepted neurotransmitters with a morphinelike action.[50] This modulation of pain perception and analgesia has been associated with the analgesia of electrical brain stimulation and acupuncture.[51]

Exercise results in elevated adrenocorticotropic hormone (ACTH), cortisol, and catecholamine levels. These are the precursors of beta endorphins. Many athletes experience decreased pain perception that allows them to make maximum effort "in spite of pain"; they even claim to reach an emotional "high" after extreme physical activity.[52]

Naloxone, a narcotic antagonist that competes for endorphin-binding sites, has altered pain perception experienced after running.[53] This substantiates endorphin action in the athlete. After 30 minutes of strenuous exercise, athletes may have an elevation of plasma endorphins.[54] However, further studies have found that mood changes attributed to endorphins after a 10-mile run were evident with and without naloxone.

After studying the effects of emotions and endorphins in stressful exercise, Pitts[55] postulated that the accumulated lactate from maximum exercising induces anxiety, which has a mood-induced endorphin effect. This again has been refuted in the finding that elevated endorphins after stressful exercise may be noted without significant elevation of lactates.[56]

Mayer and colleagues[57] revealed that they found no analgesic effect from exercise, but that an analgesic effect came from the pain "pretesting" itself. In this experiment their subjects were exposed to pain pretesting; those tested exhibited analgesia from the test alone. Exercise following the test did not alter the analgesia.

The relationship of endorphins to mood. changes, analgesia, and strenuous exercise is not yet clear, but there is value in further studies. What appears apparent, so far, is that exercise must be strenuous to be analgesic and therefore its role in pain treatment will depend on the physical and psychologic ability of the afflicted patient to implement this modality when confronted with persistent and/or chronic pain.

Until recently pain suppression producing analgesia (SPA) was derived from studies of the factors considered to be the responsible stimulation. Electrical stimulation of the midbrain periaqueductal gray area and other portions of the midbrain (Chapter 1) were found to cause profound analgesia without causing significant deficits in other sensory or motivational functions.[58,59] This pain SPA also acted at the dorsal horn level.[60]

All this SPA function was dependent on specific neurotransmitters acting at the synapses of the transmission system. This SPA function operated in the same way as opiate drugs.[58]

It has become the objective of pain suppression studies to elicit the environmental stimuli that initiate SPA.[61] Because the pituitary-adrenal axis has an adaptive response to stress, its role is apparent in pain modification. Intervention of this axis (adrenalectomy, adrenal demedullation, and adrenal denervation) affects the opioid form of stress analgesia. A relationship is implied.

The neurochemistry of nonopioid stress analgesia remains elusive, but studies implicate serotonin, norepinephrine, dopamine agonists, and histamine.[62] Stimulation of the pituitary-adrenal and sympathetic-adrenal systems with the release of adrenaline, noradrenaline, and corticol excretion have been thought to be related to distress and effort, as both systems are involved in strenuous exercise.[63] It remains evident, therefore, that exercise can be involved in pain management.

Exercises have a well-documented place in the physical treatment of most painful disabling neuromusculoskeletal conditions and will be discussed under this concept in subsequent chapters dealing with specific musculoskeletal conditions and particularly in Chapter 8.

TRANSCUTANEOUS ELECTRICAL NERVE STIMULATION

In the physical treatment of pain, transcutaneous electrical nerve stimulation (TENS) has been well accepted. Its neurophysiologic basis has also been established.

Pain mediation through the unmyelinated C fibers and the lightly myelinated A-alpha fibers has been established (Chapter 1). Large-diameter myelinated fibers transmit mechanoreceptor impulses and have a lower threshold at their synapse at the dorsal horn. As they transmit at a faster speed than those of the unmyelinated or lighter-myelinated fibers, they arrive at the gate earlier. The gate concept (Chapter 1) implies that these impulses block subsequent pain-producing impulses.

Low-frequency, high-intensity TENS of less than 10 Hz has been clinically shown to create analgesia.[65] Endorphins have been created in the absence of pain,[66] and the effect of TENS has been eliminated by simultaneous use of nalaxone, an indication of a neurochemical basis.[67]

Two questions have been raised: Is there an increase in endorphins from TENS? And what is the appropriate frequency of the TENS to elevate this opium peptide in the cerebral spinal fluid (CSF)?[68] It was determined that low-frequency (2 Hz) stimulation caused an elevation of Met-enkephalin-Arg-Phe-dynorphin, an opioid peptide in the CSF. Higher-frequency TENS (100 Hz) caused a lesser elevation of a different opioid. This indicates that there is an elevation of opioid when the TENS application is effective. It also accentuates the need to determine which frequency is the most effective and which opioid is liberated.

Electrical stimulation has been shown to increase levels of dopamine epinephrine and serotonin, which are established algogens.[69] Electrical stimulation has been shown to decrease nerve action potential of A-delta fibers, which are the pain mediators.[70] All these factors confirm a physiologic basis for effective pain modulation.

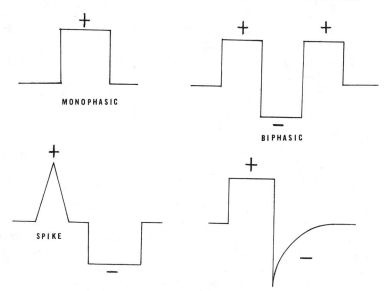

Figure 4–2. Waveforms of TENS.

The manner, site, and type of TENS is vital for effective pain modulation. TENS is most effectively applied proximally in nerve injuries, and the precise site of application must be clinically ascertained. The current wavelength must be determined (Fig. 4–2), as well as its form (Fig. 4–3). A recent report advocated greater relief from the use of ultralow-frequency TENS (0.66 Hz) in contradiction to the currently advocated strengths.[71]

The efficacy of TENS in treating chronic pain has varied from 12 to 60

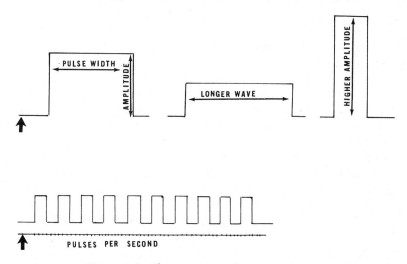

Figure 4–3. Characteristics of TENS application.

percent depending on the reporter.[72] Patients whose pain is complicated by significant depressive illness receive significantly less benefit from the use of TENS, so TENS cannot be considered to effect pain modulation through its psychotherapeutic benefit.

ACUPUNCTURE

Derived from ancient Eastern medicine, acupuncture has evolved in current Western medicine for the treatment or prevention of pain. The modality of acupuncture treatment is essentially the insertion of small, thin, solid needles into the skin, immediate subcutaneous, muscular tissues in regions called "meridians."[73]

Chinese medicine considered human health as the result of conflicting forces of nature, termed *yin* and *yang*.[74] When these forces were out of harmony, "disease" resulted. Vascular and neurologic energy flowed through meridians. These meridians allegedly followed a circadian rhythm, and each was directly associated with an organ system.[75]

The meridians were interconnected within the vital life energy *chi*. Allegedly, a deficiency of *chi* caused pain. Pain could thus be modified by inserting needles into the meridians that rebalanced energy flows. More recent concepts associate the meridian process with the autonomic nervous system.[76,77]

There are numerous techniques for inserting acupuncture needles that have not been officially recognized. The angle and depth of the insertion varies, and numerous techniques exist such as "twirling," twisting the inserted needle, pressing down on the needle, or applying a ball of herbs at the base and igniting the ball.

The site of insertion appears to be the major basis for success. The site of "trigger points" or motor points has been postulated as the optimum site for acupuncture.[78]

The physiologic basis for acupuncture remains unconfirmed.[79] Its efficacy and validity as an accepted medical modality remains ambiguous by Western medical standards. In 1981, the American Medical Association concluded that acupuncture had no more effect on pain than placebo or sham acupuncture.[80]

Animal studies are themselves inconclusive because stress is imparted to the animal during the acupuncture experiment, and stress itself is analgesic.[81] The results of animal studies cannot be translated to humans. Human studies are also nonspecific although there is evidence that endorphins are elevated in the plasma.[82] The transfer of these endorphins to the central nervous system remains unclear, however.

Clinical studies of acupuncture are subjective, as are most pain studies. The mere belief that acupuncture can be effective influences the degree of patient's relief from pain.[83] Studies have revealed that acupuncture is no more effective than TENS at the same tissue site.[84] The effect of cultural background on experienced benefit from acupuncture has been studied and found not to be a significant factor.[85]

SPINAL CORD STIMULATION

Spinal cord stimulation has evolved over the past 20 years as being effective for treatment of intractable chronic pain.[86] This has been considered as last resort, but in properly selected patients it has been effective when all other modalities have failed.

Success for this has been the interruption of the central ascending pain pathways at the spinal cord level (Chapter 1). The implant of a stimulator followed the claim that electrical stimulation applied via intracutaneous needles could produce local analgesia.[87] During the following years implant of transcutaneous nerve stimulation equipment (TENS) was considered diagnostic for future implant, but the TENS implant itself became an accepted procedure.[88]

The duration and efficacy of this dorsal column stimulation (DCS) vary.[89] Duration of pain relief persists after cessation of the stimulation. The exact sites on the spinal column remain unconfirmed.[90] This latter fact does not invalidate the use of DCS but does call into question the precise knowledge of the neurophysiology of pain transmission. The possibility of distal influence, for example, on the thalamic tracts and the thalamus, via a "loop," has been postulated.[91] Of the many concerns regarding the basis for DCS effectiveness is the experimental finding that sections of the dorsal column caudal to the site of DCS stimulation abolish the benefits of the DCS.[92] The reader is advised to review a summary of current concepts.[93]

DCS relief is found in neurogenic conditions, that is, conditions resulting from injury to the nervous system.[94] Pain resulting from pathologic processes in nonnervous cell tissues—such as in myofascial, skeletal, and inflammatory conditions—are less likely to respond to DCS. Thalamic pain and other pains of supraspinal origin also benefit less from DCS. It can be concluded that patients who benefit from TENS and/or acupuncture are more apt to be candidates if the pain is excruciating and severely disabling.

Long-term results are in the range of 50 percent: that is, 50 percent of patients receive 50 percent reduction in their pain ratings.[95] The techniques for implant are beyond the scope of this text but are discussed in current literature.[96]

INTRACEREBRAL STIMULATION

Electrical stimulation at higher levels is termed intracerebral stimulation (ICS) or deep-brain stimulation (DBS). This concept received its impetus from the finding that stimulation of the periaqueductal gray matter in rats could produce powerful analgesia.[97]

This finding specifically confirmed that the periaqueductal-periventricular gray (PAG-PVG) regions of the brain are important in pain transmission and their stimulation could interrupt pain. The PAG-PVG region in the brainstem is an endogenous pain-controlling system in the transmission system—the first synaptic relay from the tract ascending from the dorsal horn in the spinal cord. Clinically interrupting this synapse offers great possibilities in pain control.

Hormonal release from this stimulation has enhanced our knowledge of pain mechanisms. Stimulation of the PAG-PVG regions causes an increase of beta endorphins in the ventricular CSF.[98] However, naloxone, which normally blocks endorphin action, was not evident in this study, calling into question the validity of beta endorphin as a pain reliever, even though stimulation of the PAG-PVG region was effective.[99] A different mechanism apparently operates in this modality.

In neuropathic pain, stimulation of the sensory thalamus or the PAG-PVG area is indicated when there has been damage or loss of peripheral nerve tissue in the dorsal root, the spinal ganglia, or the cord; under these circumstances, DCS is not feasible. When pain is attributed to a thalamic lesion (thalamic pain), stimulation of the sensory limb of the internal capsule may be beneficial.[100]

In the management of intractable chronic pain, neurosurgical intervention is becoming more relevant. The selection of the appropriate patient for any of these procedures is pertinent as the procedures are time-consuming, expensive, and not available in every medical community. The clinical diagnosis must ascertain that the pain is neurogenic.[96]

Patients with a large psychologic overlay, drug addiction, low mentality, secondary gains, and hysteroid personalities have been stated to be poor candidates. Patients failing to receive benefit from morphine are also considered undesirable as the benefit from central nervous system stimulation apparently operates along the same lines. In the case of cancer and mechanical pain problems, such as failed low back surgery, clear indication is needed that the patients are suitable candidates.

The future of pain relief from surgical intervention has enhanced pain research and offered success for long-lasting relief of the severely debilitated patient with long-term intractable pain. Both the duration of benefit and the precise technique to be used yet remain to be confirmed.[101] The promise is on the horizon.

REFERENCES

1. Bonica, JJ: The Management of Pain, ed 2. Lea & Febiger, Philadelphia, 1990, pp 651–1621.

2. Thomas, CL (ed): Taber's Cyclopedic Medical Dictionary, ed 16. FA Davis, Philadelphia, 1989.
3. Sherrington, CS: The Integrative Action of the Nervous System. Yale University Press, New Haven, 1906/1947.
4. Bonica, JJ: Management of Pain. Lea & Febiger, Philadelphia, 1953.
5. Cailliet, R: Head and Face Pain Syndromes. FA Davis, Philadelphia, 1992.
6. Michlovitz, SL: Thermal Agents in Rehabilitation, ed. 2. FA Davis, Philadelphia, 1990.
7. Ciccone, CD and Wolf, SL: Pharmacology in Rehabilitation. FA Davis, Philadelphia, 1990.
8. Gennaro, AR (ed): Remington's Pharmaceutical Sciences, ed 18. Mack Publishing Company, Easton, PA, 1990.
9. Iggo, A, Guilbaud, G, and Tegner R: Sensory mechanisms in arthritic rat joints. In Kruger, L and Liebeskind, JC (eds): New York, Raven Press, 1984, pp 83–93.
10. Menetrey, D and Besson, JM: Electrophysiological characteristics of dorsal horn cells in rats with cutaneous inflammation resulting from chronic arthritis. Pain 13:343, 1982.
11. Gautron, M and Guilbaud, G: Somatic responses of ventrobasal thalamic neurons in polyarthritic rats. Brain Res 237:459, 1982.
12. Ochoa, J: The newly recognized painful ABC syndrome: Thermographic aspects. Thermology 2:65, 1986.
13. Dubner, R and Bennett, GJ: Spinal and trigeminal mechanisms of nociception. Annu Rev Neurosci 6:381, 1983.
14. Lynn, B: The detection of injury and tissue damage. In Wall, PD and Melzack, R (eds): Textbook of Pain. Churchill-Livingstone, New York, 1984, pp 19–33.
15. Travell, J: Myofascial trigger points: Clinical view. In Bonica, JJ and Able-Fessard, DG (eds): Advances in Pain Research and Therapy, Vol 1. Raven Press, New York, 1976, pp 919–926.
16. Goldscheider, A: Veber den Schmertz in Physiologischer und Klinischer Hensicht. Hirschwald, Berlin, 1894.
17. Gammon, GD and Starr, I: Studies on the relief of pain by counter-irritation. J Physiol 72:392, 1931.
18. Michlovitz, SL: Cryotherapy: The use of cold as a therapeutic agent. In Michlovitz, SL (ed): Thermal Agents in Rehabilitation, ed 2. FA Davis, Philadelphia, 1990, pp 63–87.
19. Douglas, WW and Malcolm, JL: The effect of localized cooling on conduction in cat nerves. J Physiol 130:53, 1955.
20. Li, C-L: Effect of cooling on neuromuscular transmission in the rat. Am J Physiol 194:200, 1958.
21. McGown, HL: Effects of cold application on maximal isometric contraction. Phys Ther 47:185, 1967.
22. Lehmann, JF and de Lateur, BJ: Therapeutic heat. In Lehmann, JF (ed): Therapeutic Heat and Cold, ed 4. Williams & Wilkins, Baltimore, 1990.
23. Michlovitz, SL: Biophysical principles of heating and superficial heat agents. In Thermal Agents in Rehabilitation. FA Davis, Philadelphia, 1990, pp 88–108.
24. Lehmann, JD, Brunner, GD, and Stow, RW: Pain threshold measurements after therapeutic application of ultrasound microwaves and infrared. Arch Phys Med Rehabil 39:560, 1958.
25. Currier, DP and Kramer, JF: Sensory nerve conduction: Heating effects of ultrasound and infrared. Physiotherapy Canada 34:241, 1982.
26. Mense, S: Effects of temperature on the discharges of muscle spindles and tendon organs. Pflugers Arch 374:159, 1978.
27. Fischer, E and Solomon, S: Physiological response to heat and cold. In Licht, S (ed): Therapeutic Heat and Cold, ed 2. Waverly Press, Baltimore, 1965.
28. Guyton, AC: Textbook of Medical Physiology, ed 7. WB Saunders, Philadelphia, 1986.

29. Wright, V and Johns, RJ: Physical factors concerned with the stiffness of normal or diseased joints. Bull Johns Hopkins Hosp 106:215, 1960.

30. Lehmann, JF and de Lateur, BJ: Diathermy and superficial heat, laser and cold therapy. In Kotke, FJ and Lehmann, JF (eds): Krusen's Handbook of Physical Medicine and Rehabilitation, ed 4. WB Saunders, Philadelphia, 1990, pp 283–367.

31. Michlovitz, SL: Thermal Agents in Rehabilitation, ed 2. FA Davis, Philadelphia, 1990.

32. Licht, S: Physical therapy. In Rehabilitation and Medicine, Vol 10. Waverly Press, Physical Medicine Library, Baltimore, 1968, pp 16–17.

33. Cailliet, R: Soft tissue concepts. In Soft Tissue Pain and Disability, ed. 2. FA Davis, Philadelphia, pp 3–17.

34. LeBan, MM: Collagen tissue: Implications of its response to stress in vitro. Arch Phys Med Rehabil 43:461, 1962.

35. Kottke, FJ, Pauley, DI, and Ptak, RA: The rationale for prolonged stretching for correction of shortening of connective tissue. Arch Phys Med Rehabil 47:345, 1966.

36. Warren, GC, Lehmann, JF, and Koblanski, JN: Heat and stretch procedures: An evaluation using rat tail tendon. Arch Phys Med Rehabil 57:122, 1976.

37. Brena, SF, Chapman, SL, and Sanders, SH: The needle and the brain: Psychophysiological factors involved in nerve blocking for chronic pain. Clin J Pain 7:245–247, 1991.

38. Derby, R: Comment on "The needle and the brain." Clin J Pain 7:248–249, 1991.

39. Brena, SF, Wolf, SL, Chapman, SL, and Hammonds, WD: Chronic back pain: Electromyographic, motion, and behavioral assessment following sympathetic nerve blocks and placebos. Pain 8:1–10, 1980.

40. Brena, SF and Unikel, IP: Nerve blocks and contingency management in chronic pain states. In Bonica, JJ and Albe-Fessard, D (eds): Advances in Pain Research and Therapy, Vol 1. Raven Press, New York, 1976.

41. Gilberstadt, H and Duker, J: A Handbook for Clinical and Actuarial MMPI Interpretation. WB Saunders, Philadephia, 1965, p 134.

42. Fordyce, WE, Fowler, RS, Lehmann, JF, Sand, PL and Trieschmann, RB: Operant conditioning in the treatment of chronic pain. In Franks, CM and Wilson, GT (eds): Annual Review of Behavioral Therapy Theory and Practice. Brunner/Mazel, New York, 1974, pp 691–712.

43. Grabois, M: Treatment of pain syndromes through exercise. In Lowenthal, DT, Bharadwaja, K, and Oaks, WW (eds): Therapeutics Through Exercise. Grune & Stratton, New York, 1979, pp 181–185.

44. Lee, MHM, Itoh, M, Yang, G-F W, and Eason, AL: Physical therapy and rehabilitation medicine. In Bonica, JJ (ed): The Management of Pain, Vol 2, ed 2. Lea & Febiger, Philadelphia, 1990, pp 1778–1781.

45. Basmajian, JV (ed): Therapeutic Exercise, ed 4. Williams & Wilkins, Baltimore, 1984.

46. DeVries, HA: Physiology of Exercise for Physical Education and Athletics, ed 3. William C. Brown, Iowa, 1966.

47. Fordyce, WE: Exercise and the increase in activity level. In Behavioral Methods for Chronic Pain and Illness, CV Mosby, St. Louis, 1976, pp 168–183.

48. Hagberg, M and Kvarnstrom, S: Muscular endurance and electromyographic fatigue in myofascial shoulder pain. Arch Phys Med Rehabil 65 (September):522–525, 1984.

49. Francis, KT: The role of endorphins in exercise: A review of current knowledge. Journal of Orthopaedic and Sports Physical Therapy 4(3):169–173, 1983.

50. Markoff, RA, Ryan, P, and Young, T: Endorphins and mood changes in long-distance running. Med Sci Sports Exerc 14:11–15, 1982.

51. Mayer, D and Watkins, L: Role of endorphins in endogenous pain control systems. Mod Probl Pharmacopsychiatry 17:68–96, 1981.

52. Appenzeller, O: What makes us run? N Engl J Med 305:578–579, 1981.

53. Haier, R, Quaid, B, and Mills, J: Naloxone alters pain perception after jogging. Psychiatry Res 5:231–232, 1981.
54. Farrell, PA, Gates, W, Maksud, M, and Morgan, W: Increases in plasma b-endorphin/ b-lipotropin immunoreactivity after treadmill running in humans. J Appl Physiol 52:1245–1249, 1982.
55. Pitts, F: Biochemical factors in anxiety neurosis. Behav Sci 16:82–91, 1971.
56. Padawer, WJ and Levine, FM: Exercise-induced analgesia: Fact or artifact? Pain 48:131–135, 1992.
57. Mayer, DL, Wolfle, H, Akil, B, Carder, J, and Liebeskind, JC: Science 164:444, 1969.
58. Lewis, JW, Stapleton, JM, Castiglioni, AJ, and Liebeskind, JC: In Fink, G and Whalley, LJ (eds): Neuropeptides: Basic and Clinical Aspects. Proceedings of the 11th Pfizer International Symposium. Churchill-Livingstone, Edinburgh, 1982, pp 41–49.
59. Basbaum, AI and Fields, HL: Annu Rev Neurosci 7:309, 1984.
60. Terman, GW, Shavit, Y, Lewis, JW, Cannon, JT, and Liebeskind, JC: Intrinsic mechanisms of pain inhibition: Activation by stress. Science 226 (December):1270–1277, 1984.
61. Watkins, LR, Johannessen, JN, Kinscheck, IB, and Mayer, DJ: Science 290:107, 1984.
62. Lewis, JW, Terman, GW, Nelson, LR, and Liebeskind, JC: In Tricklebank, MD and Curzon, G (eds): Stress-Induced Analgesia. Wiley, London, 1984, pp 103–134.
63. Lundberg, U and Frankenhauser, M: Pituitary-adrenal and sympathetic-adrenal correlates of distress and effort. J Psychosom Res 24:125–130, 1980.
64. Albe-Fessard, A: Physiology of pain—some recent concepts. Pain Symposium. Int Rehab Med 1(3):100–105, 1979.
65. Loeser, J, Black, R, and Christman, A: Relief of pain by transcutaneous stimulation. J Neurosurg 42:308–314, 1975.
66. Salar, G, Job, I, and Mingrino, S: Effect of transcutaneous electrotherapy on CSF B-endorphine content in patients without pain problems. Pain 10:169–172, 1981.
67. Sjolund, BH and Eriksson, MBE: The influence of naloxone on analgesia produced by peripheral conditioning stimulation. Brain Res 173:295–301, 1979.
68. Han, JS, Chen, XH, Sun, SL, Xu, XJ, Yuan, Y, Yan, SC, Hao, JX, and Terenius, L: Effect of low- and high-frequency TENS on Met-enkephalin-Arf-Phe and dynorphin A immunoreactivity in human lumbar CSF. Pain 47:295–298, 1991.
69. Akil, H and Liebeskind, JC: Monoaminergic mechanisms of stimulation produced analgesia. Brain Res 94:279–296, 1975.
70. Ignelzi, RJ and Nyquist, JK: Direct effect of electrical stimulation on peripheral nerve evoked activity: Implications in pain relief. J Neurosurg 45:159–165, 1976.
71. Langberg, GJ: Ultra-low frequency TENS: A well-kept secret. Pain Management Sept-Oct:278–280, 1990.
72. Long, DM and Hagfors, N: Electrical stimulation in the nervous system: The current status of electrical stimulation of the nervous system for the relief of pain. Pain 1:109–123, 1975.
73. Vincent, C and Richardson, PH: The evaluation of therapeutic acupuncture: Concepts and methods. Pain 24:1, 1986.
74. Steiner, RP: Acupuncture-cultural perspectives, Vol 1. The Western view. Postgrad Med 74:60, 1983.
75. Winfree, AT: The timing of biological clocks. Scientific American Library/Scientific American Books, New York 1987.
76. Hyodo, M: An Objective Approach to Acupuncture. Ryodoraku (Autonomic Nerve Society), Osaka, Japan, 1975.
77. Hyodo, M: Modern scientific acupuncture, as practiced in Japan. In Liptonand, S and Miles, J (eds): Persistent Pain. Grune & Stratton, Orlando, 1985, pp 129–156.
78. Gunn, CC and Milbrandt, WE: Dry needling of muscle motor points for chronic low-back pain: A randomized clinical trial with long-term follow-up. Spine 5:279, 1980.

79. Melzack, R: Myofascial trigger points: Relation to acupuncture and mechanism of pain. Arch Phys Med Rehabil 62:114, 1981.
80. Annual Meeting Report: Acupuncture. J Tenn Med Assoc. 75:202, 1981.
81. Bodnar, RJ: Dose-dependent reductions by naloxone of analgesia induced by cold-water stress. Pharmacol Biochem Behav 8:667, 1978.
82. Chapman, CR, Benedetti, C, Colpitts, YH, and Gerlach, R: Naloxone fails to reverse pain thresholds elevated by acupuncture: Acupuncture analgesia reconsidered. Pain 16:13, 1983.
83. Norton, GR: The effects of belief on acupuncture analgesia. Can J Behav Sci/Rev Can Sci Comp 16:22, 1984.
84. Chapman, CR, Wilson, ME, and Gehrig, JD: Comparative effects of acupuncture and transcutaneous stimulation on the perception of painful dental stimuli. Pain 2:265, 1976.
85. Chapman, CR, Sato, J, Martin, RW, Tanka, A, Ozazaki, N, Colpitts, YM, Mayeno, JF, Gagliaro, GJ: Comparative effects of acupuncture in Japan and the United States on dental pain perception. Pain 12:319–328, 1982.
86. Shealy, CN, Mortimer, J, and Reswick, J: Electrical inhibition of pain by stimulation of the dorsal columns: A preliminary report. Anesth Analg 46:489–491, 1967.
87. Wall, PD and Sweet, WH: Temporary abolition of pain in man. Science 155:108, 1967.
88. Sweet, WH and Wepsic, JG: Treatment of chronic pain by stimulation of fibers of primary afferent neurons. Trans Am Neurol Assoc 93:103, 1968.
89. Erickson, DL and Long, DM: Ten-year follow-up of dorsal column stimulation. In Bonica, JJ, Lindblom, U, and Iggo, A (eds): Advances in Pain Research and Therapy, Vol 5. Raven Press, New York, 1983, pp 583–589.
90. Campbell, JN: Examination of possible mechanisms by which stimulation of the spinal cord in man relieves pain. Appl Neurophysiol 44:181, 1982.
91. Nyquist, JK and Greenhoot, JH: Responses evoked from the thalamus centrum medianum by painful input: Suppression by dorsal funiculus conditioning. Exp. Neurol 9:215, 1973.
92. Foreman, RD, Beall, JE, Coulter, JD, et al: Effects of dorsal column stimulation on primate spinothalamic tract neurons. J Neurophysiol 39:534, 1976.
93. Meyerson, BA: Electrostimulation procedures: Effects, presumed rationale, and possible mechanisms. In Bonica, JJ, Lindblom, U, and Iggo, A (eds): Advances in Pain Research and Therapy, Vol 5. Raven Press, New York, pp 495–534.
94. Lindblom, U: Assessment of abnormal evoked pain in neurological pain patients and its relation to spontaneous pain. A descriptive and conceptual model with some analytical results. In Fields, H, Dubner, R, and Cervero, F. (eds): Advances in Pain Research and Therapy, Vol 9. Raven Press, New York, 1985, pp 409–423.
95. Urban, BJ and Nashold, BS: Percutaneous epidural stimulation of the spinal cord for the relief of pain. J Neurosurg 48:323, 1978.
96. Meyerson, BA: Electrical stimulation of the spinal cord and brain. In Bonica, JJ (ed): The Management of Pain, Vol 2, ed 2. Lea & Febiger, Philadelphia, 1990, pp 1862–1877.
97. Reynolds, DV: Surgery in the rat during electrical analgesia induced by focal brain stimulation. Science 164:444, 1969.
98. Hosobuchi, Y, Rossier, J, Bloom, FE, and Guillemin, R: Stimulation of human periaqueductal gray for pain relief increases immunoreceptive beta-endorphin in ventricular fluid. Science 203:279, 1979.
99. Meyerson, BA: Biochemistry of pain relief with intracerebral stimulation: Few facts and many hypotheses. Acta Neurochir 30(Suppl):229, 1980.
100. Hosobuchi, Y: The current status of analgesic brain stimulation. Acta Neurochir 30(Suppl):219, 1980.
101. North, RB, Ewend, MG, Lawton, MT, and Piantadosi, S: Spinal cord stimulation for chronic, intractable pain: Superiority of "multi-channel" devices. Pain 44:119–130, 1991.

CHAPTER 5

Psychologic Intervention in Pain

BIOFEEDBACK

Biofeedback has recently emerged in the treatment of pain and mood disorders. The modality of feedback has been defined as "a process in which a person learns to reliably influence physiological responses of two kinds: either responses which are not ordinarily under voluntary control or responses which ordinarily are under voluntary control but which regulation has broken down due to trauma or disease."[1] The intention of this approach is to regain control of the neuromuscular and neurovascular aspects of painful disease states.[2,3]

The neuromuscular aspects of a painful state are included in the tension states (Fig. 5–1), and the headaches that respond are a combination of neurovascular and muscular tension etiology.[4] Biofeedback is recognized as a valid treatment and has been accepted by the American Association for the Study of Headache.[5] The American Psychiatric Association has given a less enthusiastic endorsement.[6]

In this chapter we are only discussing the pathomechanics of biofeedback, not the actual technical application. Suffice it to say that biofeedback uses special electronic devices to detect, record, and amplify various neuromuscular and vascular responses and convert these visual and auditory responses into a form recognized, and thus controlled, by the patient.

The neurophysiologic basis for the efficacy of biofeedback in muscle tension has been postulated as regaining control of the muscle fiber through its intervention on the muscle spindle, which is termed "the prime organ of muscle sense."[2] This author proposes that the alpha motor neuron is influenced by the gamma motor neuron, which determines the tonic stretch reflex and modifies the extent and duration of the alpha control of the extrafusal fibers via supracortical controls. Biofeedback allegedly reasserts this control, which has been impaired by emotional or systemic disease.

The control of muscle has been discussed fully elsewhere,[7] but a brief

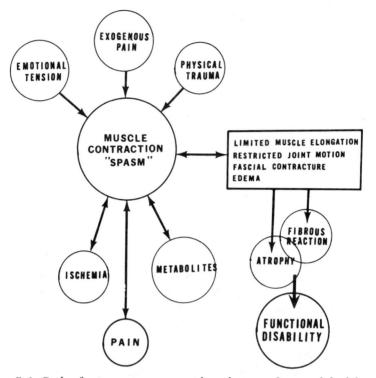

Figure 5–1. Cycle of pain causing spasm with evolution to functional disability.

review is indicated. The higher cortical control of the muscle complex is illustrated in Figure 5–2. As much of the "uncontrolled" neurologic involvement is in the autonomic system, which biofeedback attempts to control, the relationship of the autonomic and somatic nervous system must be postulated (Fig. 5–3).

The controlling innervation of the muscle occurs because of interdependence of the spindle and Golgi systems and the alpha extrafusal control system (Fig. 5–4). At the muscle fiber level the tone of the extrafusal fiber is controlled by "feedback" from the intrafusal spindle and Golgi fibers (Fig. 5–5). The coordination of this system is impaired when "perturbers" (Fig. 5–6) such as anger, anxiety, fatigue, depression, and sympatheticopenia intervene.[7]

Sympatheticopenia is depletion of all sympathetic chemical mediators: adrenaline-norepinephrine.[7]

The concept of sympatheticopenia as a factor in disease also alludes to its relationship in musculoskeletal dysfunction, which forms the basis for osteopathic manipulation therapy.

Hess described "ergotropic" function, which adjusts circulatory, metabolic, and visceral activity to postural and musculoskeletal demand.[8] This

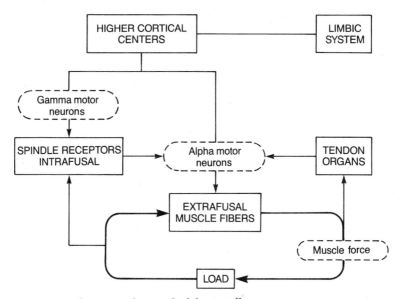

Figure 5–2. Higher cortical control of the spindle system.
The higher cortical centers indicate the intended muscular activity to perform the action. A feedback system correlates this activity. The load of the action determines the effort needed. The limbic system is the pathway of the perturbers, which are emotional and effect the effort via the limbic system.

demand implies that the sympathetic nervous system receives afferent input from the peripheral muscular system with modification from higher cortical centers. Osteopathic medicine approaches this input through the modality of vertebral manipulation on the assumption that there is a segmental vertebral and paraspinous dysfunction that influences the related neurologic control of viscera.

The sympathetic innervation of the skeletal system has an augmentary effect through the Orbeli phenomenon.[9] The muscle spindle system is directly affected by the sympathetic nervous system.[10] Any change in the autonomic nervous system alters the production of its chemical products, especially norepinephrine.

Hyperactivity or prolonged sustained sympathetic activity may lead to depletion at its synaptic terminations.[11] The continued afferent input to the sympathetic nervous system from injured peripheral tissues and their liberated algogens may result in sympatheticopenia.

The indications for biofeedback will be considered in subsequent chapters; biofeedback is predominantly indicated in tension or vascular (migraine) headaches and fibromyositic conditions.[12–14] It is also helpful in treating low back pain,[15,16] cervical tension states, and shoulder, scapular, and temporomandibular myalgia.[17,18] The use of biofeedback in neurovascular condi-

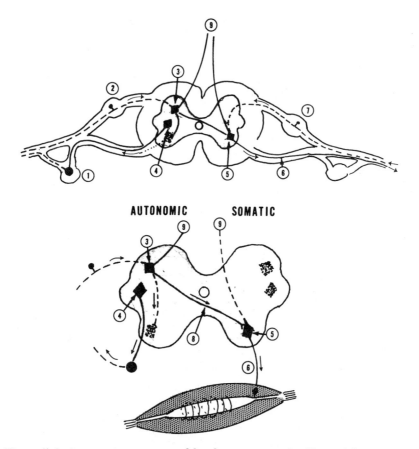

Figure 5–3. Autonomic-somatic cord level interaction. The fibers of the autonomic and the somatic nervous systems are shown: *(1)* the stellate ganglion, *(2)* the dorsal root ganglion, *(3)* sensory fiber nuclei within the gray matter, *(4)* motor cells of the autonomic system, *(5)* anterior horn (somatic motor) cells, *(6)* motor fibers to muscles, *(7)* somatic sensory fibers, *(8)* internal neuronal connections of the somatic autonomic systems, and *(9)* the cortical upper motor sensory neuronal connections. The connection *(8)* remains unproved.

tions causing chronic pain, such as reflex sympathetic dystrophy, is being studied.[19]

HYPNOSIS

For hundreds of years hypnosis has been used in entertainment, self-help, and therapy even though we do not fully understand how it works. Many terms are used to describe its workings: "absorption," "selective atten-

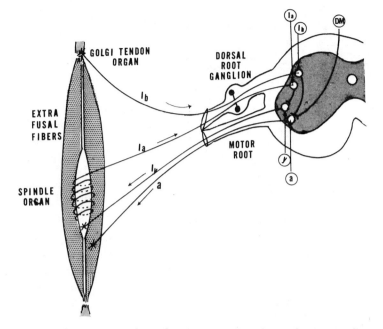

Figure 5–4. Pathways of spindle and Golgi systems to the cord. The spindle system supplies sensation to the cord via Ia fibers, the Golgi organs via Ib fibers. They end in the gray matter at cells Ia and Ib. The motor fibers to the spindle system are via I gamma fibers. These impulses "reset" the spindle system. The extrafusal fibers are innervated from the anterior horn cells *(a)* via alpha (a) fibers. Within the cord gray matter are numerous intercommunicating fibers. The upper cortical motor control is shown as *DM*.

tion," "suggestibility," and "dissociation." People under the influence of hypnosis are said to be in a trance, defined as "a sleeplike state . . . with limited sensory or motor contact with the ordinary surroundings . . . with subsequent amnesia of what has occurred during the state."[20] A few hypnotic subjects can produce vivid negative hallucinations, automatic writing, and even age regression in which they become their childhood self.

The trance can be regarded as a dissociative state in which there is a lack of integration of knowledge, memory, and voluntary control. *Hypnosis* derives from the Greek word for sleep because people in a hypnotic state walk and talk as if they are asleep. Electroencephalographic studies, however, reveal that people who are hypnotized are not asleep but are actually fully awake.

It has been estimated that about 20 percent of people are highly hypnotizable and 30 percent are not susceptible. The susceptibility is gauged as to depth of trance and ease of entering the trance state. No scale appears prevalent and there is no indication that sex, age, intellect, or education influences susceptibility. Hypnotic susceptibility requires a willingness to

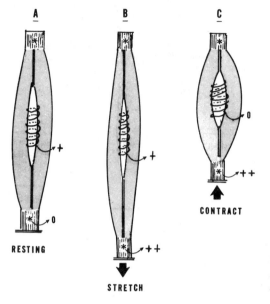

Figure 5–5. Spindle system coordination of muscular length, rate of contraction, and tension. (A) depicts resting muscle which, by its intrinsic elongation, activates the spindle system. (B) shows activity engendered in the Golgi organ by passive stretch with no spindle activity. In the actively contracted muscle (C), the spindle is relaxed and the Golgi strongly activated. The spindle and Golgi coordinate muscular action.

commit one's attention without fear of external threats, distraction, and repercussions. Schizophrenics are poor candidates as they cannot concentrate, paranoid patients are too suspicious, obsessional personalities too defensive, sociopaths too manipulative, and depressed patients too involved in their misery to become involved.[21]

Hypnosis is often portrayed as control over another person's mind, but in fact people cannot be hypnotized to perform any actions that go against their will, moral sense, or normal standards of behavior.

Hypnosis can be self-induced or induced by another person. In actuality, all hypnosis is self-induced, with the hypnotist acting as a guide or assistant.

Figure 5–6. Nervous control circuit of the muscular system. The motor cortex initiates muscular action via the somatic system (spinal cord). The Golgi organs and the spindle system act as sensors that coordinate muscular action regarding length and force for appropriate action. Perturbers are extraneous factors (such as fatigue, anxiety, fear, anger, and so forth) that upset the fine coordination.

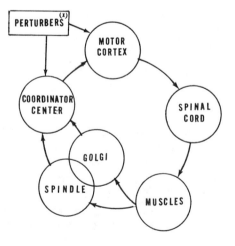

The usual method of inducing a hypnotic state is to relax the subject by directing his or her attention with a verbal, rhythmic, repetitive, and often monotonous instruction such as "Your eyelids are getting heavy," "Your legs are getting numb," or "Imagine you are on an escalator slowly ascending." Watching a swinging object, such as a watch or pendant on a thin chain, can also direct and capture the attention. The trance can be induced for seconds or for several hours and can be terminated simply by an instruction or suggestion from the hypnotist.

Trances have been induced for thousands of years; they are part of yoga meditation and many forms of religious rituals. Franz Mesmer[22] introduced this "healing" technique into Western medicine in the 18th century using the analogy of magnetic transmission as the vehicle. Hypnosis became known as "mesmerizing." In the 19th century Pierre Janet discovered that hypnotic suggestion produced forms of anesthesia,[22] and Sigmund Freud used hypnosis as a "catharsis" to eliminate traumatic memories. Freud gradually stopped using hypnosis because he felt the benefit was shallow and short-lived.[22] In 1957, the American Society for Clinical Hypnosis was founded, giving this modality formal recognition. Ultimately, the American Medical Association endorsed hypnosis as a legitimate aid to therapy.[23]

Hypnosis has various uses. In psychodynamic therapy, hypnosis induces relaxation and enables the patient to retrieve memories that may be related to his or her problem. Hypnosis is not considered useful in the treatment of severe mental disorders such as schizophrenia or major depressions. It is considered most effective in the treatment of pain syndromes, which is our current interest. Susceptibility must be determined by the therapist.[24]

The hypnotist may suggest to the patient that the painful area feels numb or less sensitive, thus allowing the patient to concentrate on other aspects of his or her body and feelings.[25] By distracting the patient, the therapist relieves anxiety.[26] In susceptible patients the perception of the "painful stimuli" may be changed, or there can be a placebo effect.

What has not yet been completely evaluated is the discovery of buried symptoms that affect the learned aspects of pain—the "value" of pain and disability to the patient. The magnitude of the pain can be diminished, allowing other forms of therapy to be instituted.[27] In certain medical conditions, such as migraine, the patient's control of an impending attack can be enhanced.[28]

In a multidiscipline pain center, hypnosis has a valid place; it can be used to determine susceptibility to suggestions, to diminish anxiety and anger, to reveal hidden psychodynamic factors that have enhanced the learned aspects of pain, to reveal childhood and familial aspects of pain behavior, and to decrease the intensity of pain sensation. Once any or all of these components of the pain are revealed, more directive therapy can then evolve. However, long-term benefit from mere suggestion during a hypnotic state has not been proven.

The patient must have confidence in the therapist before hypnosis is even attempted: The patient must not think that the therapist is using hypnosis because he or she believes that the pain is imaginary and can be overcome by exerting "mind over matter" or that the therapist can "remove" the pain by suggestion. Dependency on the therapist must be avoided or at least minimized. Suggestion is a valuable modality, but it is also powerful and must be carefully employed.

Hypnosis has been valuable in the relief of acute pain by acting as an analgesic.[29] Many surgical procedures have been performed under hypnosis.[30] Hypnotic imagery has been effective in many postoperative oncology patients to diminish their pain.[31] Dental patients have been effectively treated with hypnosis as the sole anesthetic.[32,33] Hypnosis has reduced labor pain in obstetric cases and probably plays a large role in natural childbirth.[34]

Hypnosis can possibly be considered as hypnotic analgesia by contributing to the decrease of anxiety. Although its neural mechanism is unknown, its apparent clinical benefit is not to be denied to patients that benefit from this modality.

REFERENCES

1. Blanchard, EB and Epstein, LH: A Biofeedback Primer. Addison-Wesley, Reading, MA, 1978.
2. Taylor, PL: Electromyometric Biofeedback Therapy, ed 1. Biofeedback and Advanced Therapy Institute, Los Angeles, 1981.
3. Budzynski, T: Biofeedback in the treatment of muscular-contraction (tension) headache. Biofeedback Self Regul 3:408, 1978.
4. Diamond, S, Diamond-Falk, Jr, and DeVeno, T: Biofeedback in the treatment of vascular headache. Biofeedback Self Regul 3:385, 1978.
5. American Association for the Study of Headache: Biofeedback therapy. Headache 18:107, 1978.
6. American Psychiatric Association: Task Force Report 19: Biofeedback. American Psychiatric Association, Washington, DC, 1980.
7. Korr, IM: Sustained sympathicotonia as a factor in disease. In Collected Papers of Irwin M. Korr. American Academy of Osteopathy, 1979.
8. Hess, WR: The Diencephalon-Autonomic and Extrapyramidal Functions. Grune & Stratton, New York, 1954.
9. Hutter, OF and Lowenstein, WR: Nature of neuromuscular facilitation by sympathetic stimulation in the frog. J Physiol 130:559–571, 1955.
10. Hunt, CC: The effect of sympathetic stimulation on mammalian muscle spindles. J Physiol 151:332–334, 1960.
11. Cheu, JW: Catecholamine depletion in the chronic fatigue syndrome: A pending publication. Personal communication, 1991.
12. Blanchard, EB, et al: Prediction of outcome from the non-pharmacological treatment of chronic headache. Neurology 33:1596, 1983.
13. Silver, BV, et al: Temperature biofeedback and relaxation training in the treatment of migraine headaches: One year follow-up. Biofeedback Self Regul 4:359, 1979.

14. Peck, CL and Kraft, GH: Electromyographic biofeedback for pain related to muscle tension. Arch Surg 112:889, 1977.

15. Freeman, CW, Calsyn, DA, Page, AB, and Halar, EM: Biofeedback with low back pain patients. American Journal of Clinical Biofeedback 3:118, 1980.

16. Keefe, FJ: EMG-assisted relaxation training in the management of chronic low back pain. American Journal of Clinical Biofeedback 4:93, 1981.

17. Scott, DS and Gregg, JM: Myofascial pain of the temporomandibular joint: A review of the behavioral-relaxation therapies. Pain 9:231, 1980.

18. Moss, RA, Wedding, D, and Sanders, SH: The comparative efficacy of relaxation training and masseter EMG feedback in the treatment of TMJ dysfunction. J Oral Rehabil 10:9, 1983.

19. Turk, DC, Meichenbaum, DH, and Berman, WH: Application of biofeedback for the regulation of pain: A critical review. Psychol Bull 86:1322, 1979.

20. Thomas, CL (ed): Taber's Cyclopedic Medical Dictionary, ed 15. FA Davis, Philadelphia, 1985.

21. Biofeedback: The Harvard Medical School: 7(10):1–4, 1991.

22. Hilgard, ER and Hilgard, JR: Hypnosis in the Relief of Pain. William Kaufmann, Los Altos, CA, 1975.

23. Barber, TX: Hypnosis: A Scientific Approach. Van Nostrand Reinhold, New York, 1969.

24. Weitzenhoffer, AM and Hilgard, ER: Stanford Hypnotic Susceptibility Scale, Forms A and B, and Form C. Consulting Psychologists Press, Palo Alto, CA, 1959 and 1962.

25. Dowd, E and Healy, JM (eds): Case Studies in Hypnotherapy. Guilford Press, New York, 1986.

26. Spiegel, H and Spiegel, D: Trance and Treatment: Clinical Uses of Hypnosis. Basic Books, New York, 1978.

27. Erickson, MH: An introduction to the study and application of hypnosis for pain control. In Lassner, J (ed): Hypnosis and Psychosomatic Medicine. Springer-Verlag, New York, 1967.

28. Harding, HC: Hypnosis in the treatment of migraine. In Lassner, J (ed): Hypnosis and Psychosomatic Medicine. Springer-Verlag, New York, 1967.

29. Lea, P, Ware, P, and Monroe, R: The hypnotic control of intractable pain. Am J Clin Hypn 3:3–8, 1960.

30. Esdaile, J: Hypnosis in Medicine and Surgery. Julian, New York, 1957.

31. Koulouch, FT: Hypnosis and surgical convalescence: A study of subjective factors in postoperative recovery. Am J Clin Hypn 7:120, 1964.

32. Gottfredson, DK: Hypnosis as an anaesthetic in dentistry. Diss Abstr Int B 33(7):3303, 1973.

33. Barber, J: Incorporating hypnosis in the management of chronic pain. In Barber, J and Adrian, C (eds): Psychological Approaches to the Management of Pain. Brunner/Mazel, New York, 1982.

34. Zeltzer, L and LeBaron, S: Hypnosis and nonhypnotic techniques for reduction of pain and anxiety during painful procedures in children and adolescents with cancer. J Pediatr 101:1032, 1982.

CHAPTER 6

Pharmacologic Intervention in Pain

Analgesics are agents that are considered to relieve pain by acting centrally. A possible mechanism has been postulated by the discovery of opiate receptors in selected areas of the central nervous system and of endogenous substances known as enkephalins or endorphins.[1] The receptor sites have been termed μ, δ, and κ.[2]

Opiate receptors are located in the medial thalamus—the area which processes deep, chronic, burning pain—as well as in areas of the cord gray matter, dorsal columns, and Rexed layers I and II. Opiate receptors are also greatly concentrated in the amygdala, a part of the limbic system (Chapter 1).

The presence of these receptors indicates that the body is capable of manufacturing its own narcotic-like substances. Two such substances have been discovered, both pentapeptides: tyrosine-glycine-glycine-phenyl-alanine-methionine and tyrosine-glycine-glycine-phenylalanine-leucine.[3] Opium and morphine derivatives have been manufactured to be exogenous opioids.

It is hypothesized that opioids inserted at these receptor sites activate the descending pathways to the midbrain periaqueductal gray matter, which inhibits ascension of nociception from the cord level.[4,5] Pain interruption has thus been asserted at the cord level and at the dorsal root ganglia (DRG).

A recent study has postulated that opiates have their effects at the peripheral mechanism as well.[6] In this study, patients who had arthroscopic knee surgery followed by intra-articular morphine had significantly diminished postoperative pain. The mechanism remains obscure.

The primary afferent nociceptor neuron is directed centrally to the spinal dorsal horn, and its peripheral axons proceed distally to innervate the skin, muscle, and joint tissues. Opiate receptors are synthesized in the cell

92

bodies of the receptors located in the DRG and are transported distally and centrally.

In pain it is thought that many agents sensitize primary afferent nociceptors directly by activating a G protein. The G protein activates adenylate cyclase, which increases intracellular cyclic AMP.[7] Opiates acting on μ opiate receptors activate an inhibitory G protein, which, in turn, inhibits adenylate cyclase with decreased production of cyclic AMP.[8] The threshold of the nociceptor terminal is elevated and pain sensation is decreased. This action implies that pain mediation from opiates is essentially chemical intervention on the receptors of opiate action at various levels in the central nervous system: the median raphe of the midbrain, the DRG, and the peripheral nociceptor sites where initial trauma or irritation occurs.

Opioids, in addition to their direct action on the μ receptors, also act on the α and κ receptors and on the postganglionic sympathetic terminals that block release of prostanoids.[9] Prostanoids are thought to be involved in sympathetic maintained pain syndromes.

Opioids may also decrease the release of the pain-producing inflammatory mediator substance P.[10] The lymphocyte-derived opioid peptide, considered to act on peripheral opioid receptors, may be blocked by local opioid action.[11] How and if local opioids at the peripheral level influence other aspects of inflammation such as rubor, calor, and tumor remains a promising avenue for further research.

The local opioid liberated at the trauma site acting on the opioid receptor may not derive from the endogenous pituitary or the adrenal medulla, but it may actually be an opioid peptide derived from local lymphoid cells.

Therapies that aim to decrease influx of lymphoids at the trauma site may actually reduce endogenous peripheral pain-modulation opioids and increase the severity of local tissue damage.[12] This indicates the need to carefully monitor the therapies—both physical and medicinal modalities—applied to inflammatory conditions such as rheumatoid arthritis.

In treating pain from acute peripheral inflammatory conditions, particularly musculoskeletal, it may be better to use local opioids at the periphery or at the DRG rather than oral or intramuscular opioids acting at the central level. It may also be undesirable to decrease lymphoid influx at tissue trauma sites. As yet, these issues are unresolved.

Serotonin has been implicated in pain production, especially in cardiac pain from ischemic heart disease. Serotonin acts as a vasoactive agent by directly activating serotonergic and alpha-adrenergic receptors.[13]

During platelet aggregation serotonin is released and in turn furthers platelet aggregation. This serotonin binds 5-hydroxytryptamine receptors on epithelial and smooth muscle cells, causing contraction of blood vessels. If the epithelial cells are normal, neutralizing chemicals are liberated that "wash out" these accumulating agents. If the tissue is damaged, these neutralizers are absent or diminished and vasoconstriction results.[14,15]

Animal studies have enhanced the evidence of a serotonin pain-inhibitor mechanism in the central nervous system. Inhibition of serotonin synthesis by parachlorophenylalanine (pCPA) increases pain sensitivity. Administration of 5-hydroxytryptophan, a precursor of serotonin, restores the depleted serotonin and returns the pain threshold to normal.[16] Lesions in the medial forebrain also reduce serotonin levels and lower pain threshold, which can also be restored by administration of serotonin precursor.[17] Injection of serotonin into the cerebral ventricles of rats and mice have allegedly raised pain thresholds.[18]

Morphine depends on a serotonin mechanism for its effectiveness in modulating pain. Morphine decreases serotonin in the brain. This effect is modified by pCPA and reserpine and can be reversed by administration of a serotonin precursor.

As chronic pain is often associated with depression, a common mechanism regarding depletion or decrease in serotonin has been postulated.[19] Reserpine, and 5-hydroxytryptophan cause depression, and chlorimipramine (a selective serotonin-reuptake blocking agent) is an antidepressant. This supports the theory that increased serotonin increases pain tolerance and decreased serotonin decreases pain tolerance and increases depression. Depression with pain will be discussed in Chapter 11.

Opiates are markedly underused in treating pain, causing patients to suffer needlessly. This is partly due to the myth of opiate tolerance and addiction. The problem has been compounded by restrictive laws regarding opioids, with attendant social, political, and legal problems.

It must be remembered that knowledge of pain pathophysiology and the pharmacology of opioids is relatively new. It is probable that the vast majority of medical practitioners were trained to avoid narcotics. Many believe certain myths about opioids and pain treatment.[20]

- There is a maximum "safe" dose of morphine and other opioids.
- Opioids always cause addiction.
- Every user of opioids becomes tolerant and must increase his or her dosage.
- If a narcotic is used early in treating pain and fails, there remains no other medication to fall back on.
- Because opioids are potent, all pain will respond.
- Opioids inadvertently depress respiration.
- Demand for opioids indicates addiction.
- The onset of "other" pains will demand the use of narcotic.
- Parenteral opioids are more potent and effective than oral analgesics.

All these premises can be questioned and many have been refuted, but all need clarification and confirmation.

Opioid pain medication is generally underused in the treatment of acute pain and especially cancer pain.[21] The underuse of pain medication in treating children with pain will be addressed in Chapter 12.

The use of opioids in noncancer and chronic pain is a more complicated problem. Chronic pain can be effectively managed with opioids in many patients.[22] However, according to Arner and Meyerson,[23] pain management without opioids has proven effective and the use of opioids is not significantly justified. The standards for judging opioid efficacy are similar to the standards for judging the efficacy of antidepressants in treating diabetic and postherpetic neuropathies.[24] This lack of accepted standardization explains in part why medications, including opioids, are not effectively used.

Currently chronic pain management is confused, inappropriate, and not physiologically based.[25] For many years the long-term use of opioids for chronic pain was forbidden or at least contraindicated despite the fact that its use was highly effective.[26] This has been refuted.[27] There was even a plea for its use in an International Association for the Study of Pain (IASP) presidential address by Ronald Melzack.[28]

The basis for further evaluation is

• Tolerance, dependence, addiction, and adverse side-effects
• Analgesic efficacy
• Goals of therapeutic intervention

Sternbach[29] questioned the safety and "humaneness" of opioids in the light of a 5 percent iatrogenic addiction rate and minimal functional improvement that accompanied opioid therapy.

In patients with minimal and even undiscernible tissue damage, the use of long-term opioid therapy remains most controversial. This again brings up the concept that the quantity of pain must be equated with the quantity of tissue damage, an archaic and unacceptable concept.[30] As pain is subjective and is usually associated with feelings of anxiety and concern, the quantification of pain and its relief become essentially subjective. Thus the use of opioids is jeopardized.[31]

The contrast between somatogenic and psychogenic pain influences "objective" evaluation of any drug or modality, and opioids are included in this controversy. Many patients who enter chronic pain clinics have used, misused, and even abused narcotics in their quest for relief. A primary protocol of most chronic pain clinics is "the removal of all narcotic and habituating medications before further therapy."[32]

It is probable that many patients referred to chronic pain centers have tried—and failed to get relief from—drugs. Pain management involves functional, psychologic, behavioral, and other factors. These must be addressed in evaluating the efficacy of opioids and the desirability of terminating their use.

This question always arises about evaluating patients who improve in function yet retain their high pain level as compared to the patients who report no gains.[33] The patients who report a "reduction" of pain—that is, 20 to 50 percent—are difficult to statistically document. Compliance with other aspects of rehabilitation after pain reduction from the use of opioids also concerns the pain clinics, whose results cannot be documented.

The guidelines for long-term use of opioids offered by Portenoy[27] have been considered.

1. Persistent pain is the major impediment to function ("pain is disabling").
2. Psychologic problems are not present or considered pertinent.
3. All other analgesic (nonnarcotic) medications have failed.
4. There is no prior history of substance abuse.
5. A primary physician will assume responsibility in monitoring the medication and its response.

The difficulties in implementing these guidelines are as follows:

1. There are no objective criteria that pain is the sole or major impediment to function.
2. It is hard to ascertain the absence of psychologic factors or the degree to which existing psychopathology is the result of pain.
3. It is usually unclear whether depression is a factor in the pain and dysfunction and if opioids enhance or decrease this depression.
4. The previous use of nonnarcotic analgesics may not have been appropriate, proper, or of significant duration.
5. Compliance must be ascertained and ascertainable.[33]

Topical application of a drug termed capsaicin has diminished cutaneous sensitivity in painful conditions such as postherpetic neuralgia, cluster headaches, painful diabetic neuropathy, and the cutaneous sensitivity noted in sympathetic mediated pain.[34-36] These painful cutaneous states are allegedly the result of neurogenic vasodilation.

The mechanism by which topical capsaicin works is the possible desensitization of the C fiber nociceptors, which block the conduction of their axons. In conditions such as reflex sympathetic dystropy, altered processing of peripheral impulses in the central nervous system may even occur at the dorsal horn level.

Capsaicin probably interferes with peripheral nociception before it reaches the dorsal horn. It is ineffective in conditions in which the peripheral axons are intact. Benefit is usually temporary and may require repeated applications.

Pharmacologic intervention of pain, either acute or chronic, can be administered orally, by numerous injection routes (intramuscular, intradermal, epidural, dural, intra-articular), and even by mucosal routes. The numerous drugs available are discussed extensively in the literature.[37] Here we will only mention certain drugs in specific pathologic entities throughout this text.

REFERENCES

1. Pert, CB and Snyder, SH: Opiate receptors: Demonstration in nervous tissue. Science 179:1011–1014, 1973.
2. Hughes, J: Isolation of an endogenous compound from the brain with pharmacological properties similar to morphine. Brain Res 88:295–308, 1975.
3. Hughes, J: Search for the endogenous ligand of the opiate receptor. Neuroscience Research Program Bulletin 13:55–58, 1975.
4. Basbaum, AI and Fields, HL: Endogenous pain control systems: Brain stem spinal pathways and endorphin circuitry. Annu Rev Neurosci 7:309–338, 1984.
5. Yaksh, TI and Rudy, TA: Analgesia mediated by direct spinal action of narcotics. Science 192:1357–1358, 1976.
6. Stein, C, Comisel, K, Haimeri, E, Yassouridis, A, Lehrberger, K, Herz, A, and Peter, K: Analgesic effect of intracarticular morphine after arthroscopic knee surgery. New Engl J Med 325(16):1123–1126, 1991.
7. Taiwo, YO, Bjerknes, LK, Goetzl, EJ, and Levine, JD: Mediation of primary afferent peripheral hyperalgesia by the cAMP second messenger system. Neuroscience 32:577–580, 1989.
8. Levine, JD and Taiwo, YO: Involvement of the μ-opiate receptor in peripheral analgesia. Neuroscience 32:571–575, 1989.
9. Taiwo, YO and Levine, JD: κ- and α-opioids block sympathetically dependent hyperalgesia. J Neurosci 11:928–932, 1991.
10. Basbaum, AI and Levine, JD: Opiate analgesia: How central is a peripheral target? New Engl J Med 325(16):1168–1169, 1991.
11. Jessell, TM and Iversen, LL: Opiate analgesics inhibit substance P release from rat trigeminal nucleus. Nature 268:549–551, 1977.
12. Coderre, TJ, Chan, AK, Helms, C, Basbaum, AI, and Levine, JD: Increasing sympathetic nerve terminal-dependent plasma extravasation correlates with decreased arthritic joint injury in rats. Neuroscience 40:185–189, 1991.
13. Stein C, Hassan, AHS, Przewlocki, R, Gramsch, C, Peter, K, and Herz, A: Opioids from immunocytes interact with receptors on sensory nerves to inhibit nociception in inflammation. Proc Natl Acad Sci 87:5935–5935, 1990.
14. Lam, JY, Chesebro, JH, Steele, PM, Badimon, L, and Fuster, V: Is vasospasm related to platelet deposition? Relationship in a porcine preparation of arterial injury in vivo. Circulation 75:243–248, 1987.
15. Vanhoutte, PM and Shimokawa, H: Endothelium-derived relaxing factor and coronary vasospasm. Circulation 80:1–9, 1989.
16. Harvey, JA and Lints, C: Pharmacologist 10:211, 1968.
17. Akil, H, Mayer, DJ, and Liebeskind, JC: Antagonism of stimulation-produced analgesia by p-CPA, a serotonin synthesis inhibitor. Brain Res 44:692–697, 1972.
18. Calcutt, CR, Handley, SL, Sparkes, CG, and Spencer, PSJ: In Kosterlitz, HW, Collier, HOJ, and Villareal, JA (eds): Agonist and Antagonist Actions of Narcotic Analgesic Drugs. University Park Press, Baltimore, 1973.
19. Sternbach, RA, Janowsky, DS, Leighton, YH, and Segal, DS: Effects of altering brain serotonin activity on human chronic pain. In Bonica, JJ and Albe-Fessard, D (eds): Raven Press, New York, 1976.

20. Lipman, AG: Opioid use in the treatment of pain: Refuting ten common myths. Pain Management 4(4):13–24, 1991.
21. Dubner, R: A call for more science, not more rhetoric, regarding opioid and neuropathic pain. Pain 47:1–2, 1991.
22. Portenoy, RK, Foley, KM, and Inturrisi, CE: The nature of opioid responsiveness and its implications for neuropathic pain: New hypotheses derived from studies of opioid infusions. Pain 43:273–288, 1990.
23. Arner, S and Meyerson, BA: Genuine resistance to opioids—fact or fiction? Pain 47:116–118, 1991.
24. Watson, CPN: Neuropathic pain syndromes. In Max, MB, Portenoy, RK and Laska, EM (eds): Advances in Pain Research and Therapy, Vol 18: The Design of Analgesic Clinical Trials. Raven Press, New York, 1991, pp 221–231.
25. Turk, DC and Brody, MC: Chronic opioid therapy for persistent noncancer pain. Part I: Panacea or oxymoron. Pain Management 4(5):25–33, 1991.
26. Maruta, T, Swanson, DW, and Finlayson, RE: Drug abuse and dependency in patients with chronic pain. Mayo Clin Proc 54:241–244, 1979.
27. Portenoy, RK: Opioid therapy in the management of chronic back pain. In Tollison, CD (ed): Interdisciplinary Rehabilitation of Low Back Pain. Williams & Wilkins, Baltimore, 1989, pp 137–157.
28. Melzack, R: The tragedy of needless pain: A call for social action. In Dubner, R, Oebart, GF, and Bond, MR (eds): Proceedings of the 5th World Congress on Pain. Elsevier, Amsterdam, 1988, pp 1–11.
29. Sternbach, RA: Letter. Pain 29:259–260, 1987.
30. Morris, DB: The Culture of Pain. University of California Press, Berkeley, CA, 1991.
31. Arner, S and Myerson, BA: Lack of analgesic effect of opioids on neuropathic and ideopathic forms of pain. Pain 33:11–23, 1988.
32. Buckley, FP, Sizemore, WA, and Charlton, JE: Medication management in patients with chronic nonmalignant pain. A review of the use of a drug withdrawal protocol. Pain 26:153–165, 1986.
33. Turk, DC and Rudy, TE: Neglected topics in the treatment of chronic pain patients: Referral patterns, failure to enter treatment, and attrition. Pain 43:7–26, 1990.
34. Simone, DA and Ochoa, J: Early and late effects of prolonged topical capsaicin on cutaneous sensibility in neurogenic vasodilatation in humans. Pain 47:285–294, 1991.
35. Bernstein, JE: Treatment of chronic post-herpetic neuralgia with topical capsaicin. J Am Acad Derm 17:93–96, 1987.
36. Tandan, R: Topical capsaicin in painful diabetic polyneuropathy. Neurol (Suppl)1:380, 1990.
37. Gennaro, AR (ed): Remington's Pharmaceutical Sciences, ed 18. Mack Publishing, Easton, PA, 1990.

CHAPTER 7

Mechanisms of the Regional Aspects of Pain

Not only do the tissue sites of nociception need evaluation, but the precise mechanisms causing pain must be understood. Every musculoskeletal system, including disability and pain, have been discussed fully elsewhere.[1-8] The intent in this volume is to evaluate the specific mechanisms that cause pain and disability in each system. A complete understanding of the pathomechanics gained from a meaningful history and physical examination will lead to a physiologic diagnosis and a pertinent treatment approach. Thus, pain emanating from any musculoskeletal system can be addressed.

POSTURE

It is appropriate to begin a dissertation on musculoskeletal pain by discussing posture. Posture, the attitude a human being assumes in the sitting and standing position, influences every aspect of the musculoskeletal system. Faulty posture is implicated in every painful pathologic condition from injury, overuse, misuse, and aging.

The chronologic development of posture and its neurologic concepts have been evaluated elsewhere.[9] Development and modification of proper posture is also influenced by disease, trauma, and psychologic factors.[10]

Proprioceptive end organs located in the skin, joint capsules, ligaments, and muscles of the entire body send instantaneous information to the central nervous system, which initiates an appropriate musculoskeletal response. The sensory nervous system is thus the major determinant of correct evaluation of posture (Fig. 7–1).

What constitutes proper posture is ambiguous; many childhood factors

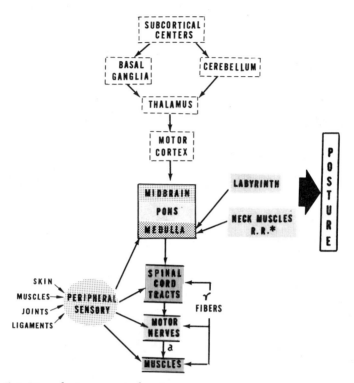

Figure 7–1. Neurologic concept of posture.

The upper neurologic pathways (subcortical centers, basal ganglia, cerebellum, thalamus, and motor cortex) are the well-documented circuits by which motor activities are initiated and coordinated.

Within the midbrain medulla are the primary righting reflex centers that receive impulses from the labyrinth and the righting reflexes (°R.R.) of the neck muscles. Posture is dependent on this medullary center and the spinal cord interneurons influencing the motor nerves that are moderated by the alpha and gamma fibers to the muscles. Each level of the central system receives and is moderated by peripheral sensory impulses from the skin, joints, capsules, ligaments, and muscles (see text).

affect this concept.[10] "Proper posture" is believed to be effortless, cosmetically correct, and pain-free. It feels good. A posture that fulfills all these criteria yet is faulty is potentially injurious to tissues, which can ultimately cause pain.

Many postural bad habits develop in childhood. A slumped posture, which may stem from peer or family pressure, anxiety, insecurity, or fear or anger in childhood, may be assumed to be "normal," as it causes no discomfort. Feldenkrais[10] suggests that many faulty postures in childhood develop from "cringing from fear of physical assault by domineering parents or siblings."

Many postures are influenced by daily activities such as hours spent at a computer or wearing bifocal glasses. [11,12] For decades, footwear was thought to affect posture. This has recently been refuted but merits evaluation. [13]

Emotions also influence posture. Essentially, we stand, sit, and walk as we feel. The depressed person exhibits depression by his posture. The angry or impatient person also depicts this feeling by her posture and actions. Body language can be very telling.

There are also organic components of abnormal posture that demand exploration. Muscle disease can cause kyphotic posture, as can fatigue of the cervical paraspinous muscles in daily posture. [14,15]

The role of the fascia in postural pain has been largely ignored. It assumes the length of the muscle it contains. It can only be influenced by external forces as it has no voluntary control. The relationship between the fascia and the forces and pressures generated by the underlying muscle contractions is poorly understood. Fasciae retract when inflamed or passively elongated and become foci of pain because of their rich nerve supply.

Posture causes a change in the mechanical aspect of both static and kinetic musculoskeletal functions. For example, the shoulder glenohumeral joint is adversely affected by a dorsal kyphotic posture, which causes impingement of the rotator cuff. The cervical spine is adversely affected by a forward head posture, which increases cervical lordosis. The lumbar spine curvature is affected by posture. Upper back pain, termed scapulocostal pain, is directly associated with posture, as is the thoracic outlet syndrome.

TRAUMA

Trauma is mentioned as a cause of pain, yet it remains undefined and unclarified. External trauma is more clearly defined; yet because it mostly affects soft tissues, which are not verifiable by objective tests, its role in pain remains obscure. Trauma of lesser force, termed microtrauma, is even less clearly understood. Microtrauma impairs muscle coordination; this results in prolonged pain and dysfunction.

Microtrauma is a perturber to coordinated neuromusculoskeletal function resulting in pain (Fig. 7–2). Normal pain-free neuromusculoskeletal coordinated action implies

- Normal intrinsic neuromuscular contraction, both concentric and eccentric
- Normal mechanical articular function

Normal neuromusculoskeletal function is dependent on sensory input with appropriate motor response. Resultant muscular contraction is a somatic nerve–controlled activity. The afferent input coordinates the efferent motor activity. [17]

"Normal" muscle contraction implies appropriate strength, timing, and

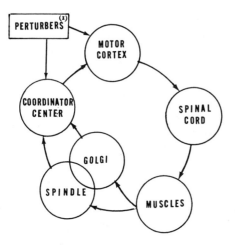

Figure 7–2. Nervous control circuit of the muscular system.

The motor cortex initiates muscular action via the somatic system (spinal cord). The Golgi organs and the spindle system act as sensors that coordinate muscular action regarding length and force for appropriate action. Perturbers are extraneous factors (such as fatigue, anxiety, fear, and anger that upset the fine coordination.

duration of contraction for the intended activity. Lifting a 20-lb object requires appropriate muscle contraction to lift that weight its appropriate distance for the duration of the lift. Excessive uncoordinated contraction leads to pain and impairment.

The neurophysiologic mechanism of muscular contraction is via the Golgi and spindle systems (Fig. 7–3). The afferent sensation of the contraction to the cord is via the Ia fibers from the spindle system and the Ib fibers from the Golgi tendon organs. These ascend through the dorsal root ganglia (DRG) to enter the dorsal horn of the cord. The alpha-motor fibers that innervate the extrafusal fibers originate at the anterior horn. They discharge the exact appropriate muscle contraction for the intended action.

The spindle and Golgi systems are "reset" instantaneously for the next contraction via the I gamma fibers (Fig. 7–4). Afferent mechanosensory fibers from the joint inform the central nervous system that the action has been accomplished. Every agonist contraction is accompanied by a commensurate antagonist relaxation mediated at the cord level (Fig. 7–5).

The neuromuscular precision to accomplish the intended task, albeit intrinsic, is influenced by extrinsic factors. When inappropriate for normal function these extrinsic factors are termed perturbers and include distraction, anger, fatigue, depression, impatience, and annoyance.

Perturber influence on neuromusculoskeletal competence causes pathologic changes in the joints, ligaments, tendons, and muscle fasciae. They liberate algogens (nociceptors), which in turn become perturbers. "Protective" muscle spasms occur, which causes further functional disability and enhances pain (Fig. 7–6). Eccentric muscle contraction is especially susceptible to trauma.[18,19] Changes seen on electron microscopy are myofibrillar necrosis, Z band changes, and sarcolemmal disruption.[20]

Neurophysiologic muscle dysfunction resulting from microtrauma has been claimed.[21] This concept implies that sudden unexpected stretching of

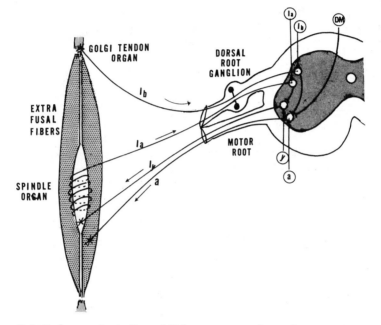

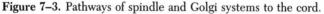

Figure 7–3. Pathways of spindle and Golgi systems to the cord.

The spindle system supplies sensation to the cord via Ia fibers; the Golgi organs via Ib fibers. They end in the gray matter at cells Ia and Ib. The motor fibers to the spindle system are via I gamma fibers. These impulses "reset" the spindle system. The extrafusal fibers are innervated from the anterior horn cells *(a)* via alpha (a) fibers. Within the cord gray matter are numerous intercommunicating fibers. The upper cortical motor control is shown as *DM*.

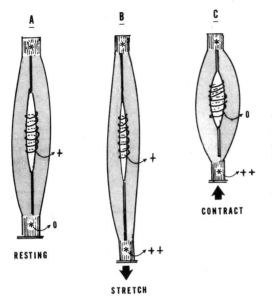

Figure 7–4. Spindle system coordination of muscular length, rate of contraction, and tension. (A) depicts resting muscle which, by its intrinsic elongation, activates the spindle system. (B) shows activity engendered in the Golgi organ by passive stretch with no spindle activity. In the actively contracted muscle (C), the spindle is relaxed and the Golgi strongly activated. The spindle and Golgi coordinate muscular action.

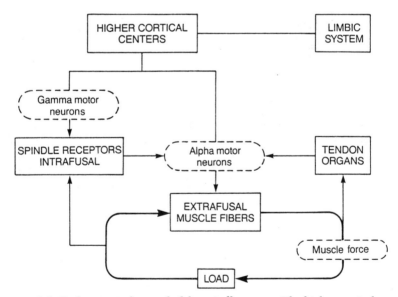

Figure 7–5. Higher cortical control of the spindle system. The higher cortical centers indicate the intended muscular activity to perform the action. A feedback system correlates this activity. The load of the action determines the effort needed. The limbic system is the pathways of the perturbers, which are emotional and effect the effort via the limbic system.

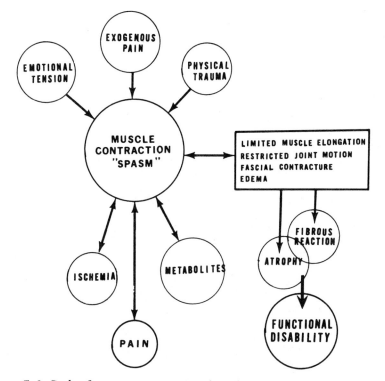

Figure 7–6. Cycle of pain causing spasm with evolution to functional disability.

an involved muscle releases a barrage of impulses from proprioceptors located within the muscle spindles and the joint capsules. These impulses allegedly impart "false" information to the spinocerebellar tracts to the midbrain and thalamic and subcortical nuclei. This results in inappropriate input to the descending tracts to the alpha and gamma motor units, which then influence the anterior horn cells and cause inappropriate muscle contractions.[22] Trauma to the spindle system now causes inappropriate neuromusculoskeletal function, which becomes a perturber, with resultant pain and dysfunction.

Sleep deprivation is another perturber as it causes fatigue and unwillingness to exercise. Inadequate physical fitness and coordination thus prediposes the individual to further microtrauma. Central fatigue causes slow-wave sleep deprivation with resultant release of muscle-derived fatigue factor (glycogen storage) and peripheral fatigue.[23]

Sympathetic maintained pain acts as a perturber of proper muscle contraction (Fig. 7–7). This autonomic involvement has an adverse effect on the microcirculation of the affected muscles.

The emotions adversely influence muscle contraction causing tension myositis syndrome.[24] Muscle relaxants have been effective in treating these

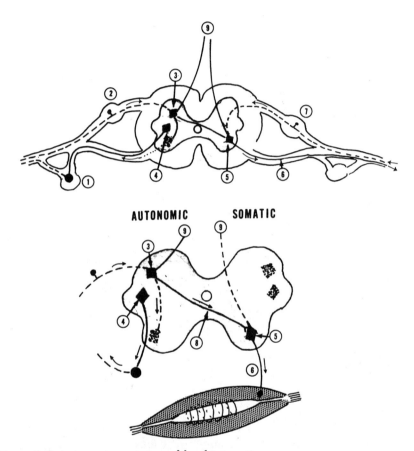

Figure 7–7. Autonomic-somatic cord level interaction.
The fibers of the autonomic and the somatic nervous systems are shown: *(1)* the stellate ganglion, *(2)* the dorsal root ganglion, *(3)* sensory fiber nuclei within the gray matter, *(4)* motor cells of the autonomic system, *(5)* anterior horn (somatic motor) cells, *(6)* motor fibers to muscles, *(7)* somatic sensory fibers, *(8)* internal neuronal connections of the somatic autonomic systems, and *(9)* the cortical upper motor sensory neuronal connections. The connection *(8)* remains unproved.

painful musculoskeletal states, but their precise mechanism has yet to be confirmed.[25]

Inner ear impairment with attendant vestibular abnormality has been noted after a cervical subluxation following a rear-end vehicular collision.

FIBROMYALGIA SYNDROMES

Fascial tissue involvement in dysfunction and pain has been mentioned. Its involvement in most painful neuromusculoskeletal syndromes justify discussing a primary myofascial pain entity.

Much has been and is being written about fibromyalgia syndrome (FS), "a syndrome characterized by chronic pain widely distributed through all the skeletal muscles and soft tissues." Its pathomechanics and neuropathology remain obscure. As all painful neuromuscular syndromes—acute or chronic—have a fibromyalgic component, a dissertation on pain and pain mechanism cannot escape addressing this entity.

This condition was written about by Hippocrates,[27] but only in the last 150 years has there been significant attention to FS as a clinical entity. Froriep[28] recognized areas of muscle "hardness" that, when palpated, elicited pain. Later Beard[29] described the syndrome, which he called neurasthenia. The term *fibrositis* originated in the literature in 1904.[30] Since then numerous diagnostic terms have been applied to the condition.[31]

The IASP classified these chronic musculoskeletal pain syndromes "without identifiable cause" as follows:[32]

1. *Primary fibromyalgia syndrome (PFS)*. Fibrositis, diffuse myofascial pain syndrome, or primary diffuse fibrositis syndrome
2. *Myofascial pain syndrome (MPS)*. Specific myofascial pain syndrome
3. *Temporomandibular pain and dysfunction syndrome (TMPSD)*

Diagnostic criteria are based on subjective evidence of long-standing musculoskeletal pain, fatigue, sleep disturbance, and the clinical findings of reproducible tender points (TP). The standard diagnostic criteria of Yunus and colleagues[33] are the most widely accepted. These include obligatory, major, and minor criteria. No objective diagnostic studies have led to a specific diagnosis.

The obligatory criteria are:

• Generalized aches and pains or prominent stiffness, involving three or more anatomic sites for at least 3 months
• Absence of traumatic injury,* structural rheumatic disease, infec-

---

*"Absence of traumatic injury" is not accepted by the author, as trauma is usually, if not universally, present.

tious arthropathy, endocrine-related arthropathy, and abnormal laboratory tests

The major criterion is:

- The presence of three or more typical and consistent TPs

The minor criteria are:

- Modulation of symptoms by physical activity
- Symptoms altered by weather changes
- Symptoms aggravated by anxiety or stress
- Poor sleep
- General fatigue or tiredness
- Anxiety
- Chronic headaches
- Irritable bowel syndrome
- Subjective swelling
- Nonradicular and nondermatomal numbness

Smythe,[34] a pioneer in the subject of fibrositis, postulated the following criteria:

- Widespread aching of more than 3 months' duration
- Local tenderness at 12 of 14 specific sites
- Skin-roll tenderness over the upper scapular region
- Disturbed sleep with morning fatigue and stiffness
- Normal estimated sedimentation rate (ESR), serum glutamate oxaloacetate transaminase (SGOT), rheumatoid factors test, antinuclear factor (ANF), muscle enzymes, and sacroiliac films

It is apparent that the diagnostic criteria are subjective and actually mandate that there be no abnormal organic tests present other than the sleep disturbance, which have been objectively ascertained.[35]

Pathophysiology

Abnormalities of the musculature have been implicated with reports of abnormal histologic findings from biopsies, yet none remain fully reproducible. Yunus[36] has speculated that all the histologic abnormalities observed could be the result of ischemia from microspasm of the musculature.

The nociceptors located in the muscles, tendons, and perivascular sites are the thin myelinated A-alpha and nonmyelinated C fibers discussed in Chapter 1. These nerve endings are inflamed by endogenous algesic chemical substances such as bradykinin, prostaglandins, leukotrienes, potassium ions, serotonin, and interleukin-1.[37,38]

Administration of two of the above algesic substances potentiates the effect at the nociceptor sites.[39] When preceded by serotonin or prostaglandin E2, the effect on the receptor of bradykinin is enhanced by 10 minutes. Bradykinin also stimulates the synthesis of prostaglandin from arachidonic acid so that the interplay of these algesic agents results in an inflammatory response.

These substances affect local microcirculation, causing vasoconstriction or vasodilation but also increasing vascular permeability; this results in extravasation and edema. Ischemia of the involved tissues results in pain. The irritating effects of algogens cause spasm, which enhances ischemia.

The hypoxia of the muscle allegedly decreases the intramuscular level of adenosinotriphosphate and phosphocreatine; this accounts for the pain.[40] Compromised capillary microcirculation in a fibrositic trapezius muscle has been found to be diminished after ultrasound treatment as compared to the increase produced in normal muscle.[41] Electromyographic studies have failed to reveal specific abnormalities that can be considered diagnostic, although fatigue in the fibrositis muscle groups has been demonstrated.[42]

Muscle strength evaluated by Cybex II dynamometer has shown weakness in involved muscles as compared to contralateral normal muscle, but the objectivity of this conclusion can be questioned as to effort expended in a painful muscle.[43,44]

Sleep disturbance in patients with fibromyalgia has been thoroughly described, yet this does not clarify the neurophysiologic basis for the syndrome.[45]

Metabolic abnormalities creating algogens in FS are promising. Serotonin, a central nervous system neurotransmitter, is being studied. Serotonin is converted from the essential amino acid tryptophan when it crosses the blood-brain barrier. The source of serotonin is considered to be the raphe nucleus in the brainstem.[46] It is well documented that depletion of serotonin decreases non-REM sleep, as well as causing symptoms of depression.[47,48] The relationship of tryptophan to symptoms of FS is questioned,[49] but recently FS patients have been found to have lower than normal levels of tryptophan as well as of six other amino acids.[50]

Benefit from the use of tricyclic drugs (amitriptyline, imipramine, cyclobenzaprine, and so on) in FS enhances the theory that they act by blocking serotonin reuptake at the synaptic cleft.[48] The precise role of serotonin is not yet confirmed.[51]

Catecholamines producing FS symptoms have also been implicated. Catecholamines are described as "biologically active amines, epinephrine and norepinephrine, derived from amino acid tyrosine. They have marked effect on the nervous and cardiovascular systems, metabolic rate, temperature and smooth muscle."[52] Serotonin is described as "a chemical (5-hydroxytryptamine) present in platelets, gastrointestinal mucosa, mast cells and carcinoid tumors. Serotonin is a potent vasoconstrictor. It is thought to be involved in neural mechanisms important to sleep and sensory perception."[52] All these have been found to be involved in FS.

FS patients have been found to have above normal urinary norepi- nephrine levels.[53] In studies making this assertion, elevated levels were also found in patients with a high level of anxiety. These high levels, incidentally, were not found in patients exhibiting depression.

Substance P, a neuropeptide considered to be an algogen, has been found to exist in virtually all neuronal structures of the central nervous system: the spinal and trigeminal ganglia, the substantia gelatinosum (layers of Rexed I and II) of the dorsal horn of the cord, as well as in higher brain centers. Their elevation or depression in the spinal fluid of FS patients has had varying results.[54,55]

Endorphins, another group of neuropeptides, have been studied in the possible mechanism of FS pain. Endorphins are endogenously produced opioid substances of complex chemical structure and action. They are located in the same regions of the central nervous system as substance P: in periph- eral nerve endings, the dorsal horn of the cord, midbrain, brainstem, and thalamus. There is speculation that endorphins modulate the transmission of pain by inhibiting substance P.

Studies suggesting that physical fitness decreases the perception of pain on the basis of endorphins were conducted.[56] Yunus[57] found no difference in serum endorphin levels between FS patients and normal controls.

Because of the similarity of FS to rheumatoid arthritis, Raynaud's syn- drome, hypothyroidism, and Sjögren's syndrome, some have thought that the immune system is involved.[58] A 30-month follow-up of FS patients, however, showed that no patient had developed systemic disease.[59] Recent interest in chronic fatigue syndrome and its relationship to FS is being explored, with some promise.[60]

One model of fibromyalgia syndrome proposed that because muscle is the end organ responsible for the syndrome, possibly microtrauma to the muscle causes the symptoms.[61] Perturber interruption of normal coordinated activities was considered a trauma.

In this proposed FS model, sleep impairment affects the growth hor- mone, which is dependent on slow-wave sleep.[62] When the patient is sleep- deprived, the suboptimal secretion of growth hormone has a negative effect on protein metabolism.[63] This may delay healing after microtrauma. Micro- trauma also impairs muscle glycogen storage, causing fatigue.[64]

An interesting sequence of pathophysiologic mechanisms tying all these concepts together has been proposed, in which the syndrome is a complex interaction of nociceptors and neuropathic dysregulatory central nervous system function is enhanced by psychosomatic mechanisms.[65]

In this concept the sensory C fibers have both sensory and neurose-

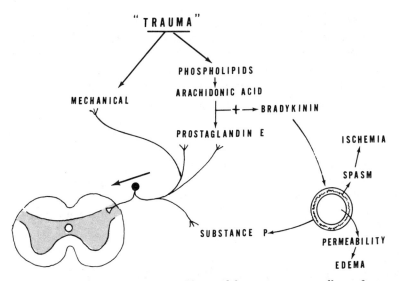

Figure 7–8. Nociceptive substances liberated by trauma. Regardless of its type, trauma may be mechanical and liberate histamines and other noxious substances. Trauma may also break down phospholipids to become arachidonic acid, which forms prostaglandin E. This end substance reacts on the end membrane of the sensory nerve fibers, initiating the sensation ultimately interpreted as pain.

Noxious substances liberated by trauma may also act on the blood vessels, causing "spasm" and may increase the permeability of these vessels, causing edema. (*Modified from* Brom, B: Neurobiological concepts of pain: Its assessment and therapy. In Brom, B (ed): Pain Measurements in Man: Neurophysiological Correlates of Pain. Elsevier Science Publishing, New York, 1984, p 18.)

cretory functions.[66] Neuropeptides released at the peripheral endings of C fibers cause vasodilation and increase capillary permeability with extravasation (Fig. 7–8). These peptides stimulate mast cells, which are related to the immune system. They also release serotonin and histamine, which act on local tissues, causing "neurogenic inflammation."[66,67] Neurogenic inflammation was elevated in fibromyalgia patients.[68]

Fifty years ago, neurogenic inflammation was termed *axon reflex* by Lewis.[69] It caused local vasodilation from increase in the microcirculation of the regional muscle.[70]

In cases diagnosed as fibromyalgia, substance P levels in the cerebrospinal fluid (CSF) was found to be high.[71] This was considered to indicate an increased production of substance P in the afferent C fibers.

Abnormal posture causing muscular hypertonus in many postural muscles may be a cause rather than a consequence of fibromyositis.[72] This is evident by the benefit gained from biofeedback in patients exhibiting low back pain even though abnormal electromyograph examinations revealing excessive "firing" have not been found in these types of patients.[73]

A central mechanism is postulated in this muscular hypertonus.[74,75] It is as yet unconfirmed, but it is accepted that algogens reaching the central nervous system are further processed in the ultimate conscious perception of pain. Dysfunction of this process may occur, resulting in the symptoms of fibromyalgia.[34] This dysfunction may be chemical, as it has been shown that substance P in the CSF is abnormally high in fibromyalgia patients.[76] This causes overactivity of excitatory transmission. The associated sleep disorder in fibromyalgia is also evidence that there is impairment of the central nervous system.

Dysfunction may occur at the dorsal horn level or as a dysfunction of the descending controls on the dorsal horn from the periaqueductal gray area.[77-79] Serotonin synthesis has a definite chemical action on this descending system.[80] A proposed deficiency of serotonin has promoted the use of L-tryptophan, a serotonin precursor, in treating chronic pain.[81]

Management of Fibromyalgia Syndromes

From the possible mechanisms of the above models it appears that management requires modifying sleep, regaining conditioning, and controlling all neuromuscular perturbers. As the painful pathology is considered to be within the muscles, all the modalities of heat, massage, ice, vasocoolant spray and stretch, exercise, posture, biofeedback, meditation, and hypnosis can be used.[82] These have been discussed in Chapters 4, 5, and 6.

Sleep abnormalities must be addressed with tricyclic drugs. Muscle relaxants (for example, cyclobenzamine) may enhance relaxation. Antidepressants have a value and should be explored.

As FS is considered a benign, self-limited entity, explanation and reassurance are therapeutic. Permanent functional disability must be avoided.

MECHANISMS OF PAIN IN SPECIFIC ANATOMIC REGIONS

In painful disabling conditions of the neuromusculoskeletal systems of the body, a basic concept is proposed that applies to any of these systems.

All human body functions respond to forces that occur within as well as without the body. These forces are specifically encountered in all motor skeletal functions. The forces generated within the skeletal structures are accepted by the precisely coordinated neuromusculoskeletal mechanisms needed to accomplish the intended act. All internal forces generated meet an opposing resistance that moderates and limits the action. The tissues involved in the action undergo "physiologic deformity" consistent with their molecular structure. These tissues have the needed flexibility, resiliency,

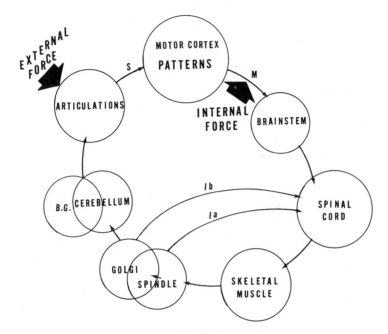

Figure 7–9. Diagram of neuromusculoskeletal control.

The neuromusculoskeletal patterns contained within the cerebral cortex and brainstem (termed neuromatrix) are activated when a physical activity is contemplated.

The motor action (M) ultimately activates the spinal cord efferents, which are monitored and controlled by the spindle system and the Golgi apparatus. The feedback mechanism to the cord is via the Ia and Ib fibers. The cerebellum and basal ganglia (BG) centrally coordinate the action.

The final motor action occurs from musculotendonous action on the articular systems of the body via lever actions. Final performance is perceived by sensory feedback (S).

Dysfunction ultimately causing pain occurs from excessive or inappropriate external or internal forces acting on this neurophysiologic system. The internal forces impose on the pattern initiation aspect, and the extrenal forces impose on the articular components.

and structural strength to accomplish the intended act and revert back to normal. A balance must exist between these generated forces, which are mediated by neuromuscular control.

A model (Fig. 7–9) depicts the neuromusculoskeletal system invoked in all human skeletal motor activities. The intended action originates at the cortical and midbrain levels where patterns exist that are inherited and developed by maturation and training. These patterns have been termed "neuromatrix" and involve many regions of the cortex.

Once generated at the cortical level they are coordinated by cerebellar

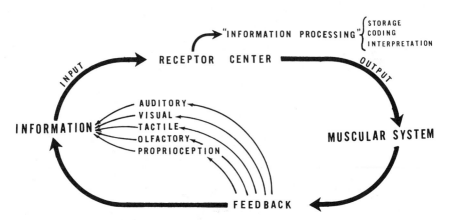

Figure 7–10. Information from internal and external environment via receptors is involved in the process of learing a skill. Almost all behavior is motor in nature; humans respond with voluntary and involuntary movements, which include posture. The learning of skills proceeds in phases. Feedback is one of the most important concepts in learning and is an important factor in the control of movement and behavior.

and basal ganglion centers and ultimately are transmitted through spinal cord pathways to end in the motor muscle systems, which act on the skeletal lever systems. The muscular action is moderated by the spindle system, which determines rate of elongation and shortening, and the Golgi apparatus, which moderates the tension generated. Both can be considered forces.

The end organs of the neuromuscular motor system are the skeletal articulations. A sensory feedback system (Fig. 7–10) "informs" the system of completion and efficacy of the action through numerous spinal and supraspinal pathways (Fig. 7–11).

External and internal forces may cause failure of these neuromusculoskeletal mechanisms leading to pain and dysfunction when they exceed normal physiologic limits. Normal external and internal forces impose a deformation of the involved tissues, which return to normal once the forces are released (Fig. 7–12). Any resultant pain from normal forces can occur from tissues being deconditioned and patterns being slightly incoordinated.

Excessive forces, either external or internal, can invoke tissue damage with the formation of nociceptors that cause pain and dysfunction (Fig. 7–13).

The external forces of gravity and inertia respond to normal physiologic actions. Excessive forces can include repetitive activities with resultant excessive flexion, extension, and/or rotation of the part; the term "excessive" applies to the temporal or weight factors. Direct trauma such as a fall or physical impact is obviously an external force.

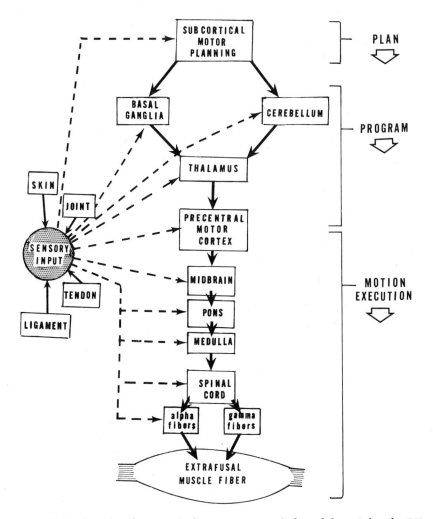

Figure 7–11. Spinal and supraspinal motor centers. (Adapted from Schmidt, RF: Fundamentals of Neurophysiology. Springer-Verlag, New York, 1978.)

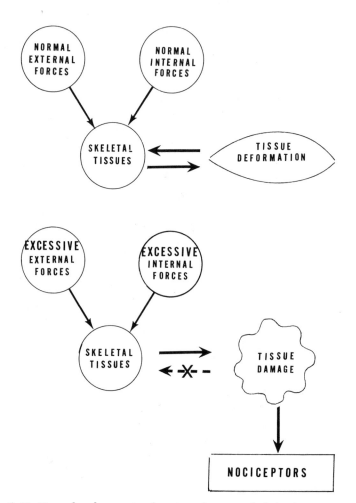

Figure 7–12. Normal and excessive forces on the musculoskeletal system.

Upper diagram: Normal external and internal forces on the skeletal tissues causing reversible tissue deformation. Resultant pain and dysfunction are not expected.

Lower diagram: Excessive forces on the skeletal tissues causing irreversible damage with the release of nociceptor elements. Pain and dysfunction result.

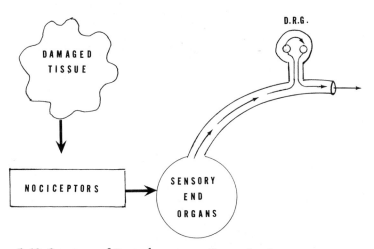

Figure 7–13. Sequence of tissue damage creating nociceptors.

The damaged tissues liberate chemical nociceptors that inflame (irritate) the sensory end organs releasing impulses to the dorsal root ganglia (DRG) via C unmyelinated and A alpha fibers, initiating ultimate pain perception.

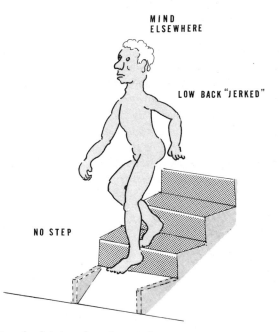

Figure 7–14. Low back injury from inattention.

With the mind elsewhere, a step down on a step not there can result in an abrupt muscular-diskal injury, causing low back ache or sciatic radiculopathy from a nuclear herniation.

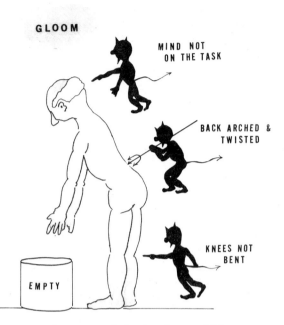

Figure 7-15. Distraction that causes faulty bending and lifting, causing low back pain.

The internal forces that may impair neuromusculoskeletal function and thus be considered excessive or improper are called "perturbers" and include fatigue, anger, depression, inattention, anxiety, poor training, and distraction. Inapropriate motor action to perform an intended act can be exemplified by the intent to lift an object anticipated as weighing 100 pounds that actually weighs only 10 pounds. The neuromusculoskeletal effort is appropriate for the 100-pound lift but is excessive for 10 pounds. Numerous similar examples can be applied to other skeletal actions (Figs. 7-14 to 7-17).

The resultant pain that is elicited from the formation of nociceptors is mediated through the pathways discussed in Chapter 8 and are summarized in Figure 7-18.

This concept of normal and excessive external and internal forces involved in musculoskeletal pain syndromes can be applied to all subsequent skeletal mechanisms discussed in Chapter 8, albeit not specified.

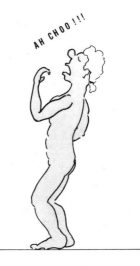

Figure 7–16. A sneeze can cause unexpected disk herniation by the combination of acute muscular contraction and an abrupt increase in spinal fluid pressure.

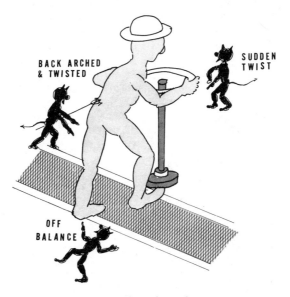

Figure 7–17. In industrial injuries a worker who makes inappropriate rotatory motion while being "off balance" causes the low back to be "twisted and arched." The position of the lumbosacral spine coupled with inappropriate rotation impose a nonphysiologic and injurious "force" on an otherwise normal spine.

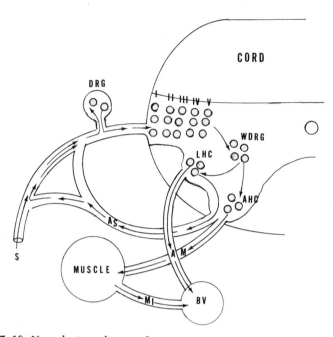

Figure 7–18. Neurologic pathways of nociception.

The sensory impulses (S) enter via afferent fibers to the dorsal root ganglion (DRG) then to Rexed layers I, II, III, IV, V, and so on. Layers I and II are the substantia gelatinosum. Intraneural fibers then transfer impulses to the lateral spinothalamic tracts (not shown) to the hypothalamus, thalamus, and cortex.

Nociceptive impulses transmit to the wide dynamic range ganglia (WDRG); to the lateral horn cells (LHC) (to initiate autonomic impulses); and to the anterior horn cells (AHC), which initiate muscular response. The efferent fibers from LHC innervate the blood vessels (BV).

Afferent autonomic fibers transmit sensation (AS) to the DRG. The skeletal muscles innervated by efferents (AM) from the AHC can cause ischemia from persistent excessive contraction causing autonomic impulses (MI) from the involved BVs. See the text for details of this pathway.

REFERENCES

1. Cailliet, R: Soft Tissue Pain and Disability, ed 2. FA Davis, Philadelphia, 1988.
2. Cailliet, R: Low Back Pain, ed 4. FA Davis, Philadelphia, 1988.
3. Cailliet, R: Neck And Arm Pain, ed 3. FA Davis, Philadelphia, 1991.
4. Cailliet, R: Shoulder Pain, ed 3. FA Davis, Philadelphia, 1991.
5. Cailliet, R: Foot and Ankle Pain, ed 2. FA Davis, Philadelphia, 1983.
6. Cailliet, R: Hand Pain and Impairment, ed 1. FA Davis, Philadelphia, 1982.
7. Cailliet, R: Knee Pain and Disability, ed 3. FA Davis, Philadelphia, 1991.
8. Cailliet, R: Head and Face Pain Syndromes, ed 1. FA Davis, Philadelphia, 1992.
9. Cailliet, R: Posture. In Neck and Arm Pain, ed 3. FA Davis, Philadelphia, 1991, pp 43–50.
10. Feldenkrais, M: Body and Mature Behavior. International University Press, New York, 1973.

11. Cailliet, R and Gross, L: The Rejuvenation Strategy: A Complete Fitness Program for Everyone 35 and Over. Pocket Books, New York, 1987, pp 58–60.

12. Cailliet, R: Abnormalities of the sitting postures of musicians. Medical Problems of Performing Artists 5(4):131–135, 1990.

13. DeLateur, BJ, Giaconi, RM, Questad, K, Ko, M, and Lehmann, JF: Footwear and posture: Compensatory strategies for heel height. Am J Phys Med Rehabil 70(5):246–254, 1991.

14. Simmons, EH, Graziano, GP, and Heffner, R: Muscle disease as a cause of kyphotic deformity in ankylosing spondylitis. Spine (Suppl) 16(8):S351–S360, 1991.

15. Gogia, PP and Sabbahi, MA: Changes in fatigue characteristics of cervical paraspinal muscles with posture. Spine 16(10):1135–1140, 1991.

16. Garfin, SR, Tipton, CM, Mubarek, SJ, Woo, SL, Hargens, AR, Akeson, WH: Role of fascia in maintenance of muscle tension and pressure. J Appl Physiol 51:317–320, 1981.

17. McMahon, TA: Muscle, Reflexes, and Locomotion. Princeton University Press, Princeton, NJ, 1984.

18. Bowers, WD, Hibbard, RW, Smoake, JA, Daume, RC, and Nilson, E: Effects of exercise on the ultrastructure of skeletal muscle. Am J Physiol 227:313–316, 1974.

19. Dennett, X and Fry, HJH: Overuse syndrome: A muscle biopsy study. Lancet, 1:905–908, 1988.

20. Newham, DJ, Mills, KR, Quigley, BM, and Edwards, RHT: Ultrastructural changes after concentric and eccentric contractions. Clin Sci 64:129–131, 1982.

21. Elson, LM: The jolt syndrome: Muscle dysfunction following low velocity impact. Pain Management pp 317–326, 1990.

22. Edgely, SA and Janowska, E: Information processed by dorsal horn spinocerebellar tract neurones in the cat. J Physiol 397:81–97, 1988.

23. O'Reilly, KP, Warhol, MJ, Fielding, RA, Frontera, WR, Meredith, CN, and Evans, WJ: Eccentric exercise induced muscle damage impairs muscle glycogen repletion. J Appl Physiol 63:252–256, 1987.

24. Sarno, J: Mind over Back Pain. William Morrow, New York, 1984.

25. Bennett, RM, Gatter, RA, Campbell, SM, Andrews, RP, Clark, SR, and Scarola, JA: Comparison of cyclobenzaprine and placebo in the management of fibrositis: A double-blind controlled study. Arthritis Rheum 31:1535–1542, 1988.

26. Chester, JB: Whiplash, postural control and the inner ear. Spine 16(7):716–720, 1991.

27. Chadwick, J and Mann, WN (trans): The Medical Works of Hippocrates. Blackwell, Oxford, 1950.

28. Simons, DG: Muscle pain syndromes, Part 1. Am J Phys Med 54:289–311, 1975.

29. Beard, GM: A Practical Treatise on Nervous Exhaustion (Neurasthenia). William Wood, New York, 1880.

30. Gowers, WR: Lumbago: Its lesions and analogues. BMJ 1:117–123, 1904.

31. International Association for the Study of Pain, Subcommittee of Taxonomy: Chronic pain syndromes and definition of pain terms. Pain (Suppl) 3:S1–S225, 1986.

32. Yunus, MB, Masi, AT, Calabro, JJ, Miller, KA, and Feigenbaum, SL: Primary fibromyalgia (fibrositis); Clinical study of 50 patients with matched normal controls. Semin Arthritis Rheum 11:151–171, 1981.

33. Smythe, HA: "Fibrositis" as a disorder of pain modulation. Clin Rhem Dis 5:823–832, 1979.

34. Moldofski, H: Sleep and musculoskeletal pain. Am J Med 81(Suppl 3A):85–89, 1986.

35. Yunus, MB and Kalyan-Ramon, UP: Muscle biopsy findings in primary fibromyalgia and other forms of nonarticular rheumatism. Rheum Dis Clin N Am 15:115–134, 1989.

36. Berberich, P, Hoheisel, U, Mense, S, and Skeppar, P: Fine muscle afferent fibers and inflammation: Changes in discharge behaviour and influence on gamma-motoneurones. In Schmidt, RF, Schaible, H-G, and Vahle-Hinz, C (eds): Fine afferent nerve fibers in pain. VCH-Verlag, Weinheim, 1987, pp 165–175.

37. Diehl, B, Hoheisel, U, and Mense, S: Histological and neurophysiological changes induced by carrageen in skeletal muscle of cat and rat. Agents Actions 25:210–213, 1988.

38. Mense, S: Sensitization of group IV muscle receptors to bradykinin by 5-hydroxytryptamine and prostaglandin E2. Brain Res 225:95–105, 1981.

39. Bergtsson, A and Hendriksson, KG: The muscle in fibromyalgia: A review of Swedish studies. J Rheumatol 16(Suppl 19):144–149, 1989.
40. Klemp, P, Staberg, B, Korsgard, J, Vagn Nielson, H, Crone, P: Reduced blood flow in fibromyotic muscles during ultrasound therapy. Scand J Rehab Med 15:21–23, 1982.
41. Hagsberg, M and Kvarnstrom, S: Muscular endurance and electromyographic fatigue in myofascial shoulder pain. Arch Phys Med Rehabil 65:522–525, 1984.
42. Jacobsen, S and Danneskiold-Samsen, B: Isometric and isokinetic muscle strength in patients with fibrositis syndrome. Scand J Rheumatol 16:61–65, 1987.
43. Ferraccioli, G, Ghirelli, L, Scita, F, Nolli, M, Mozzani, M, Fontanba, S, Scorsonelli, M, Tridenti, A, and DeRisio, C: EMG-biofeedback training in fibromyalgia syndrome. J Rheumatol 14:820–825, 1987.
44. Moldoksky, H, Scaris brick, P, England, R, and Smythe, H: Musculoskeletal symptoms and non-REM sleep disturbance in patients with "fibrositis syndrome" and healthy subjects. Psychosom Med 37:341–351, 1975.
45. Morgane, PJ: Serotonin twenty-five years later: Monoamine theories of sleep. Psychopharmacol Bull 17:13–17, 1981.
46. Moldofsky, H: Rheumatic pain modulation disorder: The relationship between sleep, CNS serotonin and pain. In Critchley, M, and Friedman, A (eds): Headache: Physiopathological and Clinical Concepts. Raven Press, New York, 1982, pp 51–57.
47. Bowden, CL, Michalek, J, Fletcher, F, and Hester, GA: Imipramine receptor density on platelets of patients with fibrositis syndrome: Correlation wth disease severity and response to therapy. Arthr Rheum (abstr) 30:S63, 1987.
48. Moldofsky, H and Warsh, JJ: Plasma tryptophan and musculoskeletal pain in nonarticular rheumatism. Pain 5:65–71, 1978.
49. Russell, IJ, Michalek, JF, Vipraio, GA, Fletcher, FM, and Wall, K: Serum amino acids in fibrositis/fibromyalgia syndrome. Arthr Rheum (abstr) 32:S24, 1989.
50. Rice, JR: "Fibrositis" syndrome. Med Clin N Am 70:455–468, 1986.
51. Thomas, CL (ed): Taber's Cyclopedic Medical Dictionary, ed 15. FA Davis, Philadelphia, 1985.
52. Feldman, RS and Quenzer, LF: Fundamentals of Neuropsychopharmacology. Sinauer, Sunderland, MA, 1984.
53. Almar, BGL, Johansson, F, Von Knorrng, L, Le Greves, P, and Terenius, L: Substance P in CSF of patients with chronic pain syndromes. Pain 33:3–9, 1988.
54. Vaeroy, H, Halle, R, Forre, O, Kass, E, Terenius, L: Elevated CFS levels of substance P and high risk incidence of Raynaud's phenomenon in patients with fibromyalgia: New features for diagnosis. Pain 32:21–26, 1988.
55. McCain, GA: Role of physical fitness training in fibrositis/fibromyalgia syndrome. Am J Med (Suppl 3A) 81:73–77, 1986.
56. Yunus, MB, Denko, CW, and Masi, AT: Serum beta-endorphin in primary fibromyalgia syndrome: A controlled study. J Rheumatol 13:183–189, 1986.
57. Goldenberg, DI: Fibromyalgia syndrome: An emerging but controversial condition. JAMA 257:105–115, 1987.
58. Dinerman, H, Goldenberg, DL, and Felson, DT: A prospective evaluation of 118 patients with fibromyalgia syndrome: Prevalence of Raynaud's phenomenon, sicca syndrome, ANAs low complement, and IG deposition at the dermal-epidermal junction. J Rheumatol 13:368–373, 1986.
59. Cheu, JW and Findley, T: Integrated Parallel-Cycle Model of Chronic Fatigue Syndrome. University of Medicine and Dentistry, New Jersey, 1991.
60. Bennett, RM: Beyond fibromyalgia: Ideas on etiology and treatment. J Rheumatology 16(Suppl 19):185–191, 1989.
61. Friden, J, Sjostrom, M, and Ekblom, B: A morphological study of delayed muscle soreness. Experientia 37:506–507, 1981.

62. Newham, DJ, Mills, KR, Quigley, BM, and Edwards, RHT: Ultrastructural changes after concentric and eccentric contractions. Clin Sci 64:129–131, 1982.

63. Nimmo, MA and Snow, DH: Time course of ultrastructural changes in skeletal muscle after 2 types of exercise. J Appl Physiol 42:910–913, 1982.

64. Zimmermann, M: Pathophysiological mechanisms of fibromyalgia. Clin J Pain 7(Suppl 1):S15, 1991.

65. Chahl, LA, Szolcsanyi, J, and Lembeck, F (eds): Antidromic vasodilation and neurogenic inflammation. Akademiai Kiado, Budapest, 1984.

66. Lembeck, F and Gamse, R: Substance P in peripheral sensory processes. In Porter, R and O'Connor, M (eds): Substance P in the nervous system. Ciba Foundation Symposium 91. Pitman, London, 1982, pp 35–49.

67. Littlejohn, GO, Weinstein, C, and Helme, RD: Increased neurogenic inflammation in fibrositis syndrome. J Rheumatol 14:1022–1025, 1987.

68. Lewis, T: Pain. Macmillan, London, 1942.

69. Ohlen, A, Lindbom, L, Hokfelt, T, Hedquist, P, and Staines, W: Effects of substance P and calcitonin gene-related peptide on the skeletal muscle microcirculation. In Henry, JL, Couture, R, Cuello, AC, Pelletier, G, Quirion, R, and Regoli, D (eds): Substance P and Neurokinins. Springer-Verlag, New York, 1987, pp 192–194.

70. Duggan, AW and North, RA: Electrophysiology of opioids. Pharmacol Rev 35:219–281, 1984.

71. Flor, H and Truk, DC: Etiological theories and treatments for chronic back pain. I. Somatic models and interventions. Pain 19:105–121, 1984.

72. Zidar, J, Backman, E, Bengtsson, A, and Henriksson, KG: Quantitative EMG and muscle tension in painful muscles in fibromyalgia. Pain 40:249–254, 1990.

73. Devor, M: Central changes mediating neuropathic pain. In Dubner, R, Gebhart, GF, and Bond, MR (eds): Proceedings of the 5th World Congress on Pain. Pain research and clinical management, Vol 3. Elsevier, Amsterdam, 1988, pp 114–128.

74. Zimmermann, M: Central nervous mechanisms modulating pain-related information: Interaction with peripheral input. In Casey, KL (ed): Pain and Central Nervous System Disease: The Central Pain Syndromes. Raven Press, New York, 1991, pp 183–199.

75. Vaeroy, H, Helle, R, Forre, O, Kass, E, and Terenius, L: Elevated CFS levels of substance P and high incidence of Raynaud's phenomenon in patients with fibromyalgia: New features for diagnosis. Pain 32:21–26, 1988.

76. Willis, WD: Control of nociceptive transmission in the spinal cord. Springer, Berlin, 1982.

77. Zieglgansberger, W: Central control of nociception. In Mountcastle, VB, Bloom, FE, and Geiger, SR (eds): Handbook of Physiology. The Nervous System, IV. Williams & Wilkins, Baltimore, 1986, 581–645.

78. Basbaum, AI and Fields, HL: Endogenous pain control systems: Brainstem spinal pathways and endorphin circuitry. Annu Rev Neurosci 7:309–338, 1984.

79. Carstens, E, Fraunhoffer, M, and Zimmermann, M: Serotonergic mediation of descending inhibition from midbrain periaqueductal gray, but not reticular formation, of spinal nociceptive transmission in the cat. Pain 10:149–167, 1981.

80. Seltzer, S, Marcus, R, and Stoch, R: Perspectives in the control of chronic pain by nutritional manipulation. Pain 11:141–148, 1981.

81. Vecchiet, L, Giamberardino, MA, and Saggini, R: Myofascial pain syndromes: Clinical and pathophysiological aspects. Clin J Pain 7(Suppl 1):S16–S22, 1991.

CHAPTER 8

Mechanisms of Pain in Specific Anatomic Regions

HEAD AND FACE PAIN

The anatomy, physiology, and pathophysiology of head and face pain has been discussed thoroughly in the literature.[1] The mechanisms therefore can be deduced from these studies that explain the symptoms, findings, and indications for the prescribed treatment protocols.

To determine the source of pain emanating from the head and face we must ascertain the nerve pathways of the painful stimulus and the chemical and hormonal nociceptor algogenic agents. There are many nerves in the head, neck, and face that are considered sensory pathways, but only the major nerves will be discussed. For more detailed information, the reader may refer to the literature.[1-3]

Pain is transmitted via the somatic system, but more recent theories suggest that the sympathetic nervous system is a more prominent pathway. The pathophysiology of migraine, for example, has been ascertained to be vascular, but there is now debate as to whether migraine is essentially nerve-mediated rather than vascular. As the vascular system is controlled by the sympathetic nervous system, there is a direct relationship between the two. A semantic as well as conceptual difference exists.

Pain is known to be transmitted via somatic sensory nerves, a small portion of motor nerve fibers, and a significant portion via the sympathetic nerves. All systems must be understood and their involvement discerned in the mechanisms of head and face pain.

Trigeminal Nerve

Pain in the intracranial and extracranial structures is subserved by cranial and upper cervical nerves. The trigeminal nerve is the Vth cranial nerve.

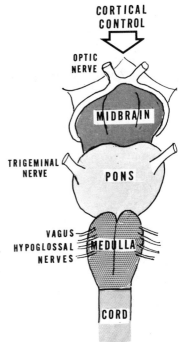

Figure 8–1. Midbrain, pons, medulla and cord. The midbrain and the site of emergence of the trigeminal nerve from the pons is shown.

It is the principal innervator of the facial skin, cornea, oral and nasal mucosa, tongue, teeth, masticatory muscles, and meningeal lining.

The trigeminal nerve, the largest cranial nerve, is a mixed somatic sensory and motor nerve. It is a short nerve emanating from the ventrolateral surface of the pons (Fig. 8–1) and proceeding in an anterolateral direction to the apex of the petrous portion of the temporal bone (Fig. 8–2). At that point it expands to form the gasserian ganglion. The sensory roots are contained in this ganglion. The trigeminal nerve divides into three major branches, as shown in Figure 8–2: the ophthalmic, the maxillary, and the mandibular.

The dermatomal areas of the face served by the trigeminal nerve are the face and anterior two-thirds of the head (Fig. 8–3). The motor roots, mentioned only for completeness, are also located within the pons beneath and below the sensory fibers and emerge via the foramen ovale at the point where it joins the sensory portion of the trigeminal mandibular division to innervate the muscles of mastication (Fig. 8–3).

Ophthalmic Division. The ophthalmic division is the uppermost and the smallest arising from the gasserian ganglion. It proceeds anteriorly through the wall of the cavernous sinus and through the superior orbital fissure to reach the orbit. This division is exclusively sensory to the eye except for vision and includes the conjunctiva, the lacrimal gland, the mucous mem-

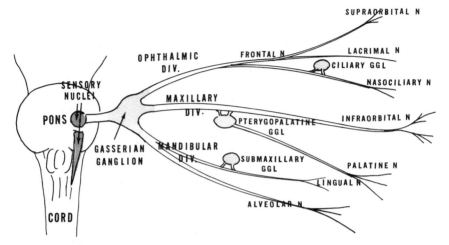

Figure 8–2. Trigeminal nerve.

The trigeminal nerve, shown schematically, has its sensory portion within the gasserian ganglion where the peripheral branches synapse to nerves entering the cord at the pons level to end in sensory nuclei. The trigeminal nerve branches into three major divisions: the ophthalmic, the maxillary, and the mandibular. The sensory areas supplied by the trigeminal nerve are the face and the anterior two thirds of the head.

brane of the nose and paranasal sinuses, and the skin of the forehead, eyelids, and nose.

The ophthalmic division of the trigeminal nerve ultimately divides into three branches: the lacrimal, the frontal, and the nasociliary. The *lacrimal branch* supplies the lacrimal gland and the conjunctiva. It has postganglionic

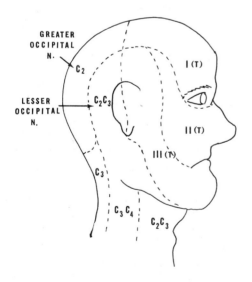

Figure 8–3. Sensory nerve supply to the head and face.

The branches of the trigeminal division, the occipital nerves through their branches, and the frontal nerves supply the skin of the head and the face. The trigeminal nerve divisions (T-I, T-II, and T-III) are shown, and the segments of the cervical plexus (C-2, C-3, and C-4) are conveyed through the occipital branches.

parasympathetic branchings, which are secretory motor fibers to the glands, and a significant sympathetic nerve supply. Any involvement of this division causes excessive lacrimation (tearing) and nasal congestion. The lacrimal branch anastomoses to the frontal nerve and the zygomatic branch of the maxillary division.

The *frontal branch* is the largest of the ophthalmic division. It enters the orbit via the superior orbital fissure. It supplies sensory input to the skin of the mesial lower portion of the forehead. Via its continuation as the supraorbital nerve, the frontal nerve supplies the upper lid and the mucous membrane of the frontal sinus. Involvement of this branch is probably the basis for many so-called sinus conditions. The frontal branch also supplies a portion of the scalp.

The *nasociliary branch* supplies the iris and the cornea with sympathetic supply to the dilator pupillary muscles. More precise details of these branches can be found in the medical literature.[4]

Maxillary Division. The maxillary division is the second division of the trigeminal nerve. It is entirely sensory, supplying the skin of the middle portion of the face: the lower eyelid, the side of the nose, the upper lip, and the mucous membranes of the nasopharynx, maxillary sinus, soft palate, tonsil, roof of the mouth, upper gums, and teeth (Fig. 8–3).

Near its origin it branches off to form the middle meningeal nerve, which supplies the ipsilateral middle meningeal artery and its branches to the dura mater. The dura mater is pain-sensitive within the cranium. The middle meningeal nerve divides into the infraorbital branch, which ultimately supplies the lower lid, the skin of the side of the forehead, the skin of the cheek, and the mucous membranes of the frontal, ethmoidal, and sphenoidal sinuses. One of its terminal branches, the greater palatine nerve, supplies the hard palate, the gums, the uvula, and a portion of the soft palate. The posterior superior alveolar branch supplies the gums, the mucous membrane of the cheek, and the molar teeth. Involvement of this division obviously is implicated in painful states of the midface, the lower orbit, and the nose and mouth structures.

Mandibular Division. The mandibular division is the third and the only mixed division; that is, it has both sensory and motor roots. Emerging from the pons region, the motor root passes beneath the gasserian ganglion and leaves the cranial cavity through the foramen ovale to rejoin the sensory components of the division.

The sensory fibers of the mandibular division innervate the skin of the temple area, auricula, the lower part of the face, and the external meatus of the ear, cheek, and lower lip. It also innervates the mucous membrane of the cheek, tongue, lower teeth, gums, temporomandibular joint (TMJ), and a part of the dura mater and skull.

The motor branches of the trigeminal nerve supply the muscles of mastication: the masseter, temporalis, pterygoids, myelohyoid, and digastric muscles. All of these muscles are involved in opening, closing, and trans-latory motion of the mandible. This is an important division in the identification and treatment of dental and temporomandibular arthralgia disease. These muscles also transmit pain via their sensory fibers.

The cutaneous afferent nociceptor fibers carried in the trigeminal nerve have been studied predominantly in the monkey, but a similar anatomic nerve supply has been ascertained in humans. Stimuli that damage or irritate the skin innervated by the trigeminal nerve traverse along small myelinated A-alpha and unmyelinated C fibers with free nerve endings. There are two types of A-alpha fibers: mechanosensitive receptors and A-alpha thermal nociceptor fibers.[5] The former require intense mechanical stimulus with resultant skin damage to respond. The latter respond to both mechanical and thermal stimuli, especially to noxious heat. C-fiber nerves respond to chemical, thermal, and mechanical stimuli. Superficial hyperalgesia often occurs from activation of the peripheral adrenergic receptors alpha$_1$ and alpha$_2$ following injury.

Pain occurs rapidly from noxious thermal stimuli, but a delayed pain response occurs when mechanical and chemical substances are released. Blood plasma releases pain-producing kinins, of which one is bradykinin. Bradykinin causes vasodilation and increased capillary permeability with resultant pain. Other substances are released from the extracellular fluid, including serotonin, which is algogenic. Mast cells are also released and in turn release histamine, an algogenic substance in high doses.

Trauma forms prostaglandins, which are algogens, from the breakdown of fatty acids, especially arachidonic acid. Injury also liberates algogenic substance P from cutaneous nociceptor C fibers.

Sympathetic Nervous System

The sympathetic nervous system is a major source of head and face pain; readers should refer to Chapter 2 for a discussion of the functional and physiologic anatomy of the sympathetic nervous system. At the cord level the sympathetic and somatic afferent nerves merge (Fig. 8–4). The skin of the face and scalp receives sympathetic innervation from the superior cervical ganglia via plexi extending along the branches of the external carotid artery (Fig. 8–5).

Acetylcholine and noradrenaline remain the foremost neurotransmitters of autonomic flow. The cerebral blood vessels are surrounded by nerve fibers that contain norepinephrine and neuropeptide Y, both of which cause vasoconstriction. Allegedly, the major function of these peptides is to attenuate excessive vasodilation caused by the secretion of vasodilator substance P and neurokinin A, which are secreted by trigeminal nerve.[6] Acetylcholine, which

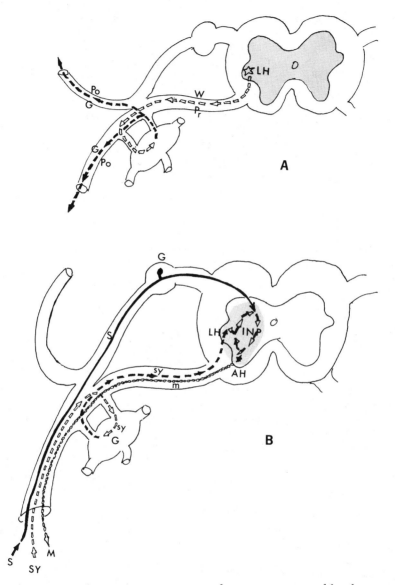

Figure 8–4. Sympathetic, somatic sensory, and motor nerve at cord level.

(A), The direction of the sympathetic fibers in a segmental peripheral nerve. The autonomic fibers originate at the lateral horn (LH) cells (see Fig. 1–4). The preganglionic myelinated white (W) nerve (Pr) and the postganglionic (Po) unmyelinated nerves leave as gray (G) fibers through the gray ramus of the ganglion (G) and proceed distally within the common peripheral nerve.

(B), The afferent pathways along the sympathetic nerve involve a cycle: the sensory nerve root (S) excites the internuncial pool (INP), which in turn excites the lateral horn cells (LH) of afferent sympathetic nerves (Sy) and afferent motor impulses (m). The motor impulses from anterior horn cells (AH) are both somatic and sympathetic.

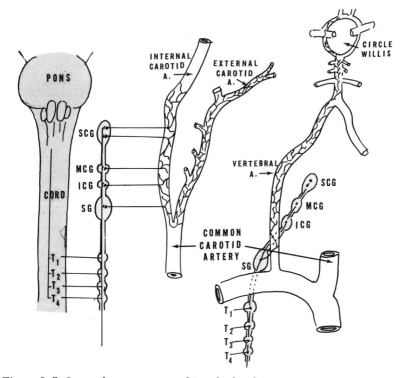

Figure 8–5. Sympathetic nerve supply to the head.

The preganglionic fibers originate from T-1, T-2, T-3, and T-4 segments of the cord and pass through white rami communicans to the paravertebral sympathetic chains where they synapse into gray rami (postganglionic) to innervate the blood vessels of the neck and head.

The sympathetic fibers transmit autonomic motor fibers to the blood vessels and carry sensation from the peripheral areas. (SCG = superior cervical ganglion; NCG = middle cervical ganglion; ICG = intermediate cervical ganglion; SG = stellate ganglion.)

is liberated by numerous nerves surrounding major cerebral arteries, also causes blood vessel dilation.[7,8]

The pain mechanism of trigeminal nerve causes the following clinical manifestations:

1. Pain resulting from involvement of the gasserian ganglion or peripheral branches
2. Loss of sensation over the sensory distribution of the nerve, including corneal anesthesia
3. Dissociated anesthesia causing loss of pain sensation but not loss of touch
4. Paresthesia

5. Paralysis of the muscles of mastication
6. Loss of jaw jerk and conjunctival and corneal reflexes
7. Impaired hearing, implying paresis of the tensor tympani
8. Trophic and salivatory disturbances

Facial Nerve

The facial nerve is a mixed nerve with a larger motor component and a smaller sensory component (Fig. 8–6). The facial nerve originates from nuclei in the caudal portion of the pons. It initially loops around the nucleus

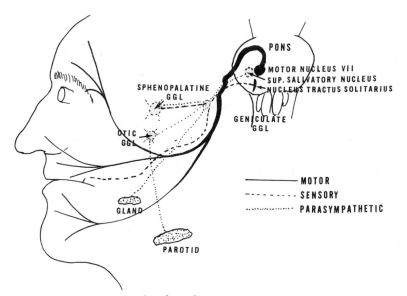

Figure 8–6. Facial nerve and its branches.

The central portion of the facial nerve (a mixed nerve in that it is sensory and principally motor) originates intracranially in the pons area. Here there exists the motor nucleus VII, the superior salivatory nucleus, and the nucleus tractus solitarius.

From the motor nucleus (*solid line*) emerge the motor nerves to the muscles of the face. From the superior salivatory nucleus emerge the parasympathetic nerves to various glands of the neck and face, such as the parotid and the salivatory glands, and to the nucleus tractus solitarius enter the sensory (*dotted lines*) from the face.

The sensory patterns served by the facial nerve are periorbital, periocular, and nasal. The sensory fibers also carry taste fibers from the tongue.

The peripheral ganglia (otic and sphenopalatines) are sites of synapsis of sensory and parasympathetic nerves that are amenable to intervention in clinical impairments of these nerve fibers.

Clinically the major pathologic aspects of facial nerve involvement are motor (facial palsy), but the sensory components are of significant clinical importance.

of the abducens and ultimately terminates to supply the stapedius muscles of the middle ear, the muscles of facial expression, the platysma, and some muscles of the scalp.

The sensory portion of the facial nerve, with which we are more specifically interested, arises from unipolar cells that are innervated by fibers from the tractus solitarius within the pons. From the geniculate ganglion the nerve immediately divides into two branches. Their peripheral branches carry taste from the anterior two thirds of the tongue via the lingual and chorda tympany nerves. The facial nerve also carries sensation from the parotid gland via the otic ganglion and the geniculotympanic nerves.

In its central connections the motor nucleus receives both contralateral and ipsilateral fibers from the corticobulbar tract, the extrapyramidal tracts, and the tectospinal tracts. The facial muscles innervated by the motor fiber of this VIIth nerve below the forehead receive contralateral cortical innervation; being bilaterally innervated, the frontalis muscle is not paretic or paralyzed by a lesion involving one motor cortex or its peripheral nerves.

Lesions of the facial nerve are primarily motor (75 percent of VIIth nerve involvements), causing a Bell's palsy (peripheral facial paralysis). The mouth droops and may be drawn toward the other side. Deep facial sensation is lost. The patient cannot whistle, wink, or close the ipsilateral eye. The forehead loses its wrinkles, and the affected eye may tear excessively. On the sensory side the taste of the anterior two thirds of the tongue is lost, as is salivation on that side. Deep pressure in the neurologic examination reveals a loss of proprioception of the facial muscles.

Lesions of the geniculate ganglion evoke an acute onset of pain behind and within the ear. Herpes is a frequent cause of this lesion. Lesions within the internal auditory canal may cause involvement of hearing (deafness) in that ear, as the VIIIth nerve is in close proximity to the VIIth nerve at this site.

Lesions of the pons (for example, meningitis) may produce lesions of the VIIth nerve as well as the adjacent Vth, VIth, VIIIth, and XIth nerves.

In a nuclear type of facial palsy there are signs of the peripheral palsy described above and also contralateral signs of hemiparesis.

There are numerous neurologic syndromes associated with facial palsy of VIIth nerve etiology that are beyond the scope of this text. Clinically, they should be referred to a neurologist for consultation.

Central Mechanism of Pain Transmission

The peripheral mechanism of pain transmission of the head involve free nerve endings, which are present in all the tissues of the face and head, including the oral mucosa, temporomandibular joint tissues, peridontium, tooth pulp, periosteum, and muscles. Pain sensations are transmitted by

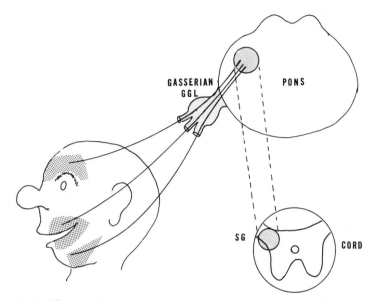

Figure 8–7. Afferents of the trigeminal nerve via the gasserian ganglion.
The sensory regions of the face enter the pons trigeminal tract V via the gasserian
ganglion (GGL).

small myelinated A-delta fibers and unmyelinated C fibers. These fibers are
stimulated after injury by virtue of production of nociceptive mechanical,
thermal, and chemical substances. The main chemical nociceptors implicated
are histamine, bradykinin, serotonin, potassium, and substance P. Tissue
breakdown of arachidonic acid into phospholipid and then into prostaglandins
is well documented in the rheumatology literature.

The peripheral nerves subserving the head and face enter the pons
region via the Vth gasserian, semilunar ganglia, facial nerve, sympathetic
nerves, and so on (Fig. 8–7). There are unmyelinated afferent fibers present
in the Vth motor nerve, but their function has not been ascertained. The
Vth nerve component within the brainstem is extensive. It is considered the
somatovisceral sensory nerve of the facial region. The afferents synapse with
the two nuclei in the pontine gray matter: the spinal nucleus and the main
sensory nucleus. The spinal nucleus corresponds to the dorsal horn of the
spinal cord, and the main sensory nucleus corresponds to the dorsal column
nuclei (Fig. 8–8). In the spinal nucleus the afferents from mechanoreceptors,
thermoreceptors, and nociceptors synapse with neurons sending axons to
the reticular formation and/or the thalamus (Fig. 8–9).

The reticular formation occupies a considerable portion of the brainstem. In addition to afferents from the Vth nerve, it receives afferents from
the spinoreticular tracts, the propriospinal tracts, and most, if not all, of the

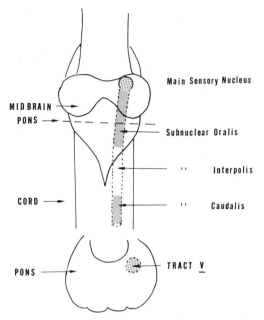

Figure 8–8. Central connections of trigeminal tract V.

The ventral connections of the trigeminal nerve are depicted extending from the main sensory nucleus in the pons area and caudally into the subnuclear oralis, subnuclear interpolaris, and subnuclear caudalis: the latter in the cord.

The nociceptive-specific (NS) neurons are located in these sites with the trigeminal subnucleus caudalis being a homolog of the spinal dorsal horn. It contains wide dynamic range (WDR) and NS neurons. The oralis and interpolaris receive afferents from the perioral and intraoral tissues. (From Yokato, T: Neural mechanisms of trigeminal pain. In Fields, HL, Dubner, R, and Cervero, F (eds): Advances in Pain Research and Therapy. Raven, New York, 1985, pp 221–232, with permission.)

cranial nerves. Efferent impulses go to the thalamus, hypothalamus, limbic system, basal ganglia, and motor cortex, all of which receive afferents.

Cerebral and Extracerebral Vasculature

Many headaches have been attributed to vascular etiology: vasodilation or vasoconstriction.[9] A century ago William Osler postulated that migraine resulted from tension of the muscles of the neck and head.[10] Pain has been elicited by stimulation of numerous extracranial and intracranial vessels, including the superficial temporal, supratrochlear, frontal, and middle meningeal vessels, the superior sagittal sinus, and the sylvian vein.[11]

There are three major vascular systems supplying the head: (1) branches of the external carotid other than to the scalp, (2) branches to the scalp, and (3) the cerebral circulation.[12]

The branches of the external carotid other than to the scalp are predominantly to the face. The arterial supply to the scalp is derived from the superficial temporal artery. The scalp also receives branches from the supraorbital, supratrochlear, and ophthalmic arteries. The superficial temporal artery is clinically the most important.

The meninges receive their blood supply from the external and internal

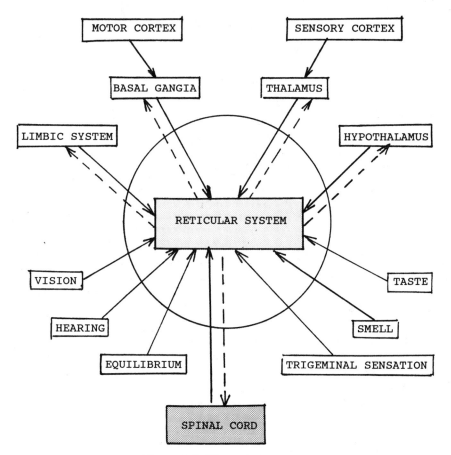

Figure 8–9. The reticular system.

carotids and the vertebral arteries. The brain receives its arterial supply from the vertebral arteries and the internal carotid arteries.

Migraine and Migraine Variants

There has been debate as to whether the etiology of migraine and migraine variant headaches is vascular, neurologic, or both. The vascular mechanism of migraine was propounded by Wolff for two reasons: (1) migraine aura can be abolished by use of amyl nitrite, a potent vasodilator, and (2) ergotamine, a vasoconstrictor, relieves migraine.[13] Laboratory studies of cerebral vascular flow did not correlate with symptomatology,[14] implying that migraine was primarily neurogenic with a secondary vascular component.[15,16]

Table 8–1. INTERNATIONAL HEADACHE SOCIETY
CLASSIFICATION OF CLUSTER HEADACHE

3.1 Cluster headache
   3.1.1. Cluster headache periodicity undetermined
   3.1.2. Episodic cluster headache
   3.1.3. Chronic cluster headache
      3.1.3.1 Chronic cluster headache unremitting from onset
      3.1.3.2 Chronic cluster headache evolved from episodic
3.2 Chronic paroxysmal hemicrania
3.3 Chronic clusterlike disorder not fulfilling above criteria

By activating the afferents, serotonin causes a retrograde (antidromal) release of substance P, which causes increased capillary permeability and ultimately edema.[17] This concept of migraine mechanism is relatively recent.

See Table 8–1 for the criteria for diagnosing migraine or migraine variants. Migraine-type headaches have been described elsewhere in the literature.[18] The mechanisms remain obscure. Prodromal symptoms, which distinguish classic from variant migraine, involve the autonomic nervous system and the somatic neuromuscular system.

Recently, the tension headache has been closely associated with the migraine headache as well as being considered a separate entity. The peripheral mechanisms of headaches include the muscles as well as the blood vessels but also invoke a central monitoring.[19]

A proposed model, termed *myofascial supraspinal myogenic (MSV) model* attempts to correlate the vascular and muscular components of migraine head pain (Fig. 8–10).[20]

The wide dynamic range (WDR) neurons of the trigeminal ganglion have connections with the intracranial and extracranial blood vessels and receive noxious stimulation from the pericranial myofascial tissues.[21] This further ties together the vascular and the muscular component of migraine. Trigger-point injection of the pericranial muscles have aborted migraine attacks.[22]

The VSM model suggests treatment that includes a combination of medication and myofascial and psychologic intervention.

Cluster Headaches

Cluster headaches have been formally recognized by the Headache Classification Committee of the International Headache Society (Table 8–2). They occur predominantly in men and, as their name implies, come in clusters: one to two per year.

Pathophysiology of Cluster Headaches. Some researchers consider cluster

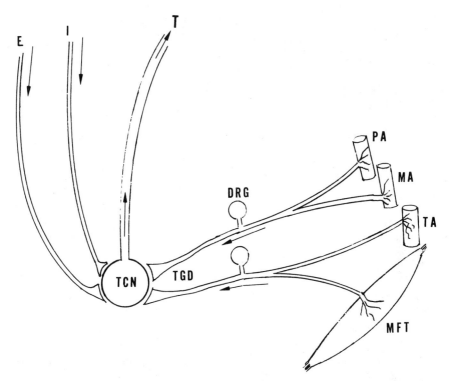

Figure 8–10. Myofascial supraspinal vascular (MSV) model of pain pathways.

The input into the pain neural pathways are depicted in this MSV model. The afferent impulses originating from the pial arteries (PA), meningeal arteries (MA), and the temporal arteries (TA), compete with the nociceptive impulses of the myofascial tissues (MFT).

All impulses converge through their dorsal root ganglia (DRG) to the trigeminal ganglion (1st) division nucleus (TCN). Modulation of these impulses that ultimately enter the thalamus (T) occurs from descending excitatory (E) and inhibitory (I) fibers from cortical levels.

headache to be vascular,[23] yet enhanced intraocular pulsations during a cluster headache has not been observed,[24] and abnormal regional blood flow studies have not been informative.[25]

The cluster headache nerve distribution is in the region of the trigeminal nerve, with vasodilation considered secondary to neuronal discharge. The vascular system of the trigeminal nerve has also been implicated.[26]

The periodicity of the cluster headache implies a circadian periodicity, invoking the suprachiasmic nuclei.[27]

Management of Cluster Headaches. The management of cluster headaches is similar to that of migraine. However, because of the severity of the headaches, the patient lives in fear of recurrence.

Oxygen normally produces cerebral vasoconstriction. Immediate relief

**Table 8–2. INTERNATIONAL HEADACHE SOCIETY
CRITERIA FOR MIGRAINE**

A. At least two attacks fulfilling B
B. At least three of the following characteristics:
  1. One or more fully reversible aura symptoms, indicating cerebral cortical and/ or brainstem dysfunction.
  2. At least one aura symptom develops gradually over more than 4 minutes or two or more symptoms occur in succession.
  3. Aura symptom lasts less than 60 minutes (if more than one aura symptom is present, accepted duration is proportionally increased).
  4. Headache follows aura with a free interval of less than 60 minutes. (It may also begin before or simultaneously with the aura.)
C. History and examination do not suggest an organic or metabolic disorder or the latter is ruled out by appropriate investigations or the migraine attacks do not occur for the first time in close temporal relation to an organic or metabolic disorder.

of a cluster headache is obtained by the inhalation of oxygen, which apparently corrects the abnormal reaction to oxygen noted in patients having cluster headaches.[28]

Ergotamine has proven effective but only if administered in a manner that gives immediate absorption, that is, via inhalation (Midhaler Ergotamine-Riker) or suppository.

A multidisciplinary approach in the management of cluster headaches is required, including vascular, muscular, life-style, and psychologic approaches.

Neurologic Aspects of Headache

There are numerous causes of headaches (Tables 8–3 and 8–4), all of which have their specific mechanisms. The clinical aspects of head and face pain are summarized as follows:

Trigeminal neuralgia. Sudden, severe, brief, lancinating pain provoked by touch or movement of the areas within the face innervated by the trigeminal nerve.
  • *Ophthalmic division.* Pain in forehead and supraorbital region and nose.
  • *Maxillary division.* Pain in the upper lip, cheek, side of nose, upper jaw, and teeth. Site of provocation is the upper lip and occasionally the upper gums.
  • *Mandibular division.* Pain in mandibular region, lower lip, chin, jaw, gums, and ear. Site of provocation is the lower lip.

Table 8–3. PARTIAL LIST OF CAUSES OF HEADACHES

Intracranial Causes

A. Toxic
  Carbon monoxide
  Toxic fumes
  Side effects of drugs: NSAIDs,
    antihypertensive, etc.
  Heavy metals
  Withdrawal headache from habitual
    uses

B. Metabolic
  Febrile illness
  Hepatic disease
  Renal disease
  Endocrine imbalance
  Cushing's disease
  Hypoparathyroidism
  Postseizure headache
  Hypothyroid and hyperthyroid
    disease

C. Infectious Diseases
  1. Meningeal acute bacterial
      meningitis
    Acute viral meningitis
    Spirochetal meningitis (syphilis,
      etc.)
  2. Parenchymal
    Syphilis
    Viral encephalitis (chronic)
    Viral encephalitis (acute)
    Toxoplasma

Extracranial Causes

A. Infectious
  Sinusitis ⎫
  Mastoiditis ⎬ bacterial, fungal, etc.
  Tonsillitis ⎭
  Herpetic

B. Vascular
  Vasculitis
  Carotid dissection
  Carotid occlusion (thrombus)
  Paget's disease

C. Dental
  Pulpitis
  Periodontitis
  Dentinal
  Cemental
  Odontalgia (atypical)

D. Bone and Joint
  Temporomandibular
  Osteomyelitis
  Eagle's syndrome
  Metastasis (skull)

E. Tumor
  Carcinoma
  Lymphoepithelioma

F. Cranial Neuralgias
  Trigeminal neuralgia
  Glossopharyngeal neuroma
  Occipital neuralgia
  Atypical facial pain

G. Vascular
  Temporal arteritis
  Stroke TIA
  Infectious vasculitis (herpes
    zoster, simplex, etc.)
  Granulomatous arteritis

H. Increased Intracranial Pressure
  Tumor
  Abscess
  Hematoma (subdural, epidural,
    parenchymal, etc.)

I. Decreased Intracranial Pressure
  CSF leak; postspinal tap

J. Tumor Invasion of Peripheral
  Nerves

K. Posttrauma Headache
  Postconcussion

TIA = transient ischemic attack; CSF = cerebrospinal fluid.

Table 8–4. FUNCTIONAL IDIOPATHIC HEADACHES

I. Vascular Headache
  A. Migraine
  B. Migraine variant
  C. Exertional headache
  D. Postcoital headache
  E. Post-cold ingestion headache (ice cream)
II. Cluster Headache
  A. Acute cyclical cluster headache
  B. Chronic cluster headache
  C. Cluster headache variants
    1. Cluster migraine
    2. Chronic paroxysmal hemicrania
III. Cervicogenic Headache (of questionable etiology)
IV. Tension Headache
V. Chronic Daily Headache (idiopathic or of numerous etiologies)

Genicular neuralgia. Tic douloureux type of pain deep in ipsilateral ear and postauricular area. Area of provocation is the inner ear, occasionally incited by swallowing.

Glossopharyngeal neuralgia. Severe piercing pains in the tonsillar or pharynx area and back of tongue. Area of provocation is the throat; hence, it is incited by swallowing and talking.

Occipital neuralgia. Continuous aching, throbbing pain in the suboccipital area, that is, the posterior and lateral scalp. Occasionally there is pain in the retroorbital region. There is no specific area of provocation other than from deep pressure in the suboccipital area near the mastoid process.

Migraine headache. Throbbing, pulsating, pressing usually unilateral headache (75 percent of cases). Often preceded by prodromal symptoms.

Migraine variant. Similar to migraine with predominance of neurologic symptoms related to a specific cranial artery. No regional area of provocation.

Cluster headache. Sudden unexpected unilateral aching or "burning" pain in ocular, frontal, and temporal area. No area of provocation.

Acute headache. Severe, continuous, generalized headache with associated other symptoms. Provoked or initiated by meningitis, subarachnoid hemorrhage, cerebral vascular accident, or postspinal puncture headache.

Musculoskeletal headache. There are two main types.
  • *Temporomandibular arthralgia.* Dull aching pain in the muscles of mastication provoked by movement of the jaw.

• *Myofascial pain syndrome.* Dull, aching, deep muscular pain located within specific muscle groups. Provoked by pressure on trigger point in that muscle.

Ocular or Periorbital Pain.

• *Ocular pain.* Deep, dull aching pain often with "foreign body" sensation.

• *Periorbital pain.* Deep, dull aching pain in orbit, often with lid edema.

Ear, Nose, and Throat Pain. Pain located in the specific organ (ear, nose, throat, paranasal or frontal sinuses). Local pain and tenderness of the region with associated symptoms of disease. Often evidence of inflammation or infection.

Psychogenic pain. Pain described in bizarre symptoms, vague etiology, poor neurologic demarcation, and associated with other psychologic factors.

Temporomandibular Joint Pain

Temporomandibular joint pain, termed TMJ syndrome, is a prominent impairing and disabling condition.[29,30] The mechanisms causing pain will be discussed here.

The International Association for the Study of Headache has included temporomandibular disorders in the classification of atypical odonyalgia (Table 8–5).[31] The subdivisions of this classification relate principally to deviations of the disk, which includes perforation, elongation, and narrowing with or

Table 8–5. TEMPOROMANDIBULAR DISORDERS

Deviation in form
Disk displacement with reduction
Disk displacement without reduction
Inflammation
Hypermobility
Osteoarthritis
Osteoarthropathy
Polyarthritides and connective tissue disorders
    Rheumatoid arthritis
    Psoriatic arthritis
    Ankylosing arthritis
    Systemic lupus erythematosus
    Scleroderma
Fibrous ankylosis
Bony ankylosis
Dislocation

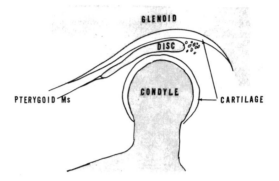

Figure 8–11. Temporomandibular joint.

The concavity of the glenoid fossa differs from the convexity of the mandibular condyle, forming an incongruous joint. Both are covered with cartilage that physiologically deforms during motion. The disk is fibrocartilaginous in structure and is held and elongated by the pterygoid muscle.

Behind the disk are numerous blood vessels, lymphatics, and connective tissue fibers *(dotted area).*

without associated pain (Fig. 8–11). Only the type with pain will be discussed here.

Pain can result from impairment of the tissues within the TMJ and from the numerous muscles that operate the jaw. Muscular disorders of the TMJ are more common (see Table 8–6).

The nerves that supply the TMJ articulation are the auriculotemporal nerve with contribution from the masseter and deep posterior temporal nerve branches of the third (mandibular) division of the trigeminal nerve. These afferents convey pain from the TMJ.

The TMJ is a diarthrodal synovial joint. The motions of the TMJ are permitted, directed, and limited by the articular surfaces, the menisci, the ligaments, the capsular tissues, and the muscles. TMJ syndrome may exist without organic joint disease or articular dysfunction; hence, the condition is more appropriately termed "myofascial pain dysfunctional syndrome of the temporomandibular articulation."

Numerous proprioceptive nerves in the ligaments and joint structure of the TMJ can become involved in the pathologic mechanisms; they are therefore pertinent in diagnosis and rehabilitation "reeducation."

Table 8–6. MUSCLE DISORDERS

Myositis
Myofascial pain
Splinting/trismus
Contracture
Hypertrophy

Figure 8–12. Deformation of the disk in jaw opening and closing. The disk deforms rather than moves with the condyle as the jaw opens and closes. The drawing shows movement but the disk essentially deforms, being held between the glenoid fossa and the moving condyle. The cartilage of the condyle (not shown) also deforms during movement.

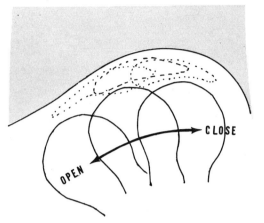

Within the joint the cartilages of the glenoid fossa are fibrocartilaginous and deform during joint motion (Figs. 8–12 and 8–13). A faulty action of the jaw may cause the disk to tear from the underlying condyle, allowing it to dislocate anteriorly from action of the lateral pterygoid muscle (Fig. 8–14). Initially, damage to the meniscus causes dysfunction of the joint but not necessarily pain. Crepitation and bruxism may occur. Pain occurs when the related muscles react to this mechanical dysfunction, as in any condition of acute synovitis.

Pain may be either intracapsular or extracapsular. Intracapsular pain results from subluxation of the joint, causing a "locked" joint, or from degenerative articular changes. Extracapsular pain is predominantly muscular.[32]

Meniscal damage varies from perforation, thinning, thickening, folding, or dislocation to ankylosis. Ultimately, capsular and cartilagenous changes lead to degenerative arthritis of the joint.

The diagnosis of the true mechanism of TMJ arthralgia is based on an accurate history and meaningful examination. Routine x-rays are of value only after the pathology is advanced. Magnetic resonance imaging (MRI) studies reveal the soft tissue pathology,[33] and computed tomography (CT) scanning reveals the site, status, and relationship of the disk as well as the status of the bony structures of the articulation.[34]

Management of TMJ syndrome involves any or all of the modalities discussed in Chapters 4 through 6, depending on the stage of development. Occlusal abnormality must be corrected, and inflammation, tension, weakness, atrophy, and contracture in the masticatory muscles must be addressed early in the treatment to prevent ultimate irreversible changes (Fig. 8–15).

Mere "clicking" usually responds to conservative measures, including an orthosis (Fig. 8–16). A locked meniscus causing symptoms must be reduced by manipulation (Fig. 8–17) followed by all other pertinent therapy modal-

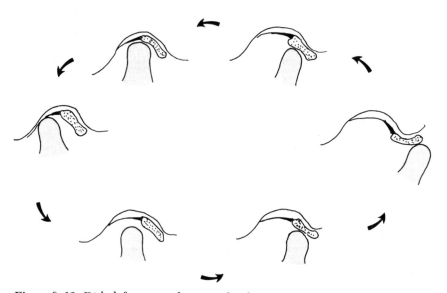

Figure 8–13. Disk deformation during cycle of jaw opening and closing.

As the jaw opens and closes, the disk deforms to accommodate the opening between the condyle and the glenoid fossa. The disk is held anteriorly by a filament to the pterygoid muscle (dark line emanating from the anterior margin of the disk). Throughout the cycle of the jaw the condyle moves anteriorly and posteriorly within the glenoid fossa (see Fig. 8–12).

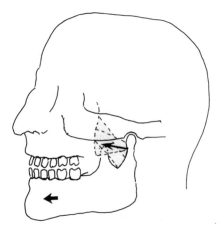

Figure 8–14. Lateral (external) pterygoid muscle.

The two divisions of the lateral pterygoid muscle lie deep to the zygomatic arch. The muscle originates from the infratemporal crest and the great wing of the sphenoid bone. It attaches to the neck of the condyle and the posterior superior aspect of the ramus of the mandible.

Its action is principally protrusion of the mandible and some lateral motion of the mandible, but it has been found to be mildly active during opening of the jaw.

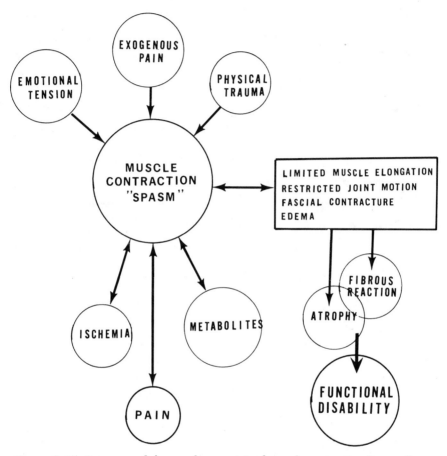

Figure 8–15. Sequence of changes from sustained muscle contraction "spasm."

Sustained muscle contraction, described as "spasm" or "tension," is caused by emotional tension, pain stimuli, and trauma. The immediate result is ischemia from compression of the internal blood vessels with accumulation of metabolites and resultant pain, which causes further contraction.

The long-range sequelae are joint limitation, muscular atrophy, and contracture. Functional disability ultimately results.

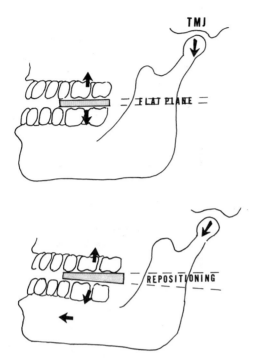

Figure 8–16. Orthosis to open, maintain opening, or reposition the mandible.

In the upper drawing the orthosis (splint) is flat planed to evenly open the bite, realign the teeth, and open the temporomandibular joint (TMJ). This may be therapeutic to open the jaw against the muscular force of the masseter and temporalis muscles.

In the lower drawing the orthosis is angled to reposition the mandible by causing it to move forward and change the bite and the opening of the TMJ. This orthosis may be used to correct the bite. The flat plane orthosis is then returned to maintain the gained TMJ opening.

Figure 8–17. Passive-active mobilization of the mandible.

(A), Finger inserted into mouth to open the jaw. This stretches the masseter and temporal muscles and their fascia and moves the temporomandibular (TMJ) anteriorly. (B), The point of resistance to strengthen the muscles that open the jaw (C) denotes anterior shear force to protrude the mandible and also anteriorly displace the TMJ.

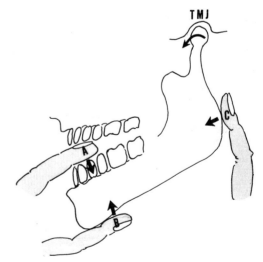

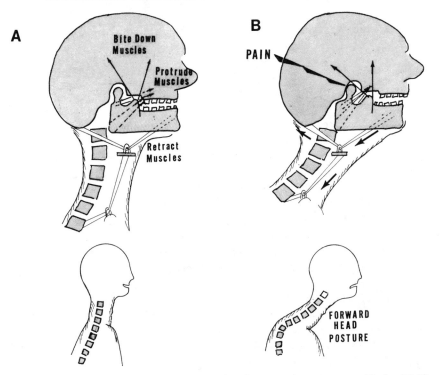

Figure 8–18. Influence of posture on dental occlusion and temporomandibular (TMJ) alignment.

(A) normal posture and its effect on the bite and TMJ alignment. In the forward head posture (B) the jaw is retracted causing malalignment of the teeth and of the TMJ, which causes disk deformation, pain, and gradual degenerative changes of the teeth and TMJ.

ities. Posture in the TMJ syndrome (Fig. 8–18) influences the pathology and must be evaluated and treated.

PAIN IN THE CERVICAL SPINE

Pain emanating from the cervical spine results from internal or external forces. When these forces are excessive and cause tissue damage, pain results.

The excessive external forces are trauma imposed on the spine, and internal excessive forces are faulty neuromusculoskeletal activities from perturber influences.

Pain from the cervical spine must be divided into upper and lower cervical segments, as each has a different functional anatomy and pain mechanism. The upper cervical segment consists of the occiput and upper three cervical vertebrae. The cervicogenic headache, emanating from the upper cervical spine,[36] is included in this area. The lower consists of vertebrae C-3 to C-7.[35]

Upper Cervical Segment Syndromes

The tissue sites of head, neck, and face pain originating from the cervical spine include the joint disks, ligaments, muscles, and nerve roots as they emerge. The major nerve carrying pain is the greater superior occipital nerve composed of roots from C-1, C-2, and C-3 (Fig. 8–19). It emerges from the cranial notch in the occipital region between the insertion of the trapezius and sternocleidomastoid muscles (Fig. 8–20).

It has been postulated that headache originates from the cervical spine with C-1 to C-2 ascending to the brainstem via the trigeminal nucleus.[37,38] The greatest influence is attributed to the C-2 component of the greater and lesser occipital nerves,[39,40] but recent observations suggest that headaches can occur from lesions of the lower cervical segments (Fig. 8–21).[41,42]

The dorsal ramus of C-2 (Fig. 8–22) innervates the disks between C-1 and C-2. The third occipital nerve (TON) is related to the C-2 and C-3 facet joint capsule; it conveys sensory fibers to the skin.

Analgesic injections of the cervical nerve C-2, which contains medial fibers from the dorsal rami of the nerve, can relieve headache.[43] Analgesic injection of the C-3 root is questionable; when effective, it may result from leakage of the agent into the facet. Analgesic injection of the facets between C-2 and C-3 gives questionable relief of headache, and injection of C-3, C-4, and C-5 fails to give relief, although there are contrary findings (Fig. 8–23).[44]

As in all musculoskeletal segments of the body, the cervical muscles (Fig. 8–24) are a source of nociception when traumatized or inflamed; this may result from both primary and referred pain from the protective spasm (Fig. 8–25).

Lower Cervical Segment Syndromes

The nociceptor tissue sites of the lower cervical spine (Fig. 8–26) are the longitudinal ligaments, dural sheaths of the nerve roots, facet capsules, posterior superficial ligaments, and erector spinae muscles. The outer annular disk fibers may also be involved.

Pain from these nociceptor tissue sites are referred to the neck and into the upper extremities. The nerve roots (Fig. 8–27) refer into their dermatomal areas, and the referred nociception from the facets refers into similar areas (Fig. 8–23). The referral sites of pain from intradiskal injections are depicted in Figure 8–28.

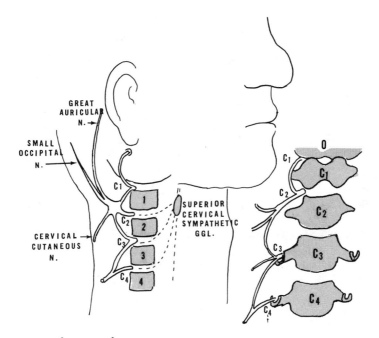

Figure 8–19. The cervical nerves.

The cervical nerves are derived from the cord segments that emerge between the occiput, the atlas (C-1), the axis (C-2), and the third cervical vertebra (C-3). C-4 emerges between the C-3 and the C-4 vertebra. These nerve roots emerge from the spinal column in an anterior lateral direction. They are contained within the gutters of the cervical vertebrae C-3 caudally. There are no gutters or intervertebral foramina in the uppermost cervical functional units.

The C-1 nerve (the suboccipital nerve) is the only branch of C-1 posterior primary division. It is mostly motor to upper cervical muscles.

C-2 nerve roots (along with a branch of C-3) form the "great occipital nerve," which is sensory to the occipital portions of the back of the ear, mastoid area, and the parotid gland. The C-3 root sends branches to the C-2 root to form the small occipital nerve (C-2 to C-3), which serves the skin of the lateral occipital portion of the scalp, the upper medial portion of the auricle, and the area over the mastoid process. It forms the third occipital branch and is sensory to a small portion of the scalp and neck. C-4 is sensory to the skin of the back and neck.

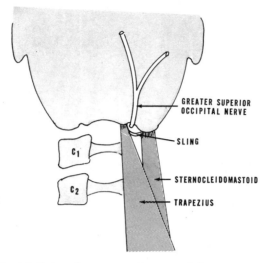

Figure 8–20. Occipital site of cranial emergence of the greater superior occipital nerve.

The greater superior occipital nerve, primarily C-2 nerve root emergence, in a groove medial to the mastoid process between the sites of attachment of the sternocleidomastoid and the trapezius muscles. A fascial sling completes the opening through which the nerve emerges.

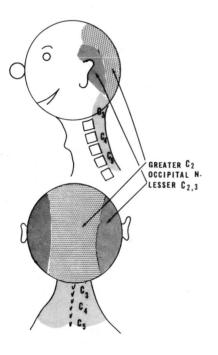

Figure 8–21. Dermatomal regions of the cervical nerves.

The dermatomal areas of all the cervical nerves from C-2 to C-5 wherein the C-2 to C-3 form the greater and lesser occipital nerves.

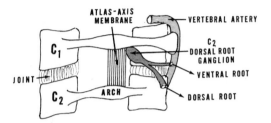

Figure 8–22. Emergence of the C-2 nerve root.

The C-2 dorsal ganglion lies under the obliquus inferior muscle (not shown), passing over the lateral atlantoaxial articulation. The C-2 nerve emerges lateral to the posterior atlas-axial membrane but does not penetrate it. It proceeds laterally to divide into a dorsal and ventral root. Its relationship to the vertebral artery is noted.

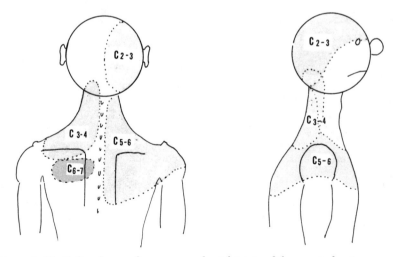

Figure 8–23. Referral areas from zygapophysial joints of the cervical spine.

The areas of referral reported by patients having neck and head pain. The area (C-6 to C-7 was not noted by the authors(*) but has been noted by this author. *Bogduk, A and Marsland, A: The cervical zygoapophysial joints as a source of neck pain. Spine 13(6):615, 1988, with permission.)

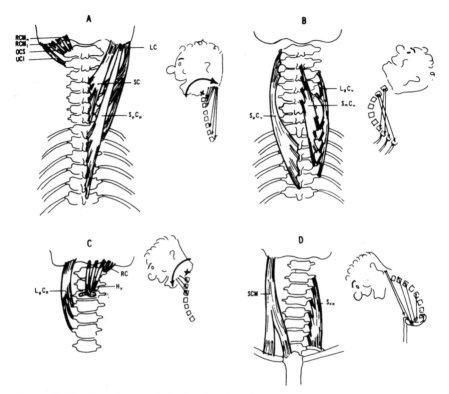

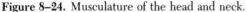

Figure 8–24. Musculature of the head and neck.

(A), The musculature of the extensor mechanism of the head and neck. The capital extensors attach to the skull and move the head on the neck (B). The cervical extensors originate and attach on the cervical spine and alter the curvature of the cervical spine (C) and (D). (C), Flexion musculature. The capital flexors attach exclusively on the cervical vertebrae and have no significant attachment to the skull. (RCMn = rectus capitis minor; RCMj = rectus capitis major; OCS = obliquus capitis superior; OCI = obliquus capitis inferior; LgCp = longus capitis; RC = rectus capitis anterior and lateral; Hy = hyoideus and suprahyoid; LC = longissimus capitis; SC = semispinalis capitis; SpCp = splenius capitis; LmCv = longissimus cervicis; SmCv = semispinalis cervicis; SCM = sternocleidomastoid; Sca = scalene medius and anticus.)

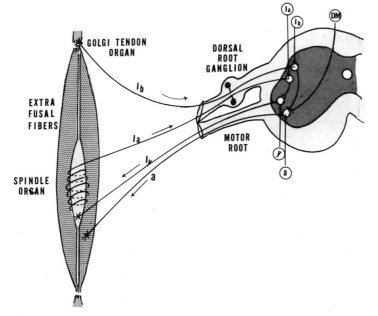

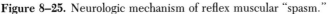

Figure 8–25. Neurologic mechanism of reflex muscular "spasm."

The extrafusal muscle fibers are kept at a specific length and tonus by a neural circuit effected by the spindle organs and tendon (Golgi) organs. Afferent impulses from these organs enter the dorsal column Ia and Ib, which has a neural contact with the anterior horn cells (a) and (y). These nuclei innervate the extrafusal muscle fibers via the Iy and a fibers to initiate an appropriate contraction or sustained tone. All afferent fibers have their nuclei in the dorsal root ganglia (DRG).

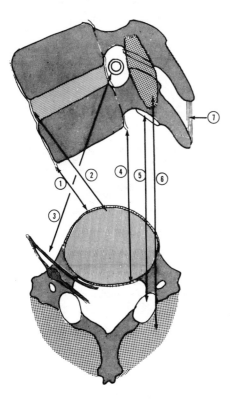

Figure 8–26. Nociceptor sites. (1 = anterior longitudinal ligament; 2 = outer annulus; 3 = dura; 4 = posterior longitudinal ligament; 5 = facet capsule; 6 = muscle; 7 = ligaments.)

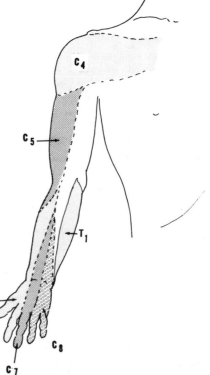

Figure 8–27. Dermatomes of cervical nerve roots C-5 to C-8.

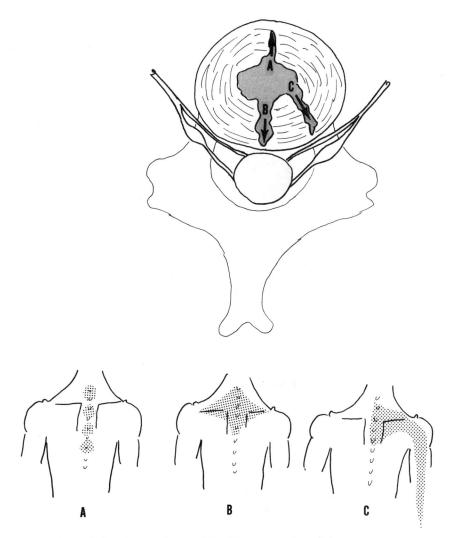

Figure 8–28. Referral sites of pain elicited by intranuclear diskograms.

(*A*), Irritation of the anterior portion of the disk refers pain to the interscapular midline. (*B*), Posterior nucleus protrusion refers pain as depicted. (*C*), Posterior lateral protrusion into the region of the intervertebral foramen causes interscapular pain plus arm radicular pain in the distribution of the nerve root dermatome.

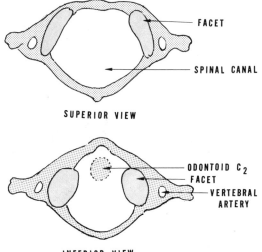

Figure 8–29. Atlas: First cervical vertebra (C-1)

The atlas (C-1) is viewed from above and below. The superior surface facets of the lateral bodies of the atlas articulate with the condyles of the occiput. The inferior facets articulate with the superior facets of the axis (C-2).

The site of the odontoid and the foramina of the vertebral arteries are depicted.

Mechanisms of Cervical Pain

How the nociceptive sites of pain in the cervical spine are provoked requires evaluation of normal cervical spine kinetics.

Upper Cervical Segment. Movement of the occipital atlas (C-1) is predominantly flexion-extension; it is limited by the capsular tissues of the facets (lateral bodies) (Fig. 8–29). Movement of the atlas (C-1) on the axis (C-2) is predominantly that of rotation. This rotation occurs about the occipital-atlas-axis ligaments (Fig. 8–30), which limit rotation and sagittal motion. Rotation about this apical ligament, which has great resiliency, causes excessive rotational motion to occur at the lateral bodies and their interposed disk (Fig. 8–31).

If the nociceptive tissues (capsules and disks) are moved beyond physiologic distance, these sensitive tissues are irritated and pain occurs. Excessive flexion-extension and rotation are the motions causing nociception, usually from an external force.[45]

Lower Cervical Segment. Each functional unit moves during neck flexion-extension (Fig. 8–32), lateral flexion, and rotation, causing foraminal opening and closing (Fig. 8–33). Physiologically this can occur without trauma to the nerve roots or any of the adjacent nociceptive tissues.

Faulty movement from perturbers or from external forces can exceed

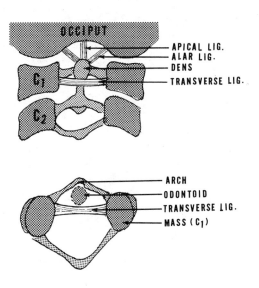

Figure 8–30. Occipital-atlas-axis ligaments.

The apical and alar ligaments connect the tip of the dens with the occiput and limit lateral, anterior-posterior movement. They are considered also to restrict a degree of rotation.

The transverse ligament acts as a sling holding the dens against the anterior arch of the atlas (lower figure). It allows rotation of the dens but protects the cord within the spinal canal.

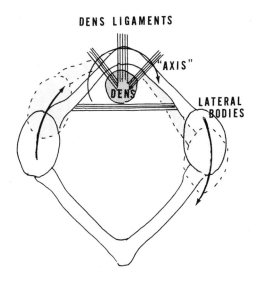

Figure 8–31. The dens as an axis of rotation.

The ligaments of the dens (odontoid process) prevent anterior-posterior and lateral movement but allow rotation of the atlas (C-1) about the axis (C-2) formed by these ligaments. In excessive external force the lateral bodies exceed their normal range of motion and cause some disruption of the intervertebral ("inter-lateral-body") disks.

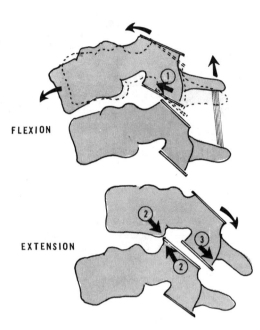

FLEXION

EXTENSION

Figure 8–32. Physiologic flexion and extension of a lower cervical functional unit.

Lower cervical units from C-3 to C-7: In flexion the facets (1) glide on each other, and the intervertebral foramina open.

In extension the posterior aspect of the vertebral body (2) impinges and stops further extension. The facets glide backward (3) and the foramina narrow.

physiologic motion (Fig. 8–34) and result in pain. In the event of stenosis of the spinal canal or the foramen, the enclosed nervous tissues lack adequate space to escape the compressive forces.

SHOULDER PAIN

Nociceptor Tissue Sites

The concept of neuromusculoskeletal reaction to external and internal forces causing pain and disability is significantly applicable to the shoulder complex. The external forces are direct trauma, and the internal forces are violation of the complex neuromusculoskeletal function applicable to the shoulder complex. Excessive force leading to tissue damage results in pain and dysfunction.

The tissues sites of possible nociception are the glenohumeral capsule,

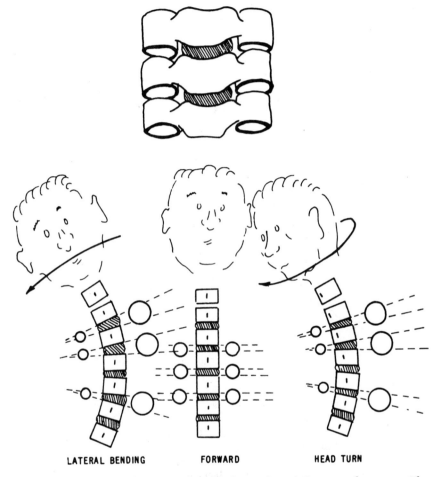

LATERAL BENDING   **FORWARD**   **HEAD TURN**

Figure 8–33. Foraminal closure in head during lateral flexion and turning. The foramina close on the side toward which the head rotates or bends laterally, and they open on the opposite side.

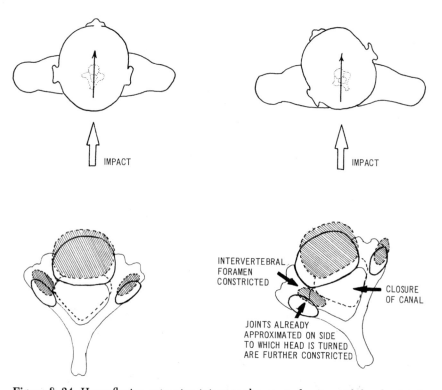

Figure 8–34. Hyperflexion-extension injury to the cervical spine with head rotated. The impact on the head in a forward direction causes a "to and fro"—flexion-extension resulting in symmetrical closing of the foramina and canal *(left)*.

With the head turned there is constriction of the intervertebral foramen on the side toward which the head is rotated. This occurs physiologically, but with impact it is excessive. The spinal canal undergoes deformation with possible cord compression *(right)*.

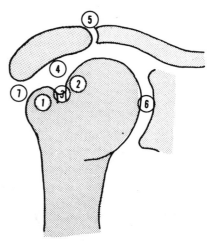

Figure 8–35. Sites of tissue pain: (1) greater tuberosity: attachment of supraspinatus tendon; (2) lesser tuberosity; (3) bicipital groove: tendon of long head of biceps; (4) subacromial bursa; (5) acromioclavicular joint; (6) glenohumeral joint and capsule; (7) subdeltoid bursa. (Modified from Steindler, A: The Interpretation of Pain in Orthopedic Practice. Charles C Thomas, Springfield, Illinois, 1959.)

the supraspinatus tendon complex, the bony and periosteal structures of the humerus and scapula, and the associated muscles (Fig. 8–35).

The nerve supply to the shoulder is from C-5 and C-6 nerve roots, which form the suprascapular, axillary (circumflex), and lateral pectoral nerves. Sensory nerves are accompanied by sympathetic nerves emanating from the cervical and stellate ganglia. They descend in the adventitia of the subclavian and axillary arteries supplying the capsule and synovial membrane of that joint.

The axillary nerve is derived from spinal segments C-5 and C-6 (Fig. 8–36). It leaves the distal part of the posterior cord of the brachial plexus, passes laterally through the axilla to bend around the surgical neck of the humerus, and ultimately innervates the deltoid muscle and its overlying skin.[46] En route it sends a branch to the teres minor muscle.

The suprascapular nerve originates from C-5 and C-6 primary rami, emerging from the upper trunk of the brachial plexus (Fig. 8–37). It descends passing through the suprascapular notch of the scapula posteriorly to the scapula to innervate the supraspinatus and infraspinatus muscle. It is primarily motor and causes pain only when normal glenohumeral function is interrupted.

The nociceptive tissues of the shoulder are the capsule, the tendons (particularly the rotator cuff tendons), the bursae, and the synovium of the glenohumeral joint.

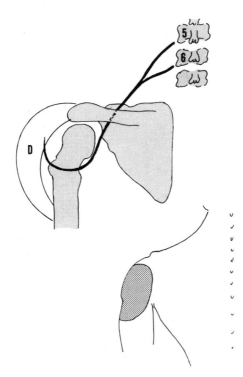

Figure 8–36. Axillary nerve.

The axillary nerve derives from C-5 to C-6 root to descend and encircle the surgical neck of the humerus. Its motor roots terminate in the deltoid muscle (D).

The sensory (dermatome) area is depicted in the lower figure at the anterolateral aspect of the shoulder area.

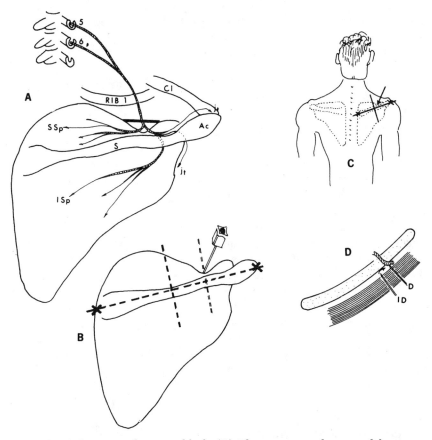

Figure 8–37. Suprascapular nerve block. *(A)*, The anatomy and course of the supra-scapular nerve, originating from C-5 to C-6. The motor nerve to the supraspinatus (SSp), and infraspinatus (ISp) and the sensory branches to the acromioclavicular joint and the shoulder joint (jt) are shown. *(B,C)*, Bisection of a line drawn along the scapular spine with the site of the groove and of needle insertion. *(D)*, The difference between direct nerve contact and indirect (ID) by infusion along the posterior portion of the scapula below the supraspinatus muscle.

Functional Mechanisms of Pain

The shoulder girdle has a primary function—to place the hand and fingers in a functional position. Neurophysiologists still do not understand exactly how the shoulder-hand-finger coordination functions to assure the appropriate steps between the decision, the initiation, and the ultimate culmination of the intended action.[47]

The central nervous system must convert information from the visual concept of the intent into initiation. This involves primarily the occipitoparietal visual system, which transforms complex neurophysiologic muscle activity.[48] It is possible that the gross musculoskeletal patterns of the upper extremity are located within the midbrain and are "modified" by upper cortical activity, which is the site of "training."[49]

The ultimate hand-finger function probably also modifies the more proximal neuromusculoskeletal patterns. The multiarticular movements motorized by numerous muscle-and-tendon structures suggest that a complex neurologic system must be postulated once the decision (goal) is made.

It is theorized that a cortical movement pattern exists because lesions in the cortex cause distinct motor deficits. Losses include spatiomotor discoordination with misreaching in lesions in the partietal cortex and deficits in learning and retrieval from lesions in the prefrontal and premotor cortex.[50–53]

The proximal upper extremity motion that places the arm, hand, and fingers in their precise positions requires appropriate distance, speed, force, and duration for that action. Upper arm motion begins with stabilization of the scapula on the thoracic wall.

The passive dependent arm is held in the glenoid fossal cavity by the supraspinatus muscle (Fig. 8–38). The scapula must be stabilized to maintain the glenoid fossa facing outward, forward, and upward.[54] This prevents the head of the humerus from sliding down and outward (Fig. 8–39). The scapula is supported isometrically by the trapezius and serratus anterior muscles. Sustained tone of these muscles is precisely directed by the spindle system (Fig. 8–40).

Shoulder Pain Mechanisms

Rotator cuff muscle failure, either from interference of the nerve supply or tear of the rotator cuff tendon, places a downward "drag" on the capsule, causing pain.

Placing the hand in a functional position requires that the scapula maintain a static position to support the shoulder action. The humerus initiates abduction and forward flexion by isokinetic contraction of the rotator cuff muscles followed by deltoid action. Abduction of the humerus gradually requires rotation of the scapula to functionally elevate the arm. This is known as the scapulohumeral rhythm (Fig. 8–41).[55]

As the humerus abducts, it must also simultaneously externally rotate to ensure the greater tuberosity passing under the overhanging acromium and the coracoacromial ligament. The same muscles that abduct also externally rotate the humerus (Fig. 8–42).

If appropriate scapulohumeral rhythm is not maintained, irritation of the nociceptive tissues in the glenohumeral joint results (Fig. 8–43). Abnormal scapulohumeral rhythm occurs when the normal range of motion is

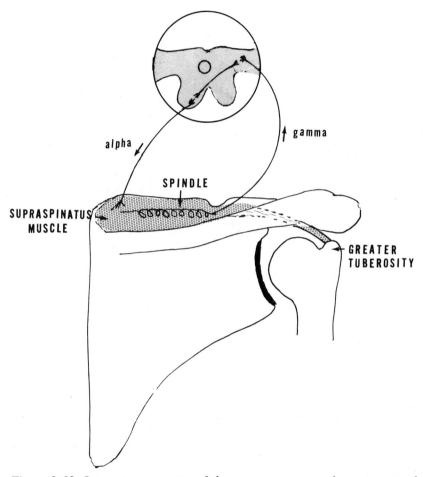

Figure 8–38. Isometric contraction of the supraspinatus muscle to maintain the humeral-glenoid relationship.

The spindle system of the supraspinatus muscle conveys to the cord via gamma fibers the exact tone (via the alpha fibers) needed to prevent the humerus from descending within the glenoid fossa.

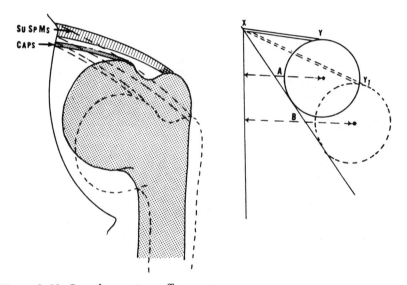

Figure 8–39. Capsular passive cuff support.

Due to the orientation of the glenoid fossa, which faces forward, upward, and outward, the superior capsule—taut in the normal position—becomes more taut as the humeral head (A) descends. (B), depicts an analogy of a ball rolling down an angled plane.

The cuff (supraspinatus muscle, Su Sp Ms) offers the major support and not the capsule (Caps).

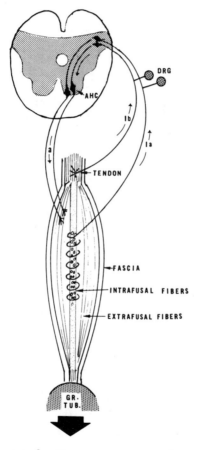

Figure 8–40. Spindle system function.

The spindle system (intrafusal fibers) is parallel with the extrafusal fibers. When stretched, they signal the cord by way of Ia (from the spindle) and Ib (from the Golgi tendon organs) through the dorsal root ganglia (DRG). An interneural connection to the anterior horn cells (AHC) causes appropriate contraction of the extrafusal fibers.

The fascia elongates according to its physiologic limits. In this illustration the muscle is the supraspinatus attached to the greater tuberosity (Gr. Tub.) of the humerus.

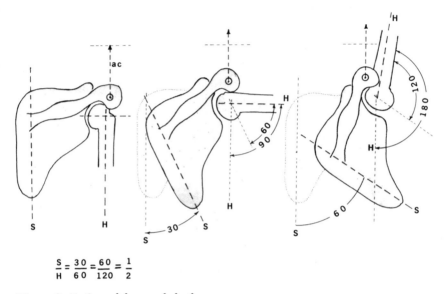

$$\frac{S}{H} = \frac{30}{60} = \frac{60}{120} = \frac{1}{2}$$

Figure 8–41. Scapulohumeral rhythm.

(Left), The scapula and the humerus at position of rest with the scapula relaxed and the arm dependent, both at position 0°. The abduction movement of the arm is accomplished in a smooth, coordinated movement during which for each 15° of arm abduction 10° of motion occurs at the glenohumeral joint and 5° occurs due to scapular rotation on the thorax. *(Center)*, The humerus (H) has abducted 90° in relation to the erect body, but this has been accomplished by a 30° rotation of the scapula and a 60° rotation of the humerus at the glenohumeral joint, a ratio of 2:1. *(Right)*, Full elevation of the arm: 60° at the scapula and 120° at the glenohumeral joint.

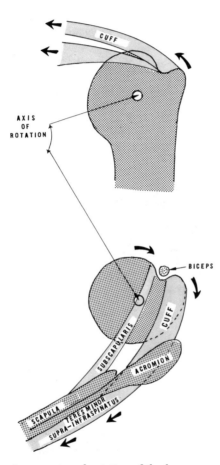

Figure 8–42. Supraspinatus external rotation of the humerus.

Superior view of the scapulocostal joint depicting the supraspinatus muscle that attaches to the greater tuberosity located lateral to the bicipital groove. Being lateral to the axis of rotation, the attachment permits the supraspinatus muscle to rotate the humerus (H) externally. Located under the scapula, the subscapularis (*dotted area*) attaches to the lesser tuberosity (medial to the bicipital groove) and thus is an internal rotator (*dotted arrow*) of the humerus. The ribs attach to the transverse processes of the thoracic vertebrae at the costovertebral (C-V) joints.

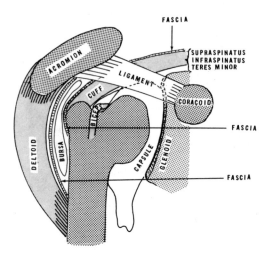

Figure 8–43. Tissues within the suprahumeral space capable of being nociceptive sites.

The following tissues within the suprahumeral space are innervated to be nociceptive sites when irritated or injured. (1) bursa; (2) capsule; (3) biceps tendon sheath; (4) fascial layers.

exceeded, when repetitive activities are continued to the point of fatigue, or when there is external trauma. Faulty posture predisposes to abnormal shoulder mechanics (Fig. 8–44). The abnormal mechanics of the shoulder irritate the sensitive tissues. Damage to normal tissues such as the rotator cuff, labrum, and subdeltoid bursa predisposes to further painful faulty motion.

PAIN IN THE ELBOW, HAND, AND FINGERS

The elbow consists of three articulations: the humeroulnar, the capitular radial (radiohumeral), and the radioulnar joints (Fig. 8–45).[56] Pain in any of these joints can occur as a result of a faulty motion that has exceeded the normal range of motion (strain-sprain); a systemic disease, such as rheumatoid arthritis, that involves the synovial system of these joints; or external trauma, such as a fall or athletic injury. Trauma is the greatest cause of elbow pain.

Posttrauma stiffness is the most devastating sequela of trauma. There are four features of the anatomy of the elbow that predispose this joint to stiffness: (1) there is significant congruity of the joints, (2) the joints are traversed by muscle rather than tendons, (3) intra-articular fractures are difficult to immobilize, and (4) the joint capsules have a unique propensity to thicken and contract.[57]

Contractures are either of soft tissue (capsular) or of bone (osseous bridging). Intrinsic contracture occurs from adhesions or avascular articular damage. Any of these can cause pain when normal range of motion is exceeded.

Deviation from normal movement is evident in the history and the clinical examination. These joints lend themselves to clinical evaluation, as all motions are in the purview of the examiner, and radiologic examinations are confirmatory.

The tissue sites of nociception are the synovial articulations, the capsules, and the ligaments. The ulnar-humeral and the radioulnar joints are involved. Periarticular tissues may become nociceptive sites where tendons attach to the periosteum. Contiguous nerves may also be sites of nociception.

Ulnar Neuritis

The ulnar nerve is superficial within the olecranon fossa and is subject to direct trauma. The groove behind the medial condyle (Fig. 8–46) contains the ulnar nerve, which is covered by a fibrous sheath. The nerve then enters the forearm between the two heads of the ulnar flexor muscle.

Resultant pain and dysfunction occur from ulnar nerve "compression"

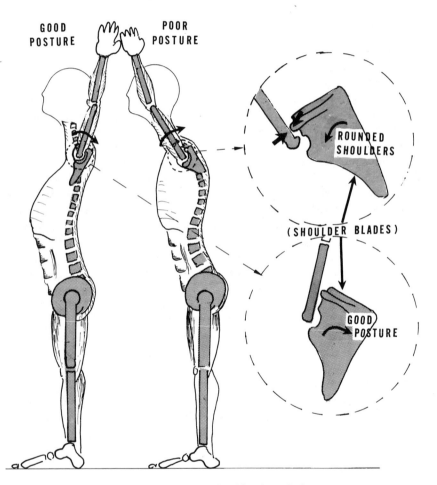

Figure 8–44. Impingement syndrome of shoulder from faulty posture.
In "good" erect posture the humerus does not impinge on the acromium in
overhead elevation. In a rounded shoulder posture the scapula is downward rotated
placing the acromium in a position on which the humerus impinges *(arrows)*.

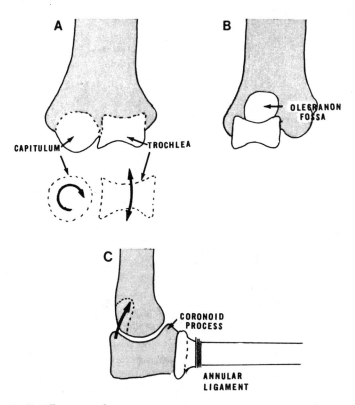

Figure 8–45. Elbow joint bony anatomy.

(A), Anterior view depicting the round sphere of the capitulum, on which the radius rotates and the spool-shaped trochlea, about which the ulna flexes and extends. (B), Posterior view of the humerus showing the olecranon fossa, into which the posterior (olecranon) portion of the radius enters on elbow extension. (C), Lateral view of the elbow joint.

or trauma. The sensory fibers of the ulnar nerve are more superficial than are the motor fibers; thus, sensory symptoms are more prevalent.[58]

Sensory symptoms occur in the following sequence:

Grade 1: Paresthesia and minor hypoesthesia.

Grade 2: Weakness and wasting of the interosseous muscles; incomplete hypoesthesia.

Grade 3: Paralysis of the interosseous muscle with atrophy of the hypothenar muscles and the adductor muscles of the thumb. (These cause "clawing" of the ring and little fingers.)

Assuming the mechanism to be compression of the nerve in the cubital canal, treatment is to diminish or minimize direct pressure. Surgical trans-

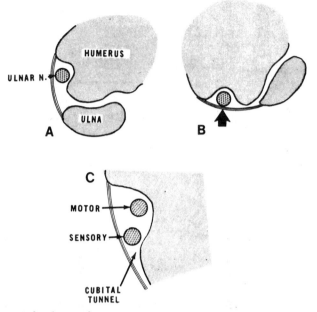

Figure 8–46. Cubital tunnel.

(A), Full supination removes the ulnar nerve from external pressure. (B), Full pronation places the nerve in position of pressure. Full flexion can also cause nerve compression between the arcuate and medial ligaments of the floor. (C), Ulnar nerve fibers are divided, with the sensory portion more superficial; thus, pressure often causes sensory changes without motor impairment.

plantation of the nerve is no longer considered to be effective.[59] Surgical decompression by tenotomy remains effective.[60]

Radial Nerve Pain

Radial nerve entrapment causes symptoms that come from the elbow but are observed in the hand. The radial nerve descends along the lateral aspect of the humerus and proceeds anteriorly in front of the lateral condyle (Fig. 8–47) between the brachialis and brachioradialis muscles. The superficial branch of the radial nerve passes through the origination of the extensor carpi radialis muscle. It is here where direct trauma is possible, with resulting pain or numbness of the lateral aspect of the forearm. Pain may be referred to the anatomic snuffbox or to the first carpometacarpal joint, and it may mimic disease in that joint.

Fracture or dislocation of the neck of the radius can cause radial nerve damage. Direct trauma can also result from violent muscular contraction of the forearm extensor muscles or from repeated pronation or dorsiflexion

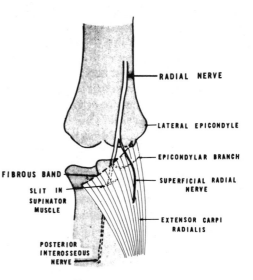

Figure 8–47. Course of the radial nerve.
The deep nerve passes under the fibrous band origin of the short radial extensor muscle. At the division just cephalad to the fibrous band, the superficial radial nerve proceeds. After entrance under the band, a small recurrent branch proceeds to the lateral epicondyle.

against resistance, as in playing tennis or wielding a heavy hammer. The diagnosis is based on eliciting a history of the offending activity and reproducing the symptoms by resisting forceful extension and/or supination of the wrist. The nerve is sensitive to direct pressure.

Treatment is to avoid the muscular mechanics. Surgical decompression is valuable if activity avoidance fails.

Epicondylitis

This frequent athletic injury is characterized by pain brought on by wrist extension with pronation or supination and forceful gripping. The pain and local tenderness is felt over the region of the lateral epicondyle.

The most frequent mechanism is microscopic tears of the wrist extensor mechanism at the lateral epicondyle (Fig. 8–48). The pain is felt when the patient extends the wrist and fingers. Repeated minor traumata probably result in the musculotendinous condition. Originally termed "tennis elbow," epicondylitis is now associated with other activities besides athletic injuries. The mechanism of pain is clarified by the history and the examination.

Management of Elbow Pain

Trauma resulting in fracture demands immediate proper reduction and rigid fixation of the involved joint but early motion of all the other elbow joints. Fixation that allows active motions of the remaining joints requires full knowledge of elbow kinetics and the involvement of a competent orthot-

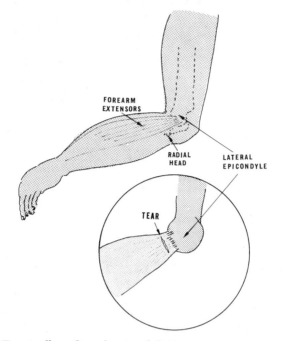

Figure 8–48. Tennis elbow (lateral epicondylitis).
The site of tennis elbow is the lateral epicondyle from which the extensor forearm muscles originate. These muscles extend the wrist and fingers. Their origin is from the periosteum and a ligament that connects with the head of the radius. Tears of the tendon or the proximal muscles are considered as the pathology.

ist.[61,62] Management of nerve compression demands that pressure be avoided by any means available. Surgical decompression is of questionable value.

Epicondylitis is also treated by splinting and extensor exercises. Some practitioners advocate local injections of an analgesic and/or steroid.

When conservative measures fail, surgical intervention may be indicated; for example:

1. Excision of the damaged portion of the extensor musculature with repair of the defect
2. Excision of the orbicular ligament, which releases the extensor musculature from the epicondyle
3. Fasciotomy distal to the extensor tendon

4. Release or lengthening of the extensor carpi radialis brevis
5. Percutaneous tenotomy[63]

HAND AND WRIST PAIN

There are relatively few causes of pain in the hand.[64] The presence of infection is usually obvious, and trauma causing fracture or dislocation can be elicited by proper history, appropriate examination, and laboratory verification. The other major causes of hand pain are articular, neurologic, or tendinous.

The hand consists of numerous joints, each containing synovial tissue, capsules, ligaments, and muscles. In 1879, Hilton aptly stated: "The same trunk of nerves, the branches of which supply the group of muscles moving any joint, furnish also a distribution of nerves to the skin over these same muscles and their insertions, and the interior of the joint receives its nerves from the same source."[65]

There are three major nerves that supply the hand: the median, ulnar, and radial nerves (Fig. 8–49, 8–50, and 8–51).[66] The articular nerve branches of these major nerves also contain vasomotor sympathetic fibers. The nerve endings are distributed in the interstitial and perivascular tissues within the subsynovial fibrous capsule, articular fat, and adventitial sheaths of the arteries and arterioles of the joint. The periosteum is innervated, but the cartilages of the joint and the subchondral bone are not innervated.

The joints are served by four types of receptors:

• Type 1 receptors are ovoid corpuscles within the fibrous joint capsule supplied by a small myelinated nerve fiber. They function as mechanoreceptors.

• Type 2 receptors are supplied by a thicker myelinated fiber with their fibrous receptors ending within the fibrous capsule. They are mechanoreceptors sensitive to rapid movement.

• Type 3 receptors resemble Golgi organs. They are supplied by thick myelinated fibers and are present in the ligaments, not the capsules. They act as slow mechanoreceptors.

• Type 4 receptors are unmyelinated fibers with abundant plexi within the fibrous capsules, the ligaments, the subsynovial capsules, and the fat pads. These fibers are the transmitter of nociception.

Rheumatoid Arthritis

Rheumatoid arthritis is a systemic inflammatory disease with early articular manifestation in the small joints of the hand; it usually spares the distal

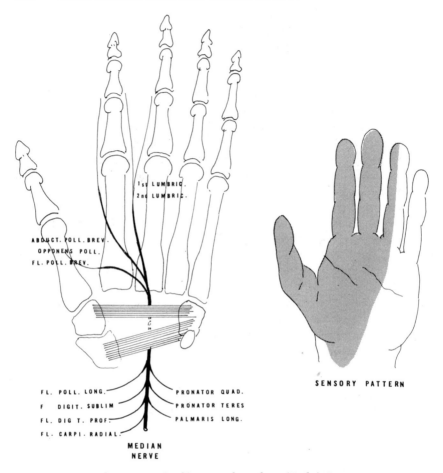

Figure 8–49. Median nerve. *(Left)*, Motor branches. *(Right)*, Sensory pattern.

finger joints. There is a proliferation of synovium, which spreads over the articular surface as a pannus and damages the cartilage, bone, and joint capsule.[67]

Inflammation is mediated by humoral and cell-mediated immunity. B cells within the synovium synthesize immunoglobulin, which forms vasoactive and chemotactic factors. The chemotactic factors phagocytize the immune complexes and secrete proteolytic enzymes. The enzymes "attack" the synovium and activate monocytes and lymphocytes, which destroy the cartilage through the produced proteases and collagenases.[68]

Alteration in the metabolism of arachidonic acid form leukotrienes and prostaglandin PGE_2. Both are vasodilators that cause smooth muscle contraction resulting in edema and pain.[69]

Treatment is aimed at preventing or minimizing tissue damage. Med-

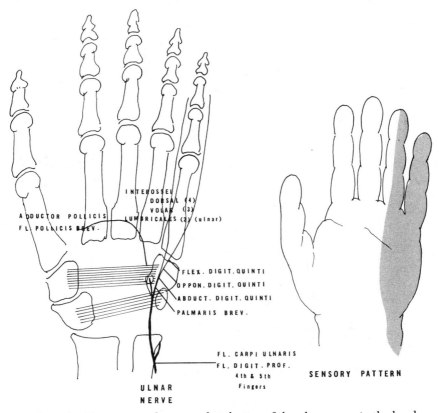

Figure 8–50. The motor and sensory distribution of the ulnar nerve in the hand.

ications remain the mainstay of treatment and consist of salicylates, non-steroidal anti-inflammatory drugs, low-dose glucocorticoids, gold salts, penicillamine, and drugs that are cytotoxic such as azathioprine and methotrexate.

Physical therapy minimizes the effects of the disease—immobilization and decalcification, joint capsular thickening, cartilage damage with joint subluxation, and muscle atrophy—which impair the patient's self-care and ability to function. All these modalities have been discussed elsewhere in the literature.

Degenerative Joint Disease

The pathology of degenerative joint disease remains unclear as to etiology and mechanism, but its clinical manifestations are well documented. There is slow, progressive loss of cartilage with gradual denuding of the bone ending in joints. Bone-to-bone contact and motion leads to pain: The cartilage

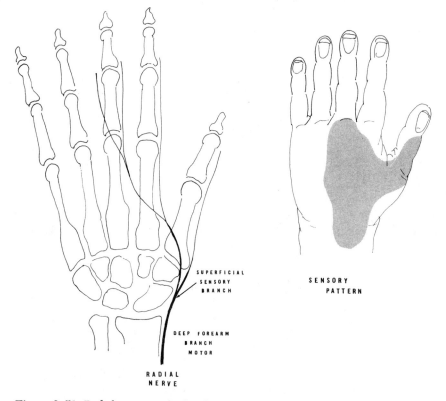

SUPERFICIAL
SENSORY
BRANCH

SENSORY
PATTERN

DEEP FOREARM
BRANCH
MOTOR

RADIAL
NERVE

Figure 8–51. Radial nerve in the hand.

The motor distribution of the nerve above the elbow supplies the triceps flexor muscle of the elbow via the brachioradial and the extensor carpi radial muscles. Below the elbow, the nerve supplies ulnar wrist extensors, extensors of the fingers, and extensors of the distal phalanx of the thumb and index finger.

and subchondral bone are not innervated, but the periosteum and the capsule are well innervated with A-alpha and C fibers.

All degenerated joints in the hand can be sites of nociception, but the joints that probably cause the most dysfunction are those at the base of the thumb, where loss of circumduction causes a loss of dexterity (Fig. 8–52). Treatment consists of splinting, intra-articular injection of analgesic drugs and steroids, and surgical fusion or replacement arthrosis.

Carpal Tunnel Syndrome

Nerve entrapments of any of the major nerves of the hand can cause pain and dysfunction. This most commonly involves the median nerve because it courses through the carpal tunnel, which also contains the flexor pollicis

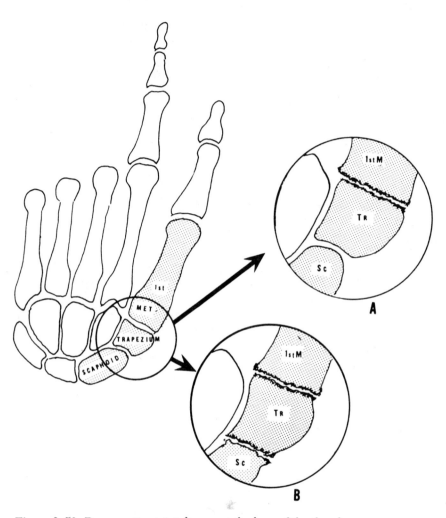

Figure 8–52. Degenerative joint disease at the base of the thumb.

(A), Degenerative arthritis of the first carpometacarpal joint responds well to treatment by splinting, injection, or surgery (excision of trapezium fusion or implant). (B), When there are arthritic changes in the trapezioscaphoid joint, arthrodesis or implant may not be of value.

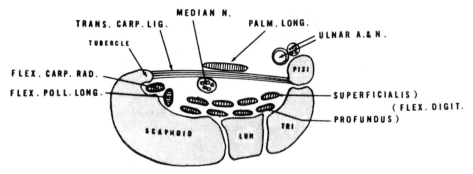

Figure 8–53. Contents of the carpal tunnel.
The tunnel described in Figure 8–54 contains the deep and superficial long finger flexor tendons, the tendons of the long flexor muscles of the thumb and of the ulnar flexor muscle of the wrist, and the median nerve.

longus tendon, four flexor digitorum superficialis tendons, and four flexor digitorum profundus tendons (Fig. 8–53). The tunnel is roofed by the two bands of the transverse carpal ligament (Fig. 8–54).

A major contributor to this syndrome is thickening of the ligament from repetitive traumata. The main symptom is paresthesia ("burning" or "tingling") in the dermatomal area of the affected hand. Confirmation is dependent on the reproduction of symptoms by Phalen test, which involves sustained forced flexion of the wrist.[70,71] Treatment is by nocturnal splinting and/or intratunnel injections of steroids, with surgical decompression as an alternative.[72]

Tendons

The hand has numerous tendons that not only form compartments containing nerves but are principally needed to perform hand-finger functions. Few muscles are contained in the hand, but many traverse the wrist and hand to serve muscular function. By their functions and superficial locations they are prone to the adverse effects of trauma, pressure, and overuse. Tendon disease or trauma results in pain and motor deficiency. Most tendons are superficial and hence can be directly palpated and observed.

Lubrication of the tendons is vital for maintained function. Many have their own sheaths (Fig. 8–55). Tenosynovitis, inflammation of the tendon sheath, is the most common cause of tendon pain in the hand. When the sheath becomes thickened or swollen and causes obstruction, it is termed stenosing tenosynovitis. Stenosing tenosynovitis often occurs at the base of

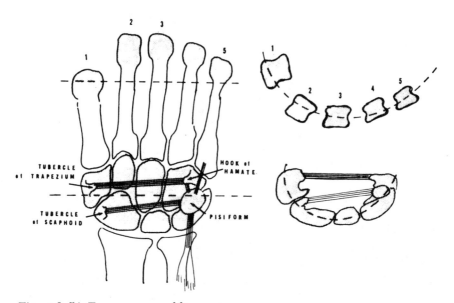

Figure 8–54. Transverse carpal ligaments.

These ligaments bridge the arch of the carpal rows and form a tunnel. The proximal band extends from the tubercle of the navicular bone to the pisiform bone; the distal band extends from the tubercle of the trapezium bond to the hook of the hamate bone.

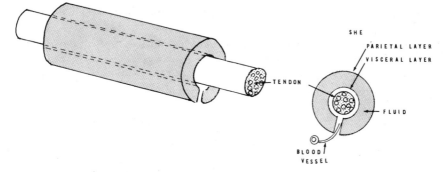

Figure 8–55. Tendon sheath (schematic).

The tendon sheath has two layers—the parietal and the visceral, between which is a synovial fluid that acts as a lubricant. The blood vessel supplying the tendon enters by way of a fold in the sheath.

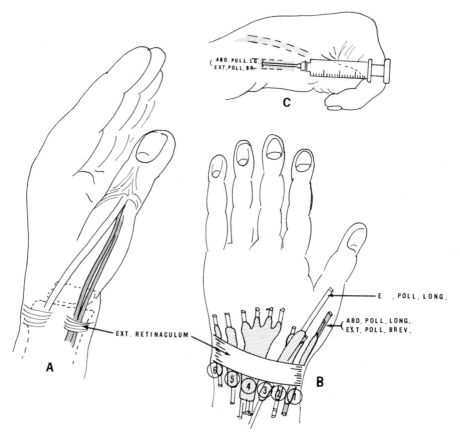

Figure 8–56. De Quervain's disease: Stenosing tenosynovitis of the extensor pollicis brevis and abductor pollicis longus.

the thumb involving the extensor pollicis brevis and abductor pollicis longus (Fig. 8–56).

A tendon may tear resulting in a tumorlike formation. The movement of a swollen tendon in its sheath may result in "snapping": This is the cause of so-called trigger finger (Figs. 8–57 and 8–58). Dysfunction and pain can be halted either by tendon sheath injection or by surgical release.[66]

THORACIC SPINE

The mechanism of chest pain varies according to the underlying pathology within the chest cavity. A thorough discussion is beyond the scope of this text. Chest pains include those of cardiac origin and those having a pulmonary etiology involving the pleura, lungs, trachea, and bronchi. The

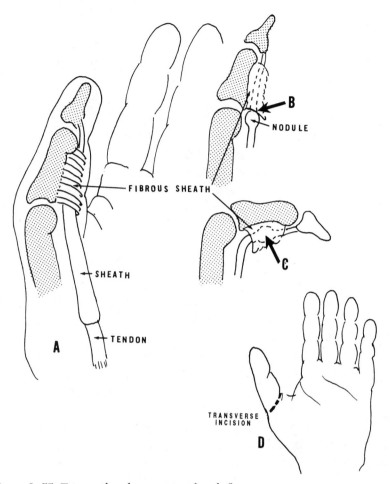

Figure 8–57. Trigger thumb, snapping thumb flexor.

(A), The relationship of the flexor tendon within its bursa sheath covered by a fibrous sheath canal. (B), A nodular thickening of the tendon prevents flexion. (C), The nodule is trapped under the sheath, and re-extension is prevented. (D), The site and direction of skin incision decompresses the tenosynovitis.

basic pathology and tissue involved determines the type of pain. The esophagus is a frequent site and source of chest pain. There are also numerous malignancies of chest cavity tissue that can cause chest pain.

Mechanisms of pain originating in or from the thoracic spine are numerous.[73] They occur primarily from stimulation of nociceptive endings in the periosteum, ligaments, and joints of the thoracic spine. Thoracic pain therefore mandates further study to elicit potential pathology such as fracture, dislocation, arthritis variants, metabolic disorder, infection, tumors, or postural disorders. Diagnosis is dependent on the history, characteristics of the

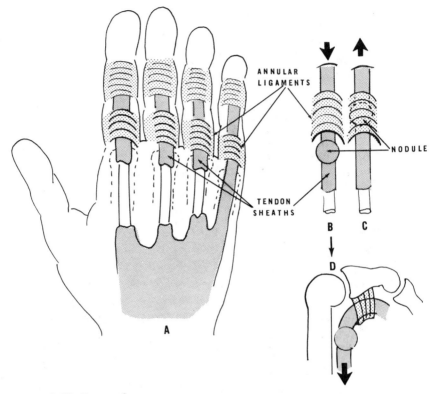

Figure 8–58. Trigger fingers.

The anatomy of the flexor region. (*A*), The flexor tendon within its synovial sheath passes under the annular ligament at the metacarpal head. (*B*), The fusiform swelling of the tendon plus thickening of the sheath proximal to the ligament. When it swells and gets in the position (*D*), re-extension (*C*) is prevented.

pain, physical examination, and laboratory tests. There is usually tenderness over the precise vertebral or involved spinal tissue when the pathology is bony, ligamentous, or articular.

Neuropathic pain from the thoracic cord must always be suspected (e.g., from intrinsic and extramedullary spinal cord lesions). Approximately 50 percent of spinal cord tumors originate in the thoracic position of the cord.[74] Of these, 25 percent are neurofibromas; 10 percent are meningiomas, sarcomas, and hemangioendotheliomas; and the remaining 15 percent[1] include tumors resulting from multiple sclerosis and syringomyelia, among others.

Pain originating within the cord is variable and vague, either constant or intermittent, occurring at rest and relieved by activity.[75] It frequently awakens the patient, forcing the patient to walk the floor or sleep in an unusual position. It recurs at the same site each time. Thoracic cord pain is often termed "lancinating" and is often aggravated by coughing or sneezing. L'Hermitte's sign may be presented. The lesion of multiple sclerosis is a sporadic patch of spinal cord demyelination, which may subside when the glia proliferate and form a scar. Other confirmatory neurologic signs include lower-extremity weakness, reduction of the visual field, scotoma, nystagmus, peripheral ataxic tremor, loss of vibration sense, reflex changes, and sphincter tone impairment.

Differential diagnosis of demyelinating disease by cerebrospinal fluid (CSF) testing reveals elevated protein. CT scanning and MRI testing may reveal a plaque.

Ankylosing spondylitis is a major form of arthritis causing thoracic pain. The initial pain is caused by inflammation of the costovertebral articulations with the aching discomfort aggravated by attempted movement of the rib cage such as by deep breathing. Intercostal neuritis may be present. X-rays and bone scanning are diagnostic.

X-ray studies may reveal Paget's disease, metastatic lesions, primary tumors, and osteoporosis with fractures. Benign musculoskeletal abnormalities causing thoracic pain include postural kyphosis (rounded shoulder posture) and thoracic scoliosis. Thoracic chest pain may result from disorders of the ribs such as fracture, posttraumatic slipping rib syndrome,[76] or costochondritis known as Tietze's syndrome.[77]

Myofascial pain frequently manifests itself in the thoracic spine musculature, as does pain referred from the shoulder.

Acute herpes zoster with postherpetic neuralgia is a severe painful condition involving the thoracic region in 50 percent of patients.[78,79] The virus migrates from the viremia of the skin to invade the dorsal root ganglion (DRG) causing an inflammatory reaction and varying degrees of degeneration, involving corresponding sensory nerves, posterior roots, posterior horn cells, and, occasionally, anterior horn cells.[80]

Before the eruptive phase, herpes zoster is suspected when the patient notes a skin lesion and experiences a "burning," aching pain in the segmental distribution, with hypersensitivity in the involved skin. Antiviral medication addresses the pain through etiologic alteration. Somatic and sympathetic nerve block interrupt neural transmission. Systemic analgesic approaches to neuritic pain are also indicated.

Trauma is usually implicated in herniated disks of the thoracic spine.[81] Central protrusions pressing on the posterior longitudinal ligament cause localized dorsal pain, whereas posterolateral protrusions cause an intercostal neuritis. A massive central protrusion on the thoracic cord can cause a myelopathy with central symptoms and findings.

Diagnostic studies such as CT scanning, MRI, and myelography will confirm the pathology, including both the level and the degree of neural compression.

Chest pain can occur from diseases of the mediastinum, the diaphragm, and the pancreas. The precise pathology can be determined by a detailed history, physical examination, and confirmatory tests.[82]

LUMBOSACRAL PAIN

Structures Producing Pain

The concept of pain and dysfunction resulting from tissue reaction to external and internal forces applies specifically to lesions of the lumbosacral spine.

External forces are less prominent than injuries so sustained by the cervical spine, but internal forces are more applicable. The normal neuro-musculoskeletal mechanisms of the lumbosacral spine violated account for the vast majority of resultant low back and diskogenic pain syndromes.

These internal forces generated by improper body mechanics result in tissue damage causing pain and disability. These "perturbers" probably are causative of the majority of low-back disorders and should receive priority when eliciting a meaningful history and creating pertinent treatment protocols.

Pain emanating from the lumbosacral spine originates from irritation of the afferent nerves contained within a functional unit (Figs. 8–59 and 8–60).

The components of the functional unit are the intervertebral disks, the anterior and posterior longitudinal ligaments, and the zygopophysial facets (Fig. 8–61). The facets provide some slight support, but essentially their function is to guide motion of the functional unit and resist rotational (torque) forces that could be imposed on the annular fibers of the disk.[83]

The recurrent nerve of Luschka is the principal nerve that supplies the tissue sites of nociception, which are the posterior and anterior longitudinal ligaments, the dura of the nerve roots, possibly the outer layer of the annulus, the facets, the posterior ligaments, and the erector spinae muscles (Fig. 8–62).[84] Pain may emanate from any of these.

Intervertebral Disks. The intervertebral disks have a multiple sensory nerve supply. The outer layers of the disk and the adjacent anterior longitudinal ligament receive their innervation from gray ramus communicantes, and the posterolateral aspects receive some innervation from the sinuvertebral nerve of Luschka. The receptors are essentially located in the outer third of the disk; most are in the lateral, fewer are in the posterior, and the least number are in the anterior portion. Their function has not been clarified, but they may have a proprioceptive and nociceptive function.[85]

The posterior longitudinal ligament has a rich nociceptive innervation, and can possibly be inflamed from chemicals liberated from the damaged disk structures.[86] Whether there are autonomous nerve fibers innervating

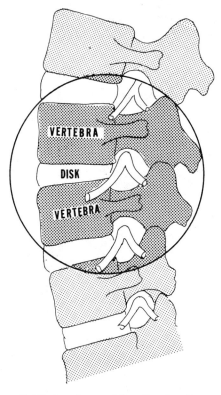

FUNCTIONAL UNIT
TWO VERTEBRAE
AND ONE DISK

Figure 8–59. Lumbosacral functional unit.
The structural components of the lumbar spine that comprise a functional unit are two adjacent vertebrae separated by the intervertebral disk.

the disk is not verified, although sweating and nausea have been reported as part of diskogenic disease.[87–88]

A high level of phospholipid A2, an inflammatory agent, has been demonstrated in excised disks.[89] Damaged disks have also shown a decrease in proteoglycan synthesis, resulting in a diminished hydrodynamic function after injury and impaired function.[90] A fibrous cap forms at the periphery of stab wounds in the disk when they heal.[91]

Annular tears fail to heal; outer annular tears lead to failure of the inner annular fibers, which do not heal.[92] This loss of normal dynamics of the intervertebral disk leads to damage of all the other components of the functional unit.[93]

Facet Joints. Each lower lumbar apophysial joint is innervated by two or three adjacent spinal nerves originating from the dorsal primary rami.[94–98] These rami also supply the deep back muscles and the intervertebral ligaments. The joint capsules are also innervated by free nerve endings, forming a dense plexus. The precise function of these nerves is still controversial.

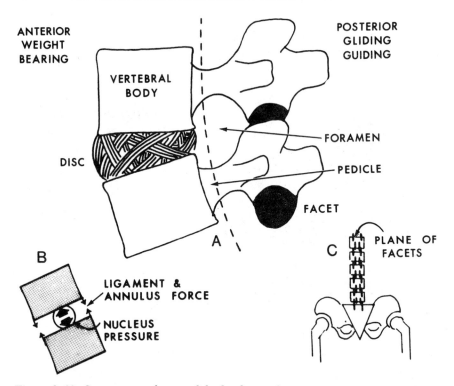

ANTERIOR
WEIGHT
BEARING

POSTERIOR
GLIDING
GUIDING

VERTEBRAL
BODY

FORAMEN

DISC

PEDICLE

FACET

A

B

C

PLANE OF
FACETS

LIGAMENT &
ANNULUS FORCE

NUCLEUS
PRESSURE

Figure 8–60. Cross-sectional view of the lumbosacral spine.
Functional unit of the spine in cross-section. Anteriorly are two vertebrae separated by the disk and lined by the longitudinal ligaments. Posteriorly is the neural arch containing the facets and forming the spinal canal and the intervertebral foramina.

They are painful when there is inflammation within the joint.[99] Wyke[100] claims there are no receptors in the synovial tissues, although Mooney, Robertson,[97,98] and Giles[101] claim the opposite.

The facets are vascular; this may contribute to their being a site of nociception. Immunohistochemical studies of degenerated facets in low back patients have revealed erosion channels extending through the subchondral bone and calcified cartilage into the articular cartilage containing substance P nerve fibers.[102] This confirms that a component of low back pain resides in the facets. How the facets impinge upon or become the site of nociception remains unclear.

Degenerative erosion of the cartilage causes inflammation, as in any synovial joint. The excessive vascularity of the facets probably leads to "over-healing," with hypertrophic changes in the joint. These may subsequently impinge on the foramen and cause irritation of the enclosed nerve root.[103]

Nerve Root. The nerve roots within the foramina are different from the

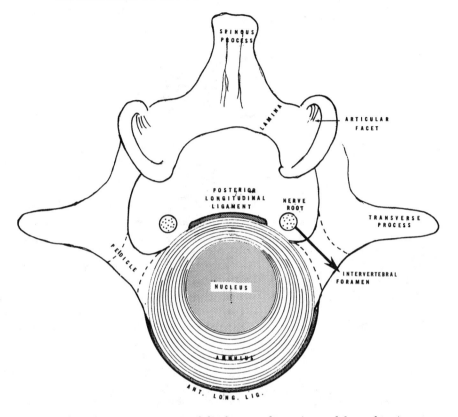

Figure 8–61. Components of the functional unit (viewed from above).

peripheral nerves. They are encased within the thin pia mater, which has no epineurium and thus cannot adequately resist mechanical stresses.[104] They receive their nutrition from CSF through the pia mater; thus, inflammation or fibrosis of this membrane can damage the encased nerve root.[105] Biochemical nociceptors released from the damaged disks or facets may result in nerve axon irritation.

Mechanical pressure on the nerve root dura in the foramen, causing axon ischemia from venous plexus compression, has been considered a cause of radiculitis.[106,107]

Dorsal Root Ganglia. With the DRG significantly involved in pain mediation (Chapters 1 and 2), their physical presence within the foramen is significant in low back pain with or without radiculitis. The sensory fibers in the DRG have been shown to discharge spontaneously from mechanical pressure, and even more after injury.[108,109]

The DRG synthesize substance P, which is transported antidromically (that is, in the opposite direction from what is considered normal) to the peripheral terminals. At the periphery the liberated substance P acts on

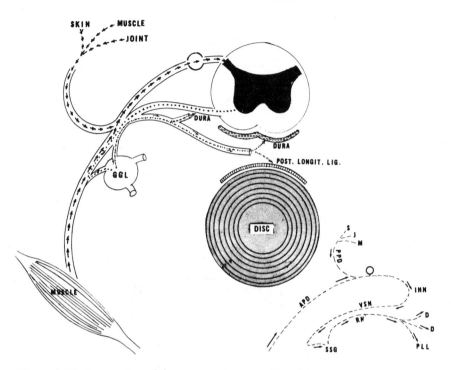

Figure 8–62. Innervation of the recurrent nerve of Luschka.
PPD = posterior primary division; APD = anterior primary division; GGL = sympathetic ganglion; INN = internuncial neurons; VSN = ventral sensory nerve (efferent); SSG = sensory sympathetic ganglion; RN = recurrent nerve of Luschka; D = to dura; PLL = posterior longitudinal ligament.

mast cells, which in turn release serotonin, histamine, and leukotrienes. These cause vasodilation, releasing nociceptor with resultant cutaneous pain and hypersensitivity at the segmental level.

It has been postulated that antidromic transportation results from intraforaminal edema pressure contrary to the concept depicted in Figure 8–63. The disk space width has an effect on the nerve root tension and must be taken into consideration.[111]

Dorsal Horn. Pain transmission from the DRG into the dorsal horn fiber terminals (laminae I and II) have been demonstrated after sciatic nerve constriction.[112] A conflict relating to pain transmission exists, as substance P does not occur in greater proportion in nociceptive fibers than in mechanosensitive fibers.[113]

There is an increase in wide range ganglia (WRG) in the cord with an increase of alpha$_2$ adrenoceptors and mucopoid receptors in the dorsal horn after a consistent bombardment at the periphery. Receptors in the cord increase with persistent peripheral and DRG inflammation.[114]

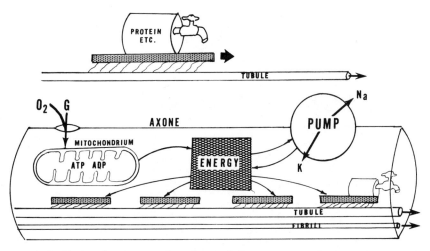

Figure 8–63. Axoplasmic neural transport: A theory.

The *flow* of protein and other derivatives begins with entry of glucose (G) into the fiber. Glycolysis and phosphorylation occur (O$_2$) in the mitochondria through metabolism of adenosine-triphosphate (ATP), which creates the energy to the sodium pump. This pump regulates balance of sodium (Na) and potassium (K) and determines nerve activity.

The transport *filaments* (F) move along the axon by oscillation and carry the nutritive protein elements along the nerve pathway. (Data from Ochs, S: Axoplasmic transport: A basis for neural pathology. In Dyck, PJ, Thomas, PK, and Lambert, EH: Peripheral Neuropathy, Vol 1. WB Saunders, Philadelphia, 1975, pp 213–230.)

Mechanisms of Low Back Pain

The mechanical basis for inflammation of nociceptive sites in the lumbosacral spine are as follows:

Static Lumbosacral Spine. Abnormal static erect spine causes low back pain, but the exact mechanism remains conjectural. Excessive lordosis was originally considered the basis of static low back pain (Fig. 8–64). This has been refuted by McKenzie, who claimed that prolonged flexion forces the nucleus posteriorly, encroaching on the posterior longitudinal ligament and possibly the nerve roots (Figs. 8–65 and 8–66).[115] Extension allegedly forces the nucleus anteriorly away from the nociceptive tissues.

In the erect static position the erector spinae muscles are inactive except for "tone." Hence, pain originating from the erector spinae muscles occurs only when the muscles have been traumatized or contracted for a prolonged period of time. If low back pain can be reproduced by initiating excessive lordosis, poor posture may be the source of the problem.

Kinetic Lumbosacral Spine. The largest incidence of low back pain occurs from faulty kinetic activity such as bending over, lifting, and so on. As the head and upper torso begin forward flexion, the erect static lumbo-

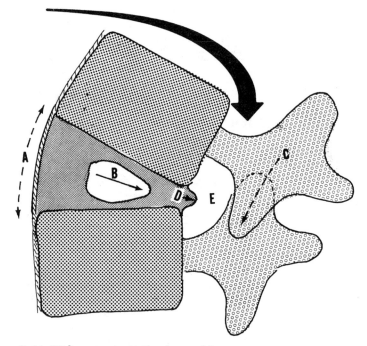

Figure 8–64. Disk protrusion in lumbosacral hyperextension.

(A), The anterior longitudinal ligament restricts further extension. (B), The nucleus has deformed to the maximum, cannot migrate further anteriorly, and thus moves posteriorly. This causes a "bulge" (D) with encroachment into the intervertebral foramen (E). The facets overlap (C), which also narrows the foramen as well as causing painful weight-bearing.

sacral spine initiates physiologic flexion. When the upper body becomes anterior to the center of gravity (Fig. 8–67), the spindle system of the erector spinae extrafusal muscles (Fig. 8–68) is activated, sending afferent impulses to the cord via Ia fibers. These impulses synapse with the motor cells of the anterior horn, instantaneously sending impulses via the A-alpha efferent fibers to the muscle cells (Fig. 8–69) that monitor the length and rate of change in length.[116,117]

In flexing the kinetic lumbosacral spine, afferent proprioceptive impulses modulate inappropriate, "eccentric" muscular contraction (Fig. 8–70); their function is to gradually elongate and decelerate forward flexion of the lumbar spine.[118]

In forward flexion the pelvis initially remains in a state of static support. The superincumbent lumbar spine changes from lordosis to kyphosis, with each lumbar functional unit flexing approximately 8 to 10° for an ultimate flexion of approximately 45°.

The first 45° of flexion is performed by the erector spinae muscles, and

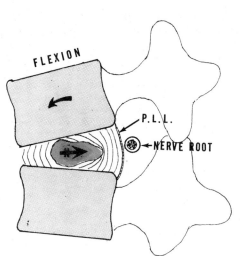

Figure 8–65. Posterior protrusion of the lumbar disk nucleus from forward flexion.

In forward flexion the disk nucleus allegedly migrates posteriorly. In this illustration the posterior annular fibers are forced posteriorly, encroaching on the posterior longitudinal ligament (PLL) and the nerve root.

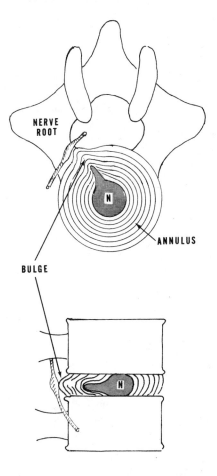

Figure 8–66. Extrusion of nucleus causing radiculitis.

Central extrusion of the nucleus in a posterolateral direction forces the intervening annular fiber to encroach on the nerve root in the foramen. The lower picture is a side view of this occurrence.

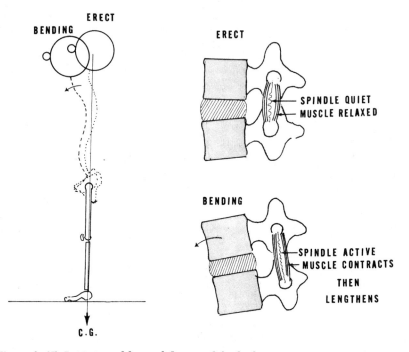

Figure 8–67. Initiation of forward flexion of the body.

Once the decision is made to "bend forward," the head goes ahead of the center of gravity (CG). The intrafusal fibers that have been inactive during the erect posture become instantaneously activated by the elongation of the erector spinae muscles. Through central neural mechanisms the erector spinae muscles now eccentrically contract and gradually elongate, allowing further forward flexion.

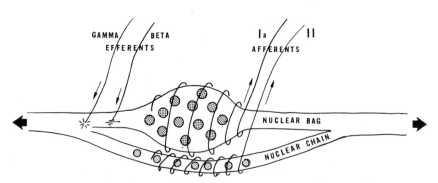

Figure 8–68. Intrafusal muscle spindle.

The intrafusal spindle system consisting of a nuclear bag (measuring tension) and nuclear chain (measuring length) has sensory afferent fibers Ia and II that ascend to the spinal cord. The motor efferents (gamma and beta) constantly "reset" the tone and length of the spindle system.

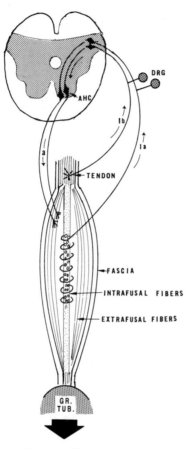

Figure 8–69. Innervation of the spindle system.

The spindle system (intrafusal fibers) is parallel to the extrafusal muscle fibers. When stretched or compressed they send signals to the cord by way of the Ia fibers (from the spindle) and the Ib fibers (from the Golgi system in the tendon) to the gray matter of the cord via the dorsal root ganglion (DRG).

An interneural synapse signals the anterior horn cell (AHC) that sends impulses via the a fibers to the extrafusal muscle fibers initiating an appropriate contraction. The muscle fascia assumes the length of the muscle fibers with limited elongation. (BA = bony attachment.)

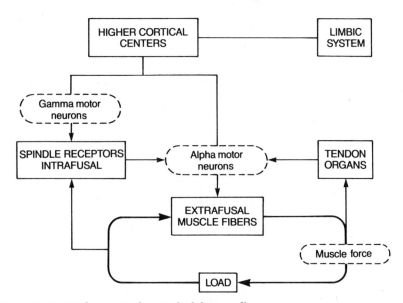

Figure 8–70. Higher cortical control of the spindle system.

The higher cortical centers indicate the intended muscular activity to perform the action. A feedback system correlates this activity. The load of the action determines the effort needed. The limbic system is the pathway of the perturbers, which are emotional and effect the effort via the limbic system.

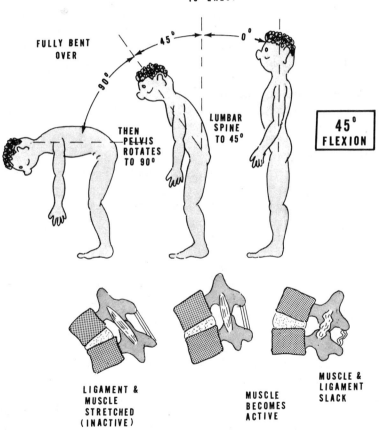

Figure 8–71. Since each functional unit opens to flex forward 8° to 10°, and there are five lumbar units, the lumbar spine bends forward about 45°.

the ligaments and fascia remain slack (Fig. 8–71). Once reaching 45° of flexion, the erector spinae muscles have been fully elongated and become passive. The ligaments and fascia, being engaged, now maintain the acquired kyphosis (Figs. 8–72 and 8–73). The pelvis now controls forward flexion.

The lumbosacral spine is supported by the lumbosacral fascia (Fig. 8–74).[119] Synchronous flexion of the lumbar spine and rotation of the pelvis constitutes lumbar pelvic rhythmn (Fig. 8–75). Normal trunk flexion mandates that the fascia, ligaments, and facet capsule have physiologic flexibility.

Obstacles to physiologic flexion causing pain are (1) limited elasticity of the soft tissues implying poor conditioning, (2) faulty rhythm coordination due to improper training, or (3) from the presence of perturbers (Fig. 8–76), such as fatigue, anger, distraction, and anxiety, which interfere with coordinated action resulting in tissue damage with resultant pain and dysfunction.[120–122]

Isokinetic trunk strength testing performed by patients under stress, anxiety, or pain coping with somatization has resulted in lower strength, diminished range of motion, and dysrhythmia (erratic neuromuscular function).

Reversed Kinetic Trunk Flexion. Faulty reextension to the erect posture is apt to result in low back pain. Reextension to the erect posture is the reverse of lumbar pelvic rhythm (Fig. 8–77). The pelvis begins derotation, while the lumbosacral spine remains kyphotic. The erector muscles retain tonus without shortening. Lumbar reextension relies on the fascia and ligaments until reaching 45° of flexion, when the erector spinae muscles contract to resume lordosis.

Reextension in the sagittal plane is accompanied by derotation. The facets (Fig. 8–78), which direct the direction of motion, must be realigned to allow derotation. This is a "coded" neuromuscular coordination, which is a learned action influenced by training and practice.

Damage to the muscle spindle nerves from inappropriate action results in atrophy of the extrafusal and intrafusal fibers. Reinnervation results in regeneration of the muscle fibers with recovery of function but impairment of coordination.[123,124] Perturbers initiate a mechanism resulting in tissue damage, causing production of chemical-mechanical nociceptors.

The role of the disk in lumbosacral and radicular pain needs clarification. As it is an inert, avascular, aneural tissue, how it affects the sensitive adjacent tissues can help to explain its mechanism of pain.

Tearing of the annular fibers with release of the contained nucleus has been postulated as the cause of low back pain with or without radiculitis. How the annular fibers tear is better understood, but how the extruded nucleus causes pain remains unanswered.

The annular tissues that contain the nucleus are oriented in sheets, with the fibers at a precise angle. The angle differs with their proximity to the nucleus (Figs. 8–79 and 8–80). Tearing of the inner fibers allows escape of

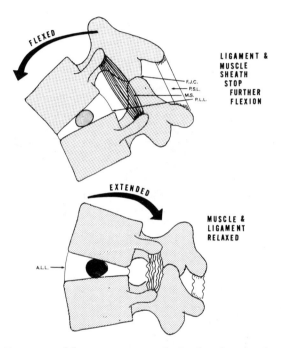

Figure 8–72. Restraints of flexion-extension of a lumbar functional unit.

Excessive flexion of a functional unit is prevented by the posterior longitudinal ligament (PLL), posterior superior ligament (PSL), the muscle fascia (MS), and possibly by the facet joint capsules (FJC).

Extension is restricted by mechanical impact of the facet joints and the anterior longitudinal ligaments (ALL).

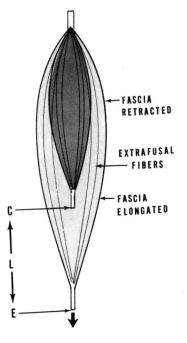

Figure 8–73. Fascial limits of muscular elongation.

A muscle bundle, the extrafusal fibers, can elongate to the length of its fascial sheath. Fascial contracture limits the flexibility of any joint subserved by the periarticular muscles and their fascia. (C = contracted length (L) of muscle; E = extended length of muscle.)

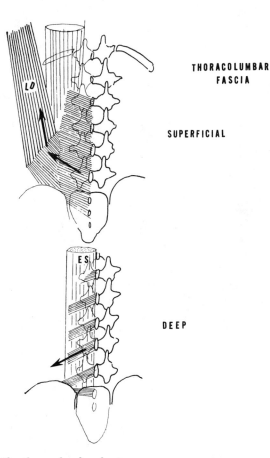

Figure 8–74. The thoracolumbar fascia.

There are three layers of thoracolumbar fascia that act through various directions of tension *(arrows)*.

The upper figure shows the superficial layers that attach at the midline of the posterior superior spines. Their tension medially is essentially lateral with a slight degree of cranial direction. The latissimus dorsi muscle and its fascia attach at the raphe and exert cranial pull, making the lateral fibers more taut (LD).

The lower figure depicts the deep-layer fibers that enclose the erector spinae muscle (ES) and exert pull caudally and laterally.

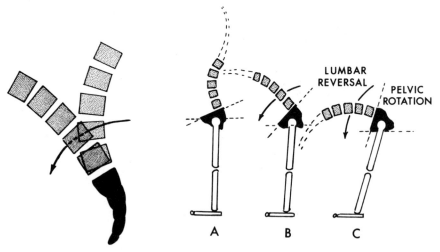

Figure 8–75. Lumbar-pelvic rhythm.

With the pelvis immobile, flexion of the lumbar spine occurs to approximately 45°; then the lumbar kyphosis remains static while the pelvis rotates.

In re-extension, the pelvis derotates first with the lumbar spine remaining flexed, and at 45° of extension the lumbar spine regains its lordosis on the static pelvis.

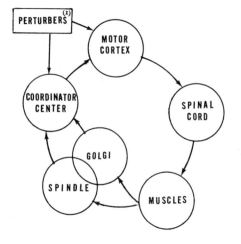

Figure 8–76. Perturber influence on neuromuscular mechanism.

The normal control of coordinated muscle activity is shown in the sequence from motor cortex through the spinal cord to the muscles where the spindle and Golgi systems operate through a coordination center that informs the cortex that the activity has been accurately accomplished.

Perturbers that upset this coordination are fatigue, anger, boredom, anxiety, compulsion, depression, and inappropriate training with practice ensuring a physiologic habit.

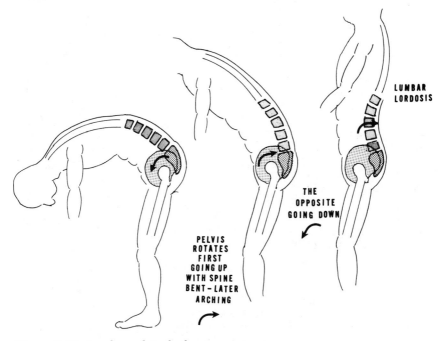

Figure 8–77. Lumbar pelvic rhythm in re-extension.

The lordosis reverses in forward flexion with simultaneous synchronous pelvic rotation. In returning to the erect position, the pelvis should "derotate" first, with the lordosis being regained when the person still flexes forward to approximately 45°.

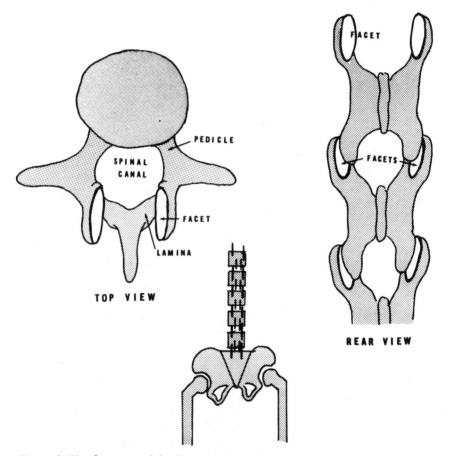

Figure 8–78. Alignment of the facets of the lumbosacral spine.

The facets (zygopophysial joints) are aligned in a vertical (sagittal) direction that allows flexion-extension but limits lateral flexion and rotation.

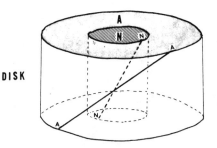

DISK

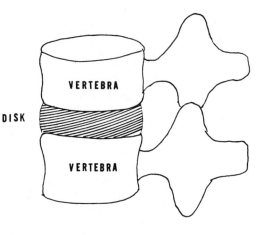

Figure 8–79. Variation of angulation of annular fibers in relationship to the nucleus.
In the periphery of the disk the annular (A) fibers angle at approximately 30° (A-A). As they approach the nucleus (N) they angle more acutely (N-N) and are shorter.

DISK

VERTEBRA

VERTEBRA

the nucleus within the confines of the annulus without encroachment on nociceptive surrounding tissues.[125]

The mechanism causing annular tears emphasizes excessive flexion and rotation, indicating that the spinal movement was inappropriate.[126–128]

Radiculopathy (sciatica) has been attributed to the mechanical pressure of the extruded disk on the nerve root and/or its dura. Only 20 percent of patients with disk protrusion presented a history of trauma.[129]

Other mechanisms than mechanical pressure on nerve roots causing low back and radicular pain have been proposed. As vertebral end plate cartilage drains via the subarticular collecting venous system directly into marrow spaces concentrated in the region of the nucleus trauma was postulated as causing drainage of irritant into the nucleus.[130] Damage to the end plate was the factor.

The role of chemical changes—for example, changes in disk hydrodynamics due to depolymerization of the polysaccharides—is being studied.[131] Substance P and phospholipase A2 have also been considered.[132–133]

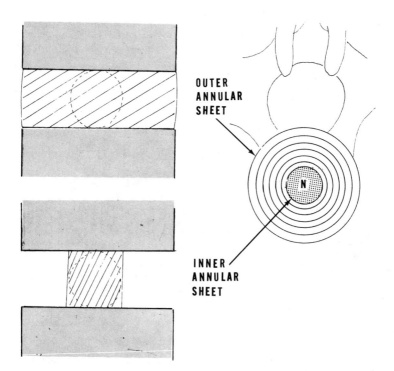

Figure 8–80. Angulation of the annular fibers: Side view.

The outer annular fibers angle at 30°, whereas those centrally, near the nucleus (N), traverse at a more acute angle.

Rotational (torque) forces would tear the more central fibers sooner because they are shorter and more acutely angled.

HIP PAIN

The hip joint is predominantly for weight bearing and ambulation. It is as congruous a joint as any in the body. The head of the femur is convex, and the opposing articular surface of the acetabulum is of a similar, concave curvature.

The horseshoe-shaped acetabulum is covered peripherally with cartilage. The shallow acetabulum is deepened by a complete ring of fibrocartilage called labrium. In the neutral leg position the head of the femur is not fully engaged in the socket because of the angle of the neck.

The femoral head is held firmly within the acetabulum by a thick capsule whose fibers are oblique and become taut when the hip is extended and rotated. Portions of the capsule are thickened to form ligaments named according to their sites of origin: the iliofemoral, pubofemoral, and ischiofemoral (Fig. 8–81).

There are four structures in the hip joint that can become sites of nociception: the fibrous capsule and its ligaments, the surrounding muscles, the bony periosteum, and the synovial lining of the joint. The articular cartilage is insensitive, but the subchondral bone has sensory nerves and becomes a site of nociception when the overlying cartilage becomes denuded.

The femoral, obturator, superior gluteal, and accessory obturator nerves supply the hip joint. The femoral nerve supplies the iliofemoral ligament, the obturator nerve supplies the medial portion of the capsule, the superior gluteal nerve supplies the fibrous region of the capsule, and the sciatic nerve supplies the posterior aspect of the capsule.

The muscles of the hip joint have the following innervation:[134]

1. Femoral nerve to the quadriceps muscle
2. Obturator nerve to the external obturator and adductor muscle groups
3. Inferior gluteal nerve to the gluteus maximus muscle
4. Sciatic nerve to the semimembranous, semitendinosus, adductor, gemellus, and quadrate muscles
5. Sacral plexus (vertebrae S-1 and S-2) to the piriformis, internal obturator, gemellus, and quadrate muscles
6. Superior gluteal nerve to the gluteus medius and minimus muscles
7. Lumbar plexus (vertebrae L-2 to L-5) to the greater psoas muscle

The nerves to the short muscles of the hip also supply the sensory fibers to the capsule. The iliohypogastric and the lateral femoral cutaneous nerves supply the anterior thigh region. The buttocks are supplied by the posterior primary division of D-12. Irritation of the hip capsule frequently refers pain to the knee region via the obturator and sciatic nerves.

Pain from the hip joint originates from the tissues supplied by sensory and sympathetic nerve fibers in their specific nerves.

Hip pain most frequently results from degenerative arthritis, acute rheu-

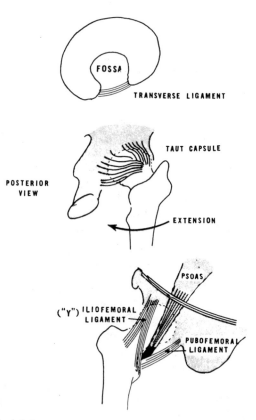

Figure 8–81. Hip joint.

(*Top*), The full articular circle of the acetabulum is completed in the inferior aspect by the transverse acetabular ligament. (*Center*), The oblique capsular fibers become taut as the hip extends. (*Bottom*), The anterior capsule is reinforced by the iliofemoral, pubofemoral, and ischiofemoral ligaments and the psoas tendon.

matoid arthritis, or fracture and dislocation. The nociceptive sites are the synovial capsule, fibrocartilaginous capsule, and the subchondral bone. If sufficient cartilage covers the femoral head, only the exposed subchondral bone becomes nociceptive.

Pain may occur in late childhood and early adolescence from femoral-head ischemia termed Legg-Calvé-Perthes disease. The early pain is probably synovial inflammation, but degenerative changes occur later from the asymmetric molding of the femoral head.[135] This condition is suggested by a limp and complaints of pain referred to the knee region. Early diagnostic physical findings are limited hip range of motion with evidence on x-ray studies of ischemic changes in the femoral head.[136]

Management resides in minimizing the effects of gravity by placing the femoral head in a position that favorably affects the molding of the head until there is epiphysial closure seen on x-rays.

Treatment of hip degenerative arthritis from Legg-Calvé-Perthes disease, as in other forms of degenerative joint disease, still invokes Blount's dictum: Don't throw away the cane.[137] Continued ambulation using a cane minimizes mechanical gravity trauma (Fig. 8–82). Nonsteroidal anti-inflammatory drugs (NSAIDs) diminish acute pain and permit exercise and ambulation. Exercises to maintain attainable range of motion should be initiated (Figs. 8–83 and 8–84).[138]

Traction has been advocated (Fig. 8–85), but its value is temporary and difficult to administer in a home environment.

In recent years, total hip replacement has been perfected and is readily available. "Cementing in" the femoral implant has been replaced by more physiologic implantation, making it available for younger surgical candidates.

KNEE PAIN AND DISABILITY

In no other skeletal system does the concept of external and internal forces causing pain and disability apply as it does in the knee joints. The knee joint(s) involve such an intricate neuromusculoskeletal mechanism invoking flexion, extension, and rotatory forces, that any violation of normal function may cause tissue damage with resultant pain and impairment.

Excessive external forces cause stresses on numerous tissues that might normally accept deformity but now respond with tissue damage. Faulty function invokes internal forces that may cause deformation of tissues with temporary dysfunction and pain but when excessive result in irreversible tissue damage and the formation of nociceptors.

Pain in the knee invokes nociceptive tissues in either the patellofemoral or the tibial-femoral articulation. The neuromusculoskeletal mechanisms of the knee joints are intricate and cause pain and malfunction when disrupted.[139]

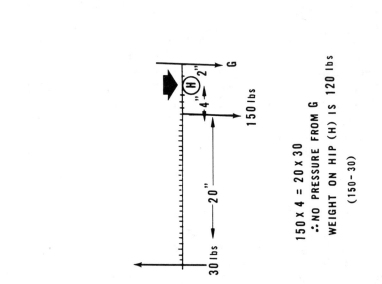
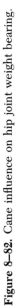
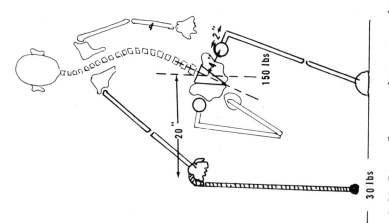

$$150 \times 4 = 20 \times 30$$
$$\therefore \text{NO PRESSURE FROM G}$$
$$\text{WEIGHT ON HIP (H) IS } 120 \text{ lbs}$$
$$(150 - 30)$$

Figure 8–82. Cane influence on hip joint weight bearing. Assuming that the cane is held 20 in from the center of gravity with 30 lb of pressure on the floor, the force on the hip is balanced, thus decreasing dependence on the gluteal muscles. A decrease of 30 lb is estimated.

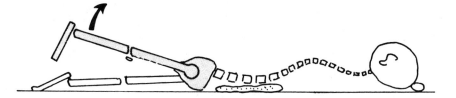

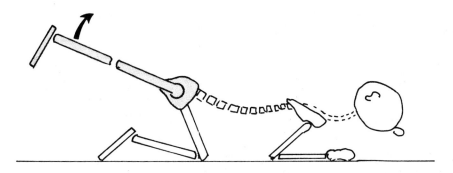

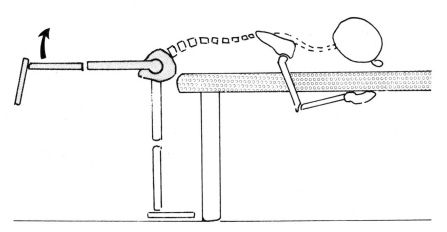

Figure 8–83. Exercises to extend hip joint: Exercises aimed to stretch the anterior hip capsule and strengthen the extensor musculature.

(*Top*), With patient prone, the leg is extended, preferably against resistance. A pillow under the abdomen decreases excessive lordosis. (*Center*), With contralateral knee flexed and bearing weight, the involved leg is extended. (*Bottom*), Exercise is similar to that in center illustration except that the patient is prone over table. The dependent leg stabilizes the pelvis, and the lumbar lordosis is decreased.

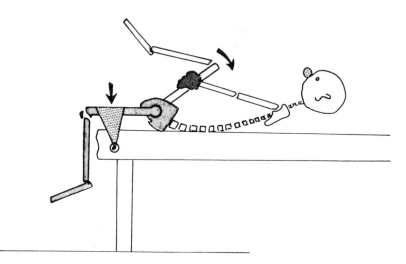

Figure 8–84. Hip flexor stretching exercise.

With patient in supine position and the normal hip held to the chest, the opposite leg by its own weight, or weighted by sandbag, is extended actively and passively.

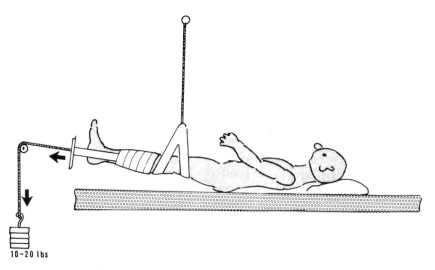

10-20 lbs

Figure 8–85. Technique of hip traction by skin application to lower leg.

The skin, synovial membranes, capsular tissues, ligaments, and muscles of the knee are richly supplied by sensory nerves. Hilton's law applies in this region, as all pertinent tissues are innervated by the same nerves.[140] Three nerves serve the knee region—the sciatic, femoral, and obturator— but the sciatic nerve plays only a minor role in knee sensation. There are numerous autonomic nerves involved in the knee structures, with most accompanying the blood vessels of the joint structures.

The cartilages of the knee joints have no sensory fibers. Only the periosteum, the synovial tissues, the capsule, and the ligaments are sensitive; the latter three are important in articular pain.

The ligaments of the knee joints are also subserved by mechanoreceptors; pain results when physiologic function is impaired. Faulty mechanisms of the knee result in inflammation of the nociceptive tissues.

Mechanisms of the Knee That Cause Pain

Flexion and extension occur with simultaneous rotation because of the configurations of the opposing articular structures, the ligaments, and the musculature[1] fibers and end organs. The cruciate ligaments, amply innervated by mechanoreceptors, are vitally involved in knee function.[141] Their role in knee function has only recently been emphasized. In 1983, a report documented that physicians failed to diagnose acutely torn anterior cruciate ligaments in 93 percent of 103 patients subsequently seen with symptomatic unstable knees.[142]

The menisci play a vital role in static and kinetic knee function. The medial meniscus is peripherally attached to the capsule, which is innervated by nociceptors. When damaged the capsule may cause painful synovitis. The resultant mechanical instability of meniscal damage leads to articular injury and degenerative changes.

A precise history and examination is mandatory in ascertaining the abnormal mechanism and hence the specific tissue causing pain. The history identifies the maneuver that caused the trauma. CT scan or MRI studies are necessary for accurate diagnosis as routine x-rays fail to implicate the offending soft tissues. Arthroscopic examinations permit direct evaluation of these intrinsic articular tissues.

Knee pain and disability results from:

1. Ligamentous injury. The collaterals are sensitive, whereas the cruciates become painful from the resulting functional impairment.
2. Injury to a meniscus that has direct connections with the capsular tissues and the collateral ligaments.
3. Injury to cartilages of both the patellofemoral and tibial-femoral joints.
4. Injury to the musculature.

The history given by the patient or spectator signifies the forces and actions leading to injury. A movement exceeding or violating normal motion is significant. The examination verifies the integrity of the ligaments (collateral or cruciate), the intactness of the menisci, or the integrity of the cartilages of the patellofemoral or femoral-tibial joints.

Evaluation of the joint fluid indicates the severity and actual tissue involvement following injury. A hemarthrosis implies structural damage to intrinsic tissues.

Management of the Painful Knee

Immediate care is directed to relief of pain and prevention of further damage to the injured tissues. Mere diminution of the pain may be counterproductive if it allows resumption of activities that could further damage the involved tissues.

Many tissues of the knee recover by rest, local modalities, and even immobilization. Rehabilitation demands restoration of muscular strength and proper neuromuscular coordination. With the advent of the MRI, soft tissue damage is now ascertainable, and arthroscopic examination permits early intervention and repair of damaged tissues with less trauma.

FOOT AND ANKLE PAIN

Foot pain occurs predominantly from extra-articular and extraskeletal soft tissues including muscles, nerves, tendons, and ligaments.[143] Skeletal, articular, and neuromusculoskeletal factors lead to these soft tissue traumata.

The foot and ankle are served by three nerves: the surae lateralis and superficial peroneal from the common peroneal nerve, the saphenous nerve from the femoral nerve, and the sural from the tibial nerve.[144]

The bones and periosteum are served essentially by the tibial nerve, and the muscles are served by the tibialis and peronei. The involved spinal segments, both sensory and motor, are L-4, L-5, S-1, and S-2.

The foot and ankle have two major functions: weight bearing and ambulation. The impaired mechanisms causing foot and ankle pain and dysfunction imply analysis of their functional anatomy.[145]

The foot presents a unique segment of human anatomy in that all its component parts are accessible to visual examination, direct palpation, and mechanical evaluation. The patient directs the attention of the examiner to the painful or disabling region of the foot and ankle. A specific functional and anatomical diagnosis evolves from this examination.

The foot has 26 bones that articulate in its weight-bearing and ambulation functions (Fig. 8–86). These articulations have precise geometric rela-

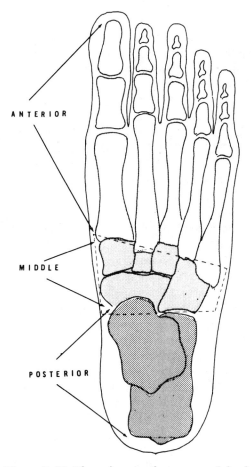

Figure 8–86. Three functional segments of the foot.

tionships and conform to physical concepts of engineering. Their congruity allows effortless weight-bearing function, and their kinetic action permits asymptomatic deformation during ambulation. These factors must be evaluated in determining the mechanism of an activity that has produced pain and dysfunction.[146]

The foot normally forms three arches: the tarsal, posterior metatarsal, and anterior metatarsal (Fig. 8–87). The tarsal and posterior tarsal arches remain firm, as the congruity of their bones form a perfect arch. The anterior metatarsal varies with kinetic function.

In normal gait the foot at heel strike of the swing phase (Fig. 8–88) is dorsiflexed and supinated. The metatarsal arch forms in the supinated position of the foot.

At midstance phase the foot pronates and remains thus through the remainder of the stance phase until heel off and toe off. In the pronated foot the metatarsal arch flattens (Fig. 8–89), with each metatarsal head becoming equally weight bearing. This is not physiologic and results in metatarsal periosteal trauma. The excessive pronation widens the forefoot, stressing the transverse metatarsal ligaments and irritating the interdigital nerves. A neuralgia can result (Fig. 8–90).

The pronated foot, besides causing a flattened metatarsal arch, also everts the hind foot to flatten the longitudinal arch (Fig. 8–91). The ligaments supporting the longitudinal arch are strained and become nociceptive sites.

The hind foot (heel) is a site of pain directly available to observation and palpation (Fig. 8–92). The plantar fascia plays a role in heel pain associated with the pronated foot (Fig. 8–93).

The mechanism of painful conditions of the toes involve the articulations: their capsules, ligaments, and cartilaginous surfaces. The alignment of the phalanges is pertinent in these mechanisms (Fig. 8–94).

The ankle articulation depends on the shape and ligamentous support of the talus and mortice (Fig. 8–95). Injury impairs the normal mechanics. A history and examination will determine the involved tissue.

Management of the Painful Foot

Having ascertained the precise articular site of the pain and thus the involved tissue, it is possible to institute appropriate treatment.

Acute care involves diminishment of pain and prevention of further trauma to the injured tissues by rest, immobilization, and appropriate modalities and medication. Correction of the improper function requires splinting, orthosis, gait correction, and restorative exercises. Surgical intervention assumes an anatomically correctible situation.

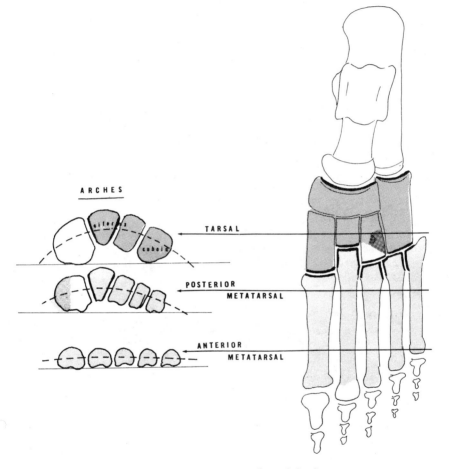

Figure 8–87. Transverse arches of the foot.

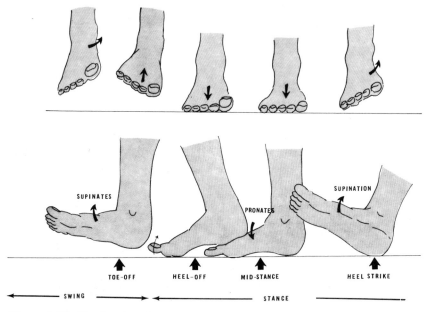

Figure 8–88. The foot in gait.

At heel strike the foot is dorsiflexed and inverted. At midstance the foot is pronated. The forefoot is "splayed" due to diminished metatarsal arch, and all metatarsal heads are weight bearing. The foot reassumes supination and dorsiflexion at the next heel strike.

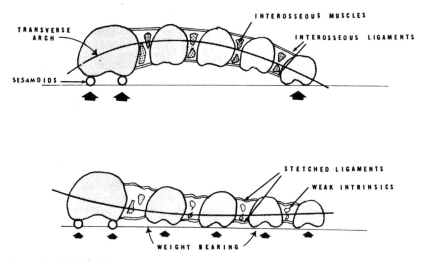

Figure 8–89. Splayfoot.

A constitutional weakness of the intermetatarsal ligament combined with weakness of the intrinsic muscles of the foot may cause the foot to spread excessively on weight bearing. Symptoms consist of pressure pain of the middle metatarsal heads with formation of bunions and calluses.

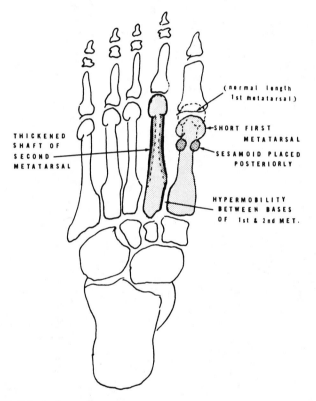

Figure 8–90. Morton's syndrome.

A short first metatarsal bone causes excessive weight to be borne by the second metatarsal.

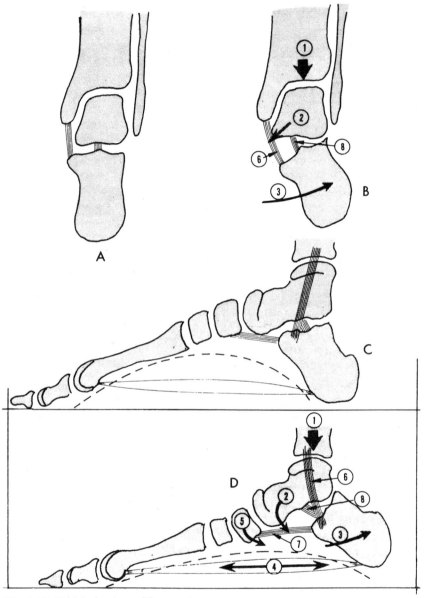

Figure 8–91. Mechanism of foot strain.

(A, C), Normal foot with proper bone and joint alignment, a central heel, and good longitudinal arch. (B, D), Stress causes malalignment of structures. Weight-bearing impact of tibia (1) on talus (2). The talus tends to slide forward and medially on the calcaneus. Under pressure, the calcaneus everts and rotates posteriorly (3), elongating the longitudinal arch and placing strain on the plantar fascia (4). The rotating calcaneus depresses the navicular bone (5) by pulling on the calcaneonavicular ligament (7), which becomes tender. The initial valgus of the heel places strain on the medial collateral ligament (6) and ultimately on the talocalcaneal ligament (8).

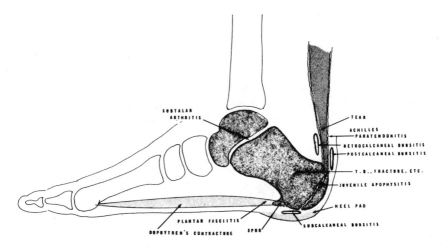

Figure 8–92. Sites of pain in the region of the heel.

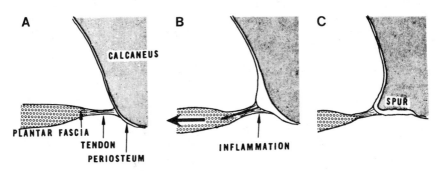

Figure 8–93. Mechanism of plantar fascitis (heel spur).

(A), Normal relationship and attachment of the plantar fascia to the calcaneus. (B), Traction on the fascial tendinous portion to the periosteum separates the periosteum from the heel, and resultant inflammation causes pain. (C), Subperiosteal invasion by inflammatory tissue and ultimate calcification into a spur. This process may be asymptomatic.

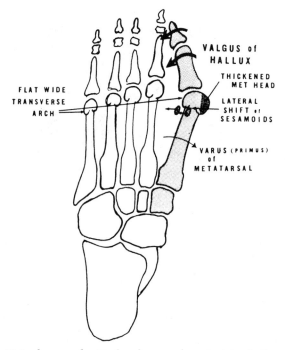

Figure 8–94. Major bony and articular changes characterizing hallux valgus.

Hallux valgus is essentially a subluxation of the two phalanges of the big toe in a valgus direction. The first metatarsal deviates in a varus direction, and the sesamoids are thus shifted laterally.

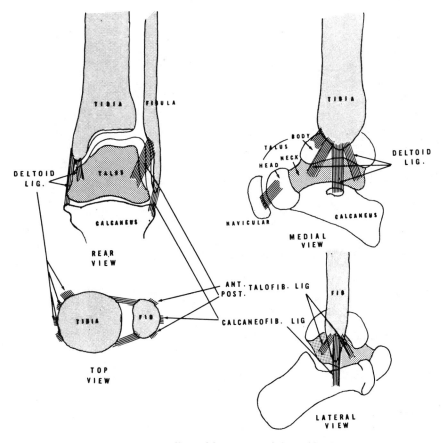

Figure 8–95. Collateral ligaments of the ankle joint.

VISCERAL PAIN

The abdomen is the most frequent site of regional pain from abdominal disorders or as a referred site of thoracic visceral diseases. The pelvis is a part of the abdominal cavity, but its referral site differs. Pain from diseases of the chest are also referred to the abdomen as both are innervated by somatic and visceral nerves that have a similar distribution in the spinal cord.

Pain is experienced from abdominal viscera when there is (1) tension or stretching of the walls of hollow viscera, (2) traction or stretching of the associated peritoneum, or (3) rapid stretching of the capsule that encloses the viscera. Examples of each depend on the organ and the cause of the dilation or stretch.

Viscera undergoing mechanical changes from bacterial, chemical, or ischemic inflammation create algogens such as bradykinin, serotonin, histamine, or prostaglandins that sensitize the sensory nerve endings. The distention of these sensitized tissues results in pain. Mechanical insult to a normal mucosa causes no pain, implying that preceding inflammation is necessary.

The origin of the nociceptive impulses determines the site and type of pain. Visceral pain is either true, referred, unreferred parietal, or referred parietal pain.

True parietal pain is dull and poorly localized; it occurs in the region of the epigastric, periumbilical, or lower midabdominal region (Fig. 8–96). The pains are often described as gnawing or cramping and are often associated with nausea, sweating, pallor, and, occasionally, vomiting.

Referred visceral pain is more precisely localized, usually in the dermatomal or myosomal regions of the same segments of the spinal cord involved.

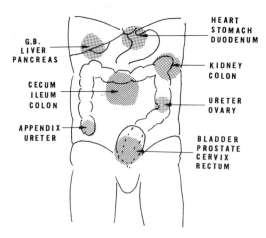

Figure 8–96. Abdominal pain according to site.

Visceral pain occurs mostly directly over the involved organs but is felt mostly in the midline, epigastric, and suprapubic areas.

Parietal pain is pain felt directly over the organ and not referred. This is the condition of acute appendicitis: Pain and tenderness are felt over the abdominal region of the right lower abdomen above the appendix.

Referred parietal pain is pain noted in a site distant from the nociceptive site. An example is pain experienced in the shoulder area during a myocardial infarct or from inflammation of the middle diaphragm.

Chronic abdominal pain remains a challenge in spite of all the recent diagnostic procedures that allow precise clinical examination, including contrast studies, endoscopy, CT scanning, MRI studies, and nuclear studies. A careful history and physical examination often suffice, and the pain sites, albeit inaccurate for precise differential diagnosis, are usually accurate enough to indicate need for further studies.

A musculoskeletal cause should always be considered in differential diagnosis of abdominal pain including pain referred from the spine or muscle wall. Patients can usually differentiate deep from superficial pain. Confusion regarding pain occurring from the abdominal wall can be dispelled by anesthetic blocking of the intercostal or paravertebral nerves. Differentiating abdominal from genitourinary pain, which blocks the celiac plexus, may be diagnostic.

There is both autonomic and somatic innervation of the abdominal viscera (Fig. 8–97). The autonomic nerve is essentially the vagus nerve supplying the parasympathetic preganglionic fibers. The sympathetic efferent nerves supplying the abdominal viscera have their cell bodies located in the T-5 to L-2 segments. They emerge through the anterior nerve roots as white rami communicantes. These nerves form numerous plexi; the celiac (solar) plexus is the most prominent. For a more detailed discussion, see Bonica.[147]

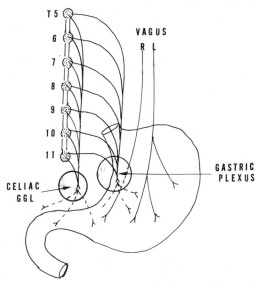

Figure 8–97. Innervation of the stomach and duodenum.

The vagus nerves, right and left, descend into the celiac plexus. The sympathetic fibers from T-5 to T-11 descend via the superior and middle thoracic splanchnic nerves to end and synapse in the celiac ganglia. (See text for details.)

There are efferent (motor) and afferent (sensory) fibers, both parasympathetic and sympathetic, devoted to the gastrointestinal tract. The vagus nerves are 90 percent afferent, of which 80 to 90 percent are nonmyelinated.[148] The remainder are A-delta, and a small proportion are A-beta. These nerves convey mechanical, chemical, thermal, and osmotic information about the viscera, which, under normal conditions, are involved in regulation of function via spinal and supraspinal reflexes.

The history is invaluable in differentiating gastrointestinal disease and indicating the appropriate procedures and tests for confirmation.

Esophageal disease usually elicits a history of heartburn: a burning or gnawing substernal discomfort. Usually the site indicated by the patient is epigastric. The pain is often felt after eating but may be related to position such as reclining or bending forward. Whether the pain is created by chemical irritation or secondary to muscle spasms remains obscure.

Stomach pain from an ulcer is felt in the epigastrium and is usually sharply localized, causing burning or gnawing pain. This pain is often felt a short while after eating or during the night. It is relieved by eating or taking antacid medication. The pain may radiate into the back at that level. The precise basis for the pain varies from irritation of the nerve endings by acid to antral spasm.

Small intestinal pain is usually crampy or colicky and felt in the periumbilical area. The cause of this pain is usually from a lesion causing distension with resultant abnormal mobility. Eating usually precipitates the pain, and defecation or fasting may afford relief. The pathology causing the pain is determined by appropriate studies.

Colon pain tends to be referred in the lower abdomen, varying according to which portion of the colon is affected. Symptoms of discomfort are often accompanied by change in bowel habits, occult blood in the stool, and so forth.

Pancreatic disease is ominous and unfortunately is difficult to diagnose. Pain originating from the pancreas is usually felt in the epigastric region and related to eating or to position. Initially relief is gained from curling into the fetal position. Progress in severity of pain implies possible cancer, usually in the head of the pancreas. Passage of a biliary stone can also be severe. It is usually felt in the right upper quadrant with radiation into the right shoulder blade and shoulder.

Liver parenchyma is insensitive to pain. Right-upper-quadrant pain from liver pathology occurs only when there is acute distension of the liver capsule.

Vascular bowel disease, termed abdominal angina, occurs as a dull periumbilical or epigastric pain. It occurs shortly after eating as the arterial supply is inadequate to meet the demands of digestion and absorption. An abdominal aneurysm presents more acutely, but a slow, expanding, leaking aneurysm may present as a dull, recurring, midepigastric pain that is relieved

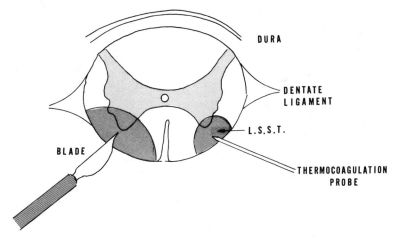

Figure 8–98. Cordotomy procedures to interrupt lateral spinothalamic tracts.
Using the guidelines of the dentate ligaments and sparing the descending motor tracts, an open cordotomy procedure uses a blade and the percutaneous procedure a thermocoagulation probe.

by sitting and leaning forward. A palpable, pulsating tender mass and a bruit are diagnostic warnings.

Pain that persists after elimination of the pathology or in an incurable gastrointestinal condition must be treated as chronic pain with all its implications.

If pharmacologic treatment of intractable abdominal pain is ineffective, a celiac anesthetic plexus block may help. It is a procedure infrequently used despite its efficacy, safety, and reasonably simple application. A local anesthetic (40–50 mL) in the retroperitoneal space at the level of the celiac plexus blocks the efferent and afferent autonomic nerves. After the effect wears off, an injection of ethanol into that area causes sclerosis of the fine autonomic nerves.[149] In a pancreatic cancer patient the benefit of these blocks is longer than the patient's lifespan.

Patients with severe intractable pain from a malignancy may benefit from other neurosurgical procedures. In recent years there has been a disturbing trend to consider neurosurgical intervention of intractable cancer pain only in the late stages of the disease when the patient is often totally debilitated and less able to tolerate the procedure. The procedures include cordotomy; open and percutaneous (Fig. 8–98); rhizotomy; and intradural or percutaneous stereotaxic cranial procedures such as periventricular gray stimulation. Epidural or intrathecal catheter (Fig. 8–99) with or without continuous infusion pump are becoming more accepted and feasible.

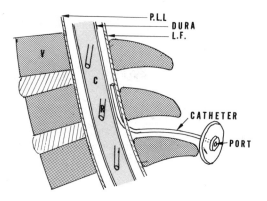

Figure 8–99. Epidural anesthesia by indwelling catheter.

The epidural catheter enters the epidural space and the distal end is connected to the abdominal wall to a sutured button the center of which is the port through which medications can be injected either as a bolus or a continuous drip.

PELVIC PAIN

The pelvis contains the urinary bladder, terminal portion of the ureters as they enter the bladder, sigmoid colon, rectum, and internal genitalia (Fig. 8–100). The pelvic viscera are supplied by sympathetic and parasympathetic nerves containing both efferent and afferent fibers. These are included in the innervation from the celiac ganglion (Fig. 8–97) and its subsidiary plexi forming the superior and inferior hypogastric plexi (Fig. 8–101).

As in other abdominal viscera the parenchyma of the organs of the pelvis is not supplied with pain receptors. The peritoneum and the arterial walls contain a rich network of nerve fibers. The sensory fibers of the viscera are transmitted via the same somatic nerves as those subserving the skin; thus, the true origin of the pain is confusing to the patient as it is experienced at a different level and poorly localized.

Pain from the fundus of the uterus is commonly felt in the hypogastrium: the lower midabdominal section. Cervical pain is commonly referred to the

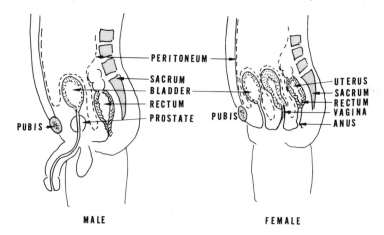

Figure 8–100. Male and female contents of pelvis.

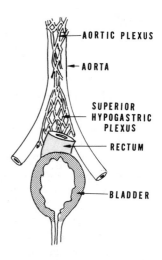

Figure 8–101. Nerve supply of the pelvis. The autonomic and somatic nerves that supply the pelvic viscera contain both afferent and efferent fibers. From the celiac plexus the nerves descend into the aortic plexus, then into the superior and inferior hypogastric plexi. The inferior hypogastric plexus is not shown in the drawing, as it resides behind the rectum and the bladder on the arterior aspect of the sacrum.

low back and sacral area as well as to the hypogastrium. Ovaries are mobile and thus ovarian pain is felt usually when there is stretching of the surrounding peritoneum to which the ovaries adhere.

Localization of the offending organ is accomplished by a careful pelvic and rectal examination. Gentleness is emphasized as the female pelvis is usually extremely sensitive and false information can be gained from rough handling.

Fortunately, there are many additional examination procedures—MRI, CT scanning, and pelvic ultrasonography—that clarify what has been revealed by manual examination. The history must never be undervalued as it differentiates functional as well as structural changes. Response to appropriate medication is diagnostic as well as therapeutic.

It has been aptly stated that the physician who examines and treats the woman with pelvic pain must be an internist, a surgeon, and a psychiatrist. Iatrogenic disease is predominant, resulting in unnecessary and ineffectual surgical intervention.

Of the many pelvic lesions causing pain, a few should be listed. Dysmenorrhea is usually cramping in nature and felt in the lower midabdominal region with radiation to the low back. Dysmenorrhea may develop at ᵗhe onset of menarche (primary) or it may occur in later life.

The cause of dysmenorrhea remains unknown, but is considered to be related to prostaglandins and hypoxia from increased intrauterine pressure.[150,151] There is a decreased uterine blood flow during menstruation. This is confirmed by the relief experienced with the administration of beta-sympathomimetics.[152] Secondary dysmenorrhea may be related to acquired pathology such as endometriosis, adenomyosis, leiomyomata, salpingitis, or cervical stenosis.

Endometriosis implies the presence of extrauterine endometrial tissue, that is, endometrial tissue outside the uterine cavity in the area of the ovaries, peritoneum, pelvic ligaments, and even the rectum or bladder. Why this occurs is not known. A theory has been expounded claiming a retroflux of menstrual blood into the pelvic cavity: a sort of "transtubal regurgitation." Other theories postulate activation of ectopic endometrium which has been dormant.

Endometriosis occurs in women between the ages of 25 and 45. There is related dysmenorrhea and often dyspareunia (painful intercourse). If the endometrium involves the gastrointestinal tract, there are gastrointestinal symptoms during the menses.

Diagnosis may be suspected by finding a relatively fixed uterus in the cul de sac and enlarged ovaries. Nodularity of the uterine ligaments is considered diagnostic. When endometriosis is strongly suspected but the examination is nonspecific, laparotomy is diagnostic. The symptoms of endometriosis stop during pregnancy. High doses of birth control pills are often used to treat endometriosis as they cause a sort of pseudopregnancy.[153]

Leiomyomata, commonly called fibroids, is the frequent condition of benign muscle tumors within the uterine wall, which may remain merely in the wall or originate in the submucosa and ultimately protrude into the uterine cavity. Pain is infrequent and, when present, implies possible concurrent pathology. Discomfort in the lower abdomen is common, and when there is compression on the bladder, leiomyomata may cause urinary tract symptoms. A rapidly enlarging myoma may cause pressure on the major blood vessels of the pelvis.

Invasion of the wall of the uterus by the endometrium, termed adenomyosis, is considered in women over 40 years of age experiencing dysmenorrhea or menorrhagia. Suspicion arises when the pelvic and rectal examination reveals an enlarged uterus with obvious nodularity.

As the pathology here is invasion of the uterine wall forming benign tumors of stroma and endometrium, treatment is symptomatic. Analgesics may be used until the women is beyond childbearing age. Simple hysterectomy is the ultimate choice of cure.

Pelvic inflammatory disease (PID) causes concern and indicates infection of the pelvic organs, especially the fallopian tubes. PID may result from gonorrhea, chlamydia, or *Mycoplasma hominis.*

Symptoms include pain and tenderness in the pelvic region, fever, chills, and a generalized sensation of depletion. Examination may reveal a purulent discharge of the cervix as well as tenderness of the adnexa.

Laboratory confirmation of leukocytosis and identification of the organism is specifically diagnostic. Laparotomy should be considered to determine the presence and extent of the infection and inflammation.[154]

Many other conditions of the pelvis are beyond the scope of this text.[155] Pelvic cancer can be insidiously evidenced by pelvic pain. Ovarian cancer is the most ominous cancer of women and should always be a concern of the examining physician.

The possibility of psychogenic pelvic pain presents a constant problem to the practitioner; too often it is a diagnosis of exclusion when "no pathology is found." When suspected and recognized, it requires comprehensive intervention.[156]

The pain of childbirth remains a universal problem that demands recognition and successful management. Analgesia and anesthesia, properly administered, present less maternal and prenatal mortality than considered.

There are considerable hemodynamic changes during pregnancy and labor that must be recognized and addressed.[157] The mechanisms of pain during labor are pressure on the nerve endings of the muscle fibers of the body and fundus of the uterus, ischemia of the myometrium during contractions, inflammation of the cervix during dilation, and hyperactivity of the sympathetic nervous system from fear and anxiety. Tension constricts the cervix, which increases pain because it obstructs the expulsing uterus. Lacerations of the perineum further the pain; hence the value of an episiotomy.

Management implies the need of a comprehensive program including prenatal information, training, and conditioning; psychologic analgesia ("natural childbirth") including hypnosis; inhalation analgesia and anesthesia; and regional analgesia and anesthesia. The latter may include pudendal block, caudal analgesia including continuous epidural blocks, and local anesthetic blocks of the perineum. Obviously, a qualified anesthesiologist is needed to determine the precise technique and indication for the specific patient and the severity of the pain.

CARDIAC PAIN

Many types of cardiac pathology produce pain, including coronary disease, valvular disease, pericardial disease, and aortic disease. Only the mechanisms can be considered in this discussion, but further study is justified by the clinician who evaluates the patient complaining of chest pain, as the significance of heart disease is formidable.[158]

The nerve supply to the heart and other thoracic viscera is complicated. The heart is richly supplied by motor and sensory myelinated and unmyelinated nerves derived from sympathetic and parasympathetic (vagal) nerves. The pertinent nerve supply must be discerned as being of the coronary arteries, the myocardium, the conducting system, and the valves. The cardiac nerve supply has been thoroughly discussed by Bonica.[159] It is simplistically illustrated in Fig. 8–102.

The coronary artery nerve supply has been considered as the richest of all the arteries of the body. The adventitia contains many myelinated and unmyelinated nerve fiber endings that accompany the arteries as they become arterioles into the myocardium. Sympathetic nerves supply the smooth muscle cells of the coronary artery media. There are sensory nerve endings in the myocardium.[160]

234 PAIN: MECHANISMS AND MANAGEMENT

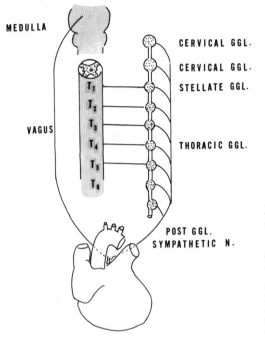

Figure 8-102. Nerve supply to the heart.

The sympathetic and parasympathetic nerve supply to the heart is shown. The afferent sensory nerves enter the thoracic spinal cord via the sympathetic chain at the T-1 to T-5 levels (GGL = ganglion).

The heart has a substantial afferent supply of A-delta and C fibers within the vagus nerves.[161] Although these fibers respond to bradykinin and ischemia, they apparently are not involved in the nociception of cardiac ischemia: Cutting the vagus nerve has no effect on the noxious stimuli.[162] Nociception is transmitted via sympathetic afferents.[163]

Sympathetic afferent activity increases when the pressure within the heart increases.[164] Algogenic substances that become nociceptive are released from ischemic myocardial muscles. Bradykinin and prostaglandins are formed by ischemic cardiac tissue, and they affect the primary nociceptive afferents, the A-delta and C fibers.

To confuse the cardiac pain concept, Malliani and associates[165] dispute the presence of specific nociceptors and claim that cardiac pain results from extreme excitation of a spatially restricted population of afferent sympathetic fibers. This concept does not refute the concept of ischemic myocardial nociception being mediated via sympathetic nerve fibers.

All cardiac pain apparently has a common denominator: ischemia.[166] The status of the blood supply, therefore, is vital in ascertaining the mechanism of cardiac disease. Cardiac pain is visceral in nature and is described by the patient in vague, diffuse, poorly localized terms; numerous other areas are often referred to. The term *angina* was initially used by Heberden, from the Latin *angor animi,* meaning "feeling of terror."[167]

The sensation is often felt in the arms as a paresthesia or sensation of

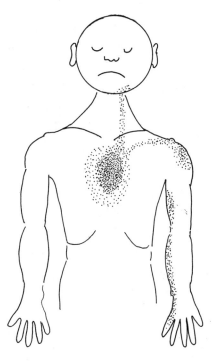

Figure 8–103. Sites of referred cardiac pain.

Ischemic cardiac pain is felt (referred) in the precordial, left shoulder region, and medial aspect of the left forearm and little finger area (C-8 dermatome).

The neural pathways are demonstrated in Figure 8–104.

weakness. There is usually a pain sensation in the sternum and substernum (Fig. 8–103). Pain is often experienced in the muscles of the chest wall. The neurologic basis for this has been postulated (Fig. 8–104). The skin hyperalgesia is often precise and sharper. The greater the degree and extent of the myocardial ischemia, the greater is the nociceptive barrage to the cord. The noxious input occurs from the myocardium, but also from the overlying skin and muscle, as all three excite the WDR cells located in laminae IV, V, and VII in the upper chest.[168] The receptive fields of these segments are the ipsilateral upper and lateral chest, which explains the radiation of cardiac ischemic pain to that region and to the ipsilateral upper extremity. Viscerosomatic convergence has been found in the somatosensory cortex.

Left thoracic vagal stimulation inhibits all of the spinothalamic cells that respond to noxious stimulation of nerve roots T-1 to T-5. This may explain the many "silent," painless myocardial ischemias noted clinically.

Management of Cardiac Pain

Once the ischemic pain has signaled myocardial ischemia, it should be relieved promptly as it then causes reflex vagal and sympathetic impulses that are detrimental to cardiac function and rhythm. The suprasegmental sympathetic reflexes and the psychologic stress combine to add to the work-

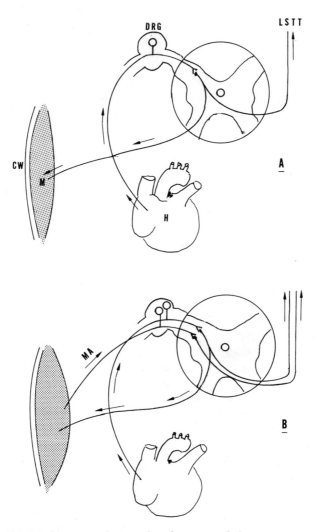

Figure 8-104. Mechanism pathways of cardiac precordial pain.

(A), The afferents from the (ischemic) heart muscle (H) enter the dorsal root ganglion (DRG) to synapse the efferents to the precordial muscle (M) and the anterior chest wall (CW). The sensory pathway ascends via the lateral spinothalamic tract (LSTT).

(B), The irritable anterior chest wall and intercostal muscles become a site of nociception entering the dorsal root ganglion via the muscle afferent (MA) fibers to also ascend to the LSTT. The LSTT enhances the cardiac pain and persists long after the ischemic cardiac nociceptive impulses have ceased.

The therapeutic basis for blocking the MA pathways is apparent.

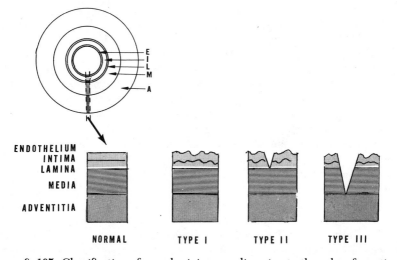

Figure 8–105. Classification of vascular injury predisposing to thrombus formation. The normal vascular levels are shown. Type I injury has merely functional alteration of the endothelial cells. Progression into type II has some denuding of the endothelial cells, but the internal elastic lamina (lamina) remains intact. As damage progresses further, type III has further denuding of the endothelium with damage into the intima and media. The adventitia remains unaffected.

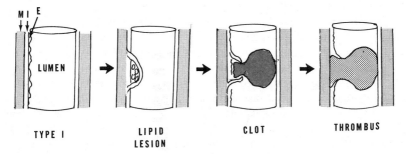

Figure 8–106. Dynamic stages of thrombus formation.

Type I depicts the endothelium (E) undergoing functional aberrations. The intima (I) and the media (M) are intact. The lumen is fully patent. As there are deposits of macrophages containing fat lobules, the lipid lesion forms an encapsulation, causing some impairment of the lumen capacity.

Blood clotting, which is pedunculated, occurs after the capsule of the lipid lesion ruptures and, depending on its size, may cause unstable angina from intermittent lumen occlusion.

As the clot organizes, a thrombus forms that may occlude the lumen partially or completely.

load of the heart and its oxygen consumption. It is therefore mandatory that cardiac ischemia be managed by oxygenation, relieving the referred pain in the muscle and skin and decreasing the anxiety.

The referred sympathetic pain may be relieved by a stellate nerve block. The referred chest wall pain can be addressed by local anesthetic nerve blocks in the region of the painful tender muscle and skin. The cardiac ischemia is relieved by nasal and mask oxygen, and the arrhythmia is relieved by appropriate medications.

Understanding the mechanism of cardiac pain explains the need for comprehensive management. The pathogenesis of coronary artery disease and the mechanism of acute coronary syndromes are beyond the scope of this dissertation.[169]

Vascular injury and thrombus formation are the basis of origin and progression of atherosclerosis that leads to acute coronary syndromes. Chronic minimal injury to the arterial endothelium seems to be caused by disturbances in the pattern of blood flow occurring in certain parts of the arterial tree such as areas of bending or branching.[169] This area of injured endothelium can be further damaged by hypercholesteremia; infections; chemical irritants, such as nicotine, smoke, and so forth.

Vascular injury is divided into three types depending on its progression.[170] Type I is basically functional alteration of the endothelial cells without significant morphologic changes. Type II undergoes endothelial denuding and intimal damage, but the internal elastic laminae remain intact. Type 3 shows damage to the intima and media as well (Fig. 8–105).

In type 1 there is an accumulation of lipids and macrophages (monocytes) within the functionally impaired area of the endothelium. The macrophages release toxins that further damage the endothelium, creating an area for platelet adhesion.[171] These platelets and other substances being released invade the intima and ultimately the blood vessel media, progressing into types 2 and 3. A proliferation of smooth muscle cells forms a fibrointimal lesion, which forms a capsule around fat cells (a lipid lesion).

This lipid capsule may rupture, forming a thrombus at the site which may progress into a fibrotic organization that partially or completely occludes the artery. This progression explains the symptoms progressing from a "silent" to an "unstable" angina to eventual stenosis. Intimal irritation in the evolution of plaque formation, along with other neurovascular factors, may cause contraction of the smooth muscles of the vessel, causing transient ischemia.

These stages (Fig. 8–106) and their detection, intervention, and prevention are beyond the scope of this text, but they lay the foundation for understanding the mechanism of cardiac pain.

REFERENCES

1. Cailliet, R: Anatomy, physiology, and pathophysiology of head and face pain. In Head and Face Pain Syndromes, ed 1. FA Davis, Philadelphia, 1992, pp 1–23.

2. Bonica, JJ: The Management of Pain, Vol 1, ed 2. Lea & Febiger, Philadelphia, 1990, pp 651–793.

3. Chusid, JG: Correlative Neuroanatomy and Functional Neurology, ed 14. Lange Medical Publishers, Los Altos, CA, 1970, pp 98–101.

4. Dubner, R, Price, DD, Beitel, RE, and Hu, JW: Peripheral neural correlates of behavior in monkey and human related to sensory-discriminative aspects of pain. In Anderson, DJ and Mathews, B (eds): Pain in the Trigeminal Region. Elsevier, Amsterdam, 1973, pp 57–66.

5. Lundberg, JM, Hokfelt, T, Anggard, A, Terenius, L, Elde, R, Markey, K, Goldstein, M, and Kimmel, J: Organizational principles in the peripheral sympathetic nervous system. Subdivision by coexisting peptides (somatostatin, avian pancreatic polypeptides, and vasoactive intestinal polypeptide-like immunoreactive materials). Proc Natl Acad Sci USA 79:1303–1307, 1982.

6. Edvinsson, L, Owman, C, Rosengren, E, and West, KA: Cholinergic mechanisms in pial blood vessels. Histochemistry, electron microscopy and pharmacology. Z Zellforsch 134:311–425, 1972.

7. Edvinsson, L, Falck, B, and Owman, C: Possibilities for a cholinergic action on smooth musculature and on sympathetic axons in brain vessels mediated by muscarine and nicotinic receptors. J Pharmacol Exp Ther 200:117–126, 1977.

8. Brayden, JE, and Bevan, JA: The autonomic innervation of the cephalic circulation. In Olesen, J and Edvinsson, L (eds): Basic Mechanisms of Headache. Elsevier, Amsterdam, 1988, pp 145–155.

9. Ad Hoc Committee on Classification of Headache: Arch Neurol 6:173–176, 1963.

10. Osler, W: The Principles and Practice of Medicine, ed. 8. Appleton, New York, 1912, pp 1092–1093.

11. Ray, BS and Wolff, HG: Experimental studies in headache. Arch Surg 41:812, 1940.

12. Dahl, E and Edvinsson, L: Anatomical organization of cerebral and extracerebral vasculature. In Olesen, J and Edvinsson, L (eds): Basic Mechanisms of Headache, Vol 2. Elsevier, Amsterdam, 1988, pp 24–47.

13. Wolff, HG: Headache and Other Head Pain. Oxford University Press, New York, 1963.

14. Olesen, J, Larsen, B, and Lauritzen, M: Focal hyperemia followed by spreading oligemia and impaired activation of RCBF in classic migraine. Ann Neurol 9:344, 1981.

15. Lashley, KS: Patterns of cerebral integration indicated by the scotomas of migraine. Arch Neurol Psychiat 46:259–264, 1941.

16. Leao, AAP: Spreading depression of activity in the cerebral cortex. J Neurophysiol 7:359–390, 1944.

17. Vanmhoutte, PM, Cohen, RA, and Van Neueten, JM: Serotonin and arterial vessels. J Cardiovasc Pharmacol 6 (Suppl 2):S422–S428, 1984.

18. Cailliet, R: Migraine and migraine variants. In Head and Face Pain Syndromes, ed 1. FA Davis, Philadelphia, 1992, pp 25–38.

19. Olesen, J and Langemark, M: Mechanisms of tension headache: a speculative hypothesis. In Olesen, J and Edvinsson, L (eds): Basic Mechanisms of Headache, Vol 2. Elsevier, Amsterdam, 1988, pp 459–461.

20. Olesen, J: Clinical and pathophysiological observations in migraine and tension-type headache explained by integration of vascular, supraspinal, and myofascial inputs. Pain 46:125–132, 1991.

21. Sessle, BJ, Hu, JW, Amano, N, and Zhong, G: Convergence of cutaneous, tooth pulp, visceral, neck muscle afferents onto nociceptive and non-nociceptive neurons in trigeminal subnucleus caudalis (medullary dorsal horn) and its implications for referred pain. Pain 27:219–235, 1986.

22. Olesen, J: Some clinical features of the acute migraine attack: An analysis of 750 patients. Headache 18:268–274, 1978.

23. Friedman, AP and Wood, EH: Thermography in vascular headache. In Uema, S (ed): Medical Thermography. Brentwood Publishers, Los Angeles, 1976, pp 80–84.
24. Horven, I, Nornes, H, and Sjaastad, O: Different corneal indentation pulse patterns in cluster headaches and migraine. Neurol 22:92–96, 1972.
25. Norris, JW, Hachinski, VC, and Cooper, PW: Cerebral blood flow changes in cluster headache. Acta Neurol Scand 54:371–374, 1976.
26. Moskowitz, MA: Neurobiology of vascular head pain. J Ann Neurol 16:157–168, 1984.
27. Kudrow, L: The cyclic relationship of natural illumination to cluster period frequency. Cephalalgia 7 (Suppl 6):76–78, 1987.
28. Kudrow, L: Response of cluster headache to oxygen inhalation. Headache 21:1–4, 1981.
29. Costen, JB: A syndrome of ear and sinus problems dependent on disturbed function of the temporomandibular joint. Ann Otol 43:1–15, 1934.
30. Cailliet, R: Temporomandibular joint pain. In Head and Face Pain Syndromes. FA Davis, Philadelphia, 1992.
31. Classification and Diagnostic Criteria for Headache Disorders: Cranial Neuralgias and Facial Pain. Cephalalgia 8(Suppl 7):1–96, 1988.
32. Hagberg, C: Electromyography and Bite Force Studies of Muscular Function and Dysfunction in Masticatory Muscles. Swedish Dental J Suppl 37:1–64, 1986.
33. Helms, CA, et al: J Craniomand Pract 2:220–224, 1984.
34. Helms, CA, et al: Radiol 145:719–723, 1982.
35. Cailliet, R: Functional anatomy. In Neck and Arm Pain, ed 3. FA Davis, Philadelphia, 1991, pp 1–24.
36. Cailliet, R: Head and neck pain from the cervical spine. In Head and Face Pain Syndromes. FA Davis, Philadelphia, 1992, pp 77–99.
37. Bovim, G, Berg, R, and Dale, LG: Cervicogenic headache: Anesthetic blockades of cervical nerve (C2–C5) and facet joints (C2/C3). Pain 49:315–320, 1992.
38. Kerr, FWL: Structural relation of the trigeminal spinal tract to the upper cervical roots and the solitary nucleus in cat. Exp Neurol 4:134–148, 1961.
39. Bovim, G, Bonamico, L, Fredriksen, TA, Lindboe, CF, Stolt-Nielsen, A, and Sjaastad, O: Topographic variations in the peripheral course of the greater occipital nerve: Autopsy study with clinical correlations. Spine 16: 475–478, 1991.
40. Keith, WS: "Whiplash"—injury of the 2nd cervical ganglion and nerve. Can J Neurol Sci 13:133–137, 1986.
41. Bogduk, N and Marsland, A: On the concept of a third occipital headache. J Neurol Neurosurg Psychiatry 49:775–780, 1986.
42. Michler, RP, Bovim, G, and Sjaastad, O: Disorders in the lower cervical spine: A cause of unilateral headache? Headache 31:550–551, 1991.
43. Sjaastad, O, Fredriksen, TA, and Pfaffenrath, V: Cervicogenic headache: Diagnostic criteria. Headache 30:725–726, 1990.
44. Bogduk, N and Marsland, A: The cervical zygapophyseal joints as a source of neck pain. Spine 13(6):610, 1988.
45. Cailliet, R: Subluxations of the cervical spine: The whiplash syndromes. In Neck and Arm Pain, ed. 3. FA Davis, Philadelphia, 1991.
46. Haymaker, W and Woodhall, B: Peripheral Nerve Injuries, ed 2. WB Saunders, Philadelphia, 1953.
47. Kalaska, JF and Crammond, DJ: Cerebral cortical mechanisms of reaching movements. Science 255:1517–1523, 1992.
48. Georgopoulos, AP, Kalaska, JF, and Caminiti, R: Exp Brain Res Suppl 10:175, 1985.
49. Thach, WT: Neurophysiology 41, 654 (1978) Normal and Abnormal Motor Activities. Raven Press, New York, 1967.
50. Talbot, RE and Humphrey, DR (eds): Posture and Movement. Raven Press, New York, 1979, pp 51–112.

51. Dum, RP and Strick, PL: In Humphrey, DR and Freund, HJ (eds): Motor Control: Concepts and Issues. Wiley, Chichester, England, 1991, pp 383–397.
52. Yahr, MD and Purpura, DP: Neurophysiological Basis of Normal and Abnormal Motor Activities. Raven Press, New York, 1967.
53. McMahon, TA: Muscles, Reflexes, and Locomotion. Princeton University Press, New Jersey, 1984.
54. Anderson, RA, Essick, GK, and Siegel, RM: Science 230:456, 1985.
55. Cailliet, R: Functional anatomy. In Shoulder Pain, ed 3. FA Davis, Philadelphia, 1991, pp 1–50.
56. Cailliet, R: Elbow pain. In Soft Tissue Pain and Disability, ed 2. FA Davis, Philadelphia, 1988, pp 209–222.
57. Morrey, BF: Posttraumatic Stiffness: Distraction Arthroplasty. Orthopedics 15(7):863–869, 1992.
58. Wadsworth, TG, Williams, JR: Cubital tunnel external compression syndrome. BMJ 3:662–666, 1973.
59. Payan, J: Anterior transposition of the ulnar nerve: An electrophysiological study. J Neurol Neurosurg Psychiatry 33:157–165, 1970.
60. Morrey, BF: Post-traumatic contracture of the elbow. J Bone Joint Surg 72A:601–618, 1990.
61. Morrey, BF and Chao, EYS: Passive motion of the elbow joint. A biomechanical analysis. J Bone Joint Surg 58A:501–508, 1976.
62. Morrey, BF, Askew, LJ, An, KN, and Chao, EY: A biomechanical study of normal functional elbow motion. J Bone Joint Surg 63:872–877, 1981.
63. Yerger, B and Turner T: Percutaneous extensor tenotomy for chronic tennis elbow: An office procedure. Orthopedics 8:1261–1263, 1985.
64. Cailliet, R: Wrist and hand pain. In Soft Tissue Pain and Disability, ed 2. FA Davis, Philadelphia, 1988.
65. Hilton, J: Rest and Pain. Wm Wood, New York, 1879.
66. Cailliet, R: Hand Pain and Impairment, ed 3. FA Davis, Philadelphia, 1982.
67. Fassbender, HB and Simmling-Annefeld, M: The potential aggressiveness of synovial tissue in rheumatoid arthritis. J Pathol 139:399, 1983.
68. Young, CL, Adamson, TC III, Vaughn, JH, and Fox, RI: Immunohistological characterization of synovial membrane lymphocytes in rheumatoid arthritis. Arthritis Rheum 27:32–39, 1984.
69. Kuehl, FA and Egan, RW: Prostaglandins, arachidonic acid, and inflammation. Science 210:978, 1980.
70. Wertsch, JJ and Melvin, J: Median nerve anatomy and entrapment syndromes: A review. Arch Phys Med Rehabil 63:623–627, 1982.
71. Gelberman, RH, Hergenroeder, PT, Hargens, AR, Lundborg, GN, and Akeson, WH: The carpal tunnel syndrome. J Bone Joint Surg 63A:380–383, 1981.
72. Garland, H, Sumner, D, and Clark, JMP: Carpal-tunnel syndrome: With particular reference to surgical treatment. BMJ March 2:581–584, 1963.
73. Bonica, JJ and Sola, AF: Chest pain caused by other disorders. In Bonica, JJ (ed): The Management of Pain, Vol 2, ed 2. Lea & Febiger, Philadelphia, 1990, pp 1114–1145.
74. Rasmussen, TB, Kernohan, JW, and Adson, AW: Pathologic classification with surgical consideration of intraspinal tumors. Ann Surg 111:513, 1940.
75. Wehrmacher, WH: Pain in the Chest. Charles C Thomas, Springfield, IL, 1964, pp 71–99.
76. Davies-Colley, R: Slipping rib. BMJ 1:432, 1922.
77. Tietze, A: Uber eine eigenartige Haufung von Fallen mit Dystrophie der Rippenknorpel. Berl Klin Wochenschr 58:829, 1921.
78. Burgoon, CF, Burgoon, JS, and Baldridge, GD: The natural history of herpes zoster. JAMA 164:265, 1957.

79. Mazur, N and Dolin, R: Herpes zoster at the NIH: A 20-year history. Am J Med 65:738, 1978.
80. Head, H and Campbell, AW: The pathology of herpes zoster and its bearing on sensory localization. Brain 23:335, 1900.
81. Arseni, C and Nash, F: Protrusion of thoracic intervertebral discs. Acta Neurochir 11:3, 1963.
82. Saibil, FB and Edmeades, J: Chest pain arising from extrathoracic structures. In Levene, DL (ed): Chest Pain: An Integrated Diagnostic Approach. Lea & Febiger, Philadelphia, 1977, p 130.
83. Bogduk, N and Long, DM: The anatomy of the so-called "articular nerves" and their relationship to the facet denervation in the treatment of low back pain. J Neurosurg 51:172, 1979.
84. Gracovetsky, S and Farfan, HF: The optimum spine. Spine 11:543, 1986.
85. Bogduk, N and Twomey, LT: Clinical Anatomy of the Lumbar Spine. Churchill-Livingstone, Melbourne, 1987, pp 139–147.
86. Giles, LGF: Anatomical Basis of Low Back Pain. Williams and Wilkins, Baltimore, 1989, pp 58–66.
87. Lipton, S: Pain: An update. In Lipton, S, (eds): Advances in Pain Research and Therapy, Vol 13. Raven Press, New York, 1990, pp 1–9.
88. Grieve, GP: Common vertebral joint problems. Churchill-Livingstone, Edinburgh, 1988, pp 319–333.
89. Saal, JS, Franson, RC, Dobrow, R, Saal, JA, White, AH, and Goldthwaite, N: High levels of inflammatory phospholipase A2 activity in lumbar disc herniations. Spine 15(7):674–678, 1990.
90. Bayliss, MT, Johnstone, B, and O'Brien, JP: Proteoglycan synthesis in the human intervertebral disc. Variation with age, region and pathology. Spine 13(9):972–981, 1988.
91. Hampton, D, Laros, G, McCarron, R, and Franks, D: Healing potential of the annulus fibrosus. Spine 14(4):398–401, 1989.
92. Osti, OL, Vernon-Roberts, B, and Fraser, RD: Annulus tears and intervertebral disc degeneration. An experimental study using an animal model. Spine 15(8):762–767, 1990.
93. Butler, D, Trafimow, JH, Andersson, GBL, McNeill, TW, and Huckman, MS: Discs degenerate before facets. Spine 15(2):111–113, 1990.
94. Keller, TS, Holm, SH, Hansson, TH, and Spengler, DM: The dependence of intervertebral disc mechanical properties on physiological conditions. Spine 15(8):751–761, 1990.
95. Bogduk, N: The innervation of the lumbar spine. Spine 8(3):286–293, 1983.
96. Bogduk, N: Lumbar dorsal ramus syndromes. In Grieve, G (ed): Modern Manual Therapy of the Vertebral Column. Churchill-Livingstone, Edinburgh, 1986, pp 396–404.
97. Mooney, V: Facet joint syndrome, In: Jayson MIV (ed): The Lumbar Spine and Back Pain, ed 3. Churchill-Livingstone, Edinburgh, 1987, pp 370–382.
98. Mooney, V and Robertson, J: The facet syndrome. Clin Orthop 115:149–156, 1976.
99. Campbell, JN, Raja, SN, Cohen, RH, Manning, DC, Khan, H, and Meyer, RA: Peripheral neural mechanisms of nociception. In Wall, PD and Melzack, R (eds): Textbook of Pain, ed 2. Churchill-Livingstone, London, 1989, pp 22–45.
100. Wyke, BD: The neurology of low back pain. In Jayson, MIV (ed): The Lumbar Spine and Back Pain, ed 2. Kent Pitman Medical, London, 1980, pp 265–339.
101. Giles, LGF: Anatomical Basis of Low Back Pain. Williams & Wilkins, Baltimore, 1989, pp 58–66.
102. Beaman, D, Glover, R, Graziano, G, and Wojtys, E: Substance P Innervation of Lumbar Facet Joints. Abstract of paper presented at the International Society for the Study of the Lumbar Spine, Chicago, IL, May 20–24, 1991.
103. Konttinen, YT, Gronblad, M, Korkala, O, Tolvanen, E, and Polak, JM: Immunohisto-

chemical demonstration of subclasses of inflammatory cells and active, collagen-producing fibroblasts in the synovial plicae of lumbar facet joints. Spine 15(5):387–390, 1990.

104. Cailliet, R: Tissue sites of low back pain. In Low Back Pain Syndrome, ed 4. FA Davis, Philadelphia, 1988, pp 66–68.

105. Mooney, V: Where is the pain coming from? Spine 12(8):749–754, 1987.

106. Yoshizawa, H, Kobayashi, S, and Kuboto, K: Effects of compression on intraradicular blood flow in dogs. Spine 14(11):1220–1225, 1989.

107. Hoyland, JA, Freemont, AJ, and Jayson, MIV: Intervertebral foramen vertebral obstruction. A cause of periradicular fibrosus? Spine 14(6):558–568, 1989.

108. Wall, PD and Devor, M: Sensory afferent impulses originating from dorsal root ganglia as well as from the periphery in normal and nerve-injured rats. Pain 17:321–339, 1983.

109. Devor, M: The pathophysiology of damaged peripheral nerves. In Wall, PD and Melzack, R (eds): Textbook of Pain, ed 2. Churchill-Livingstone, London, 1989, pp 63–81.

110. Rydevik, BL, Meyers, RR, and Powell, HC: Pressure increase in the dorsal root ganglion following mechanical compression, closed compartment syndrome in nerve roots. Spine 14(6):574–576, 1989.

111. Spencer, DL, Miller, JAA, and Bertolini, JE: The effect of intervertebral disc space narrowing on the contact force between the nerve root and a simulated disc protrusion. Spine 9:422–426, 1984.

112. Sugimoto, T, Bennett, GJ, and Kajander, KC: Transynaptic degeneration in the superficial dorsal horn after sciatic nerve injury: Effects of a chronic constriction injury, transection and strychnine. Pain 42(2):205–214, 1990.

113. Menses, S: Structure of functional relationships in identified afferent neurones. Anat Embryol (Berl) 181:1–17, 1990.

114. Simmonds, M and Kumar, S: The bases of low back pain. Neuro-Orthop 13:1–14, 1992.

115. McKenzie, RA: The Lumbar Spine: Mechanical Diagnosis and Therapy. Spinal Publications, Waikanae, NZ, 1981.

116. Hullinger, M: Mammalian muscle spindle and its central control. Rev Physiol 101:1–110, 1984.

117. Mathews, PBC: Muscle spindles and their motor control. Physiol Review 44:219–288, 1964.

118. Floyd, WF and Silver, PHS: The function of the erector spinae muscles in certain movements and postures in man. J Physiol 129:184, 1955.

119. McGill, SM and Norman, RW: Partitioning of the L4-5: Dynamic movement into disk, ligamentous and muscular components during lifting. Spine 11:666, 1986.

120. Altschule, MD: Emotion and skeletal muscle function. Med Sci 2:163, 1962.

121. Jacobson, E: Electrical measurements of neuromuscular states during mental activities: Imagination of movement involving skeletal muscles. Am J Physiol 91:567, 1930.

122. Papciak, AS and Feuerstein, M: Psychological factors affecting isokinetic trunk strength testing in patients with work-related chronic low back pain. J Occup Rehab 1(2):95–104, 1991.

123. Myles, LM and Glasby, MA: The fate of muscle spindles after various methods of nerve repair in the rat. Neuroorthoped 13:15–23, 1992.

124. Banks, RW and Barker, D: Specificities of afferents reinnervating cat muscle spindles after nerve section. J Physiol 408:345–372, 1989.

125. Crock, HV: Practice of Spinal Surgery. Springer-Verlag, New York, 1983.

126. Farfan, HF, Cossette, JW, Robertson, GH, Wells, RV, and Kraus, H: The effects of torsion on the lumbar intervertebral joints: The role of torsion in the production of disk degeneration. J Bone Joint Surg 52A:468, 1970.

127. Gunzburg, R, Hutton, WC, Crane, G, and Fraser, RD: Role of the capsulo-ligamentous structures in rotation and combined flexion-rotation of the lumbar spine. Journal of Spinal Disorders 5(1):1–7, 1992.

244   PAIN: MECHANISMS AND MANAGEMENT

128. Cailliet, R: Low Back Pain Syndrome, ed 4. FA Davis, Philadelphia, 1988.
129. Crock, HV: Internal disc disruption. Spine 11(6):650–653, 1986.
130. Crock, HV and Goldwasser, M: Anatomic studies of the circulation in the region of the vertebral end plates in adult greyhound dogs. Spine 9:702–706, 1984.
131. Naylor, A and Horton, W: Hydrophilic properties of the intervertebral disc. Rheumatism 11:32–35, 1955.
132. Weinstein, J: Mechanisms of spinal pain: The dorsal root ganglion and its role as mediator of low back pain. Spine 11:999–1001, 1986.
133. Saal, JS, Franson, RC, Dodbrow, R, Saul, JA, White, AA, and Goldwaithe, N: High levels of inflammatory phospholipase A2 activity in lumbar disc herniations. Spine 15:674–678, 1990.
134. Gardner, E: The innervation of the hip joint. Anat Rec 101:353–371, 1959.
135. Ravin, EL: Mechanical aspects of osteoarthrosis. Bull Rheum Dis 26(7):862–865, 1975–1976.
136. Trueta, J and Harrison, MHM: Normal vascular anatomy of femoral head in adult man. J Bone Joint Surg 35:442–461, 1953.
137. Blount, WP: Don't throw away the cane. J Bone Joint Surg 38A:695, 1956.
138. Cailliet, R: Hip joint pain. Soft Tissue Pain and Disability. FA Davis, Philadelphia, 1988, pp 244–265.
139. Hilton, J: Rest and Pain. Wm Wood, New York, 1879.
140. Cailliet, R: Knee Pain and Disability, ed 3. FA Davis, Philadelphia, 1992.
141. Bessette, GC and Hunter, RE: The anterior cruciate ligament. Orthopedics 13(5):551, 1990.
142. Noyes, FR, Movar, PA, Matthews, DS, and Butler, DL: The symptomatic anterior cruciate deficient knee. Part I: The long-term functional disability in athletically active individuals. J Bone Joint Surg 65A:154–162, 1982.
143. Steindler, A: Pain syndromes of foot, ankle and leg. In Lectures on the Interpretation of Pain in Orthopedic Practice. Charles C Thomas, Springfield, IL, 1959, pp 606–658.
144. Haymaker, W and Woodhall, B: Peripheral Nerve Injuries: Principles of Diagnosis, ed 2. WB Saunders, Philadelphia, 1953, pp 113–119.
145. Cailliet, R: Foot and Ankle Pain. FA Davis, Philadelphia, 1968.
146. Cailliet, R: Foot and ankle pain. In Soft Tissue Pain and Disability, ed. 2. FA Davis, Philadelphia, 1988, pp 307–365.
147. Bonica, JJ: General considerations of abdominal pain. In The Management of Pain, Vol 2, ed 2. Lea & Febiger, Philadelphia, 1990, pp 1146–1185.
148. Andrews, PLR: Vagal afferent innervation of the gastrointestinal tract. In Cervero, F and Morrison, JEH (eds): Visceral sensation. Elsevier, Amsterdam, 1986, pp 65–86.
149. Thompson, GE, Moore, DC, Bridenbaugh, LD, and Artin, RY: Abdominal pain and alcohol celiac block. Anesth Analg 56:1, 1977.
150. Chan, WY, Dowood, MY, and Fuchs, F: Prostaglandins in primary dysmenorrhea comparison of prophylactic and nonprophylactic treatment with ibuprofen and use of oral contraceptives. Am J Med 70(3):535–541, 1981.
151. Pickles, UR, Hall, WJ, Best, FA, and Smith, GV: Prostaglandins in endometrium and menstrual fluid from normal and dysmenorrheic subjects. Br J Obstet Gynaecol 72:185, 1965.
152. Hansen, MK and Seiber, NJ: Beta-receptor stimulation in essential dysmenorrhea. Am J Obstet Gynecol 121(4):566–567, 1975.
153. McArthur, JW and Ultelder, H: The effect of pregnancy upon endometriosis. Obstet Gynecol 20:709, 1965.
154. Chaparro, MV, Ghosh, S, Nashed, A, and Poliok, A: Laparoscopy for confirmation and prognostic evaluation of pelvic inflammatory disease. Int J Gynaecol Obstet 15(4):307–309, 1978.

155. Bonica, JJ: General considerations of pain in the pelvis and perineum. The Management of Pain, Vol 2, ed 2. Lea & Febiger, Philadelphia, 1990, pp 1302–1312.
156. Beard, RW: Pelvic pain in women. Am J Obstet Gynecol 128(5):566–572, 1977.
157. Bonica, JJ: Obstetric Analgesia and Anesthesia, ed 2. University of Washington Press, Seattle, 1980, pp 2–5.
158. American Heart Association: 1987 Heart Facts. American Heart Association, New York, 1986.
159. Bonica, JJ: General considerations of pain in the chest. The Management of Pain, Vol 2, ed 2. Lea & Febiger, Philadelphia, 1990, pp 973–1000.
160. Wenckebach, KF: Angina pectoris and the possibilities of its surgical relief. BMJ 1:809, 1924.
161. Agostini, E: Functional and histological studies of the vagus nerve and its branches to the heart, lung and abdominal viscera in the cat. J Physiol 135:182, 1975.
162. Brown, AM: Excitation of afferent cardiac sympathetic nerve fibers during myocardial ischemia. J Physiol 190:35, 1967.
163. White, JC: Cardiac pain. Anatomic pathways and physiological mechanisms. Circulation 16:644, 1957.
164. Malliani, A: Cardiovascular sympathetic afferent fibers. Rev Physiol Biochem Pharmacol 94:11, 1982.
165. Malliani, A: The elusive link between transient myocardial ischemia and pain. Circulation 73:203, 1986.
166. Keefer, CS and Renick, WH: Angina pectoris: A syndrome caused by anoxia of the myocardium. Arch Intern Med 41:469, 1928.
167. Heberden, W: Commentaries on the History and Cure of Diseases. Payne, London, 1802.
168. Blair, RW, Weber, RN, and Foreman, RD: Characteristics of primate spinothalamic tract neurons receiving viscerosomatic convergent inputs in T3–T5 segments. J Neurophysiol 46:797, 1981.
169. Ross, R: The pathogenesis of atherosclerosis: An update. N Engl J Med 314:488–500, 1986.
170. Fuster, V, Badimon, L, Badimon, JJ, and Chesebro, JH: The pathogenesis of coronary artery disease and the acute coronary syndromes. Mechanisms of disease. New Engl J Med 326(4):242–250, 1992.
171. Spurlock, BO and Chandler, AB: Adherent platelets and surface microthrombi of human aorta and left coronary artery: A scanning electron microscopy feasibility study. Scanning Microsc 1 :1359–1365, 1987. (Erratum. Scanning Microsc 2:1214, 1988.)

CHAPTER 9

Chronic Pain

Chronic pain is a national problem involving unnecessary suffering, overwhelming disability, personal impairment, and incredible expense. Chronic pain is no longer merely a symptom but has become a disease in its own right. The physician is responsible for recognizing, diagnosing, and treating chronic pain.

In a classic dissertation, *The Culture of Pain*, David Morris states that pain pervades all aspects of human social life and emotions and has done so since antiquity.[1] Aristotle wrote in *De Anima* that "pain upsets and destroys the nature of the person who feels it." Nevertheless, pain has been given little consideration in the training of today's physician.

Viewing pain as a "perception" rather than as a "sensation" has changed our understanding and management of the problem. Models need to be devised that fully explain the concept of pain. The biomedical model underlies traditional Western medicine. Research in neurophysiology, neuropharmacology, and hormonal studies have advanced our knowledge of pain. Great strides have been made in treating acute, recurrent, and even chronic pain.

Chronic pain from discernible causes appears better understood, but so-called benign pain—pain with no discernible cause—remains an enigma. Benign pain has become epidemic.[2] It is now open to question whether the physician is the only person who can solve this problem. Many people in society influence the life of a chronic-pain patient: psychologists, religious leaders, entertainers, and family members.

Figure 9–1 shows one way of viewing pain, postulated by Sternbach.[3] The peripheral mechanisms of pain were recognized early in the 1950s, largely owing to J.J. Bonica's seminal work, *The Management of Pain*.[4] His approach highlighted the efficacy of interrupting pain by blocking the nerve from the afflicted organ or tissue considered to be the site of pain. This

246

Figure 9–1. Pain, a concept. (Adapted from Sternbach, RA: Strategies and tactics in the treatment of patients with pain. In Crue, L: Pain and Suffering. Charles C Thomas, Springfield, Illinois, 1970, p 177.)

PAIN IS
(Choose One)

Elementary Sensation

Complex Perception

Affect (Emotion)

Neurophysiologic Activity
Neurochemical Stress Reaction

Reflex Adaptive Behavior
Result of Internal Psychic Conflict

Interpersonal Manipulation

Human Condition

"peripheral" concept of pain transmission is still considered valid in understanding and managing acute, recurrent, and even chronic pain.

Considering pain as exclusively a peripheral manifestation was questioned by Crue,[5] who, as a neurosurgeon, realized that interruption of the peripheral nerve in tic douloureux did not relieve the pain in many patients. He had observed that many acute pains neurosurgically relieved by peripheral nerve intervention persisted. He deduced that pain must originate in the brain in some way other than in the periphery. He postulated this as an illness, which he termed benign chronic intractable pain syndrome (BCIPS). Crue did not imply that pain was imagined, unreal, or "mental." He considered it to be central and added a psychologist to his team for evaluating and treating chronic pain. However, he admitted that many if not most chronic pain syndromes began as organic or traumatic peripheral injuries.

Crue's concept began the controversy of peripheralists and centralists in understanding pain. He recognized the dichotomy and stated,

> The overwhelming majority of patients we see with chronic intractable pain syndromes have had both their pain syndrome and their pain behavior iatrogenically reinforced over and over again. Many of them have been subjected to mutilating operative procedures, where the only reasonable expectation was, quite frankly, the placebo effect. It is time that neurosurgeons, orthopedists, and anesthesiologists admit that with few rare exceptions they are bankrupt when it comes to treating chronic intractable benign pain syndrome patients.[6]

See also the article by Cailliet[7] "Chronic Pain: Is it Necessary?"

Crue also brought into consideration the term *pain behavior*, which is now the mainstay in understanding chronic pain. He issued a challenge to physicians to define the term *placebo* and clarify the concept of "all in the mind" from a neurohormonal point of view.[7a]

Placebo had implied tricking the mind into believing useless admonitions. The sugar water medication "cured" the illness. Norman Cousins, suffering from a severe organic disease, wrote of the significant benefit he received from laughter incited by viewing comic movies. This benefit was attributed to the placebo effect, allegedly mind over body.[8] Plato, Socrates, and the Roman poet Horace all note the use of comic relief of pain.[1] The

English playwright Christopher Fry wrote, "In tragedy we suffer pain: in comedy pain is a fool: suffered gladly."[9]

Chronic pain evaluation and management is at a crossroads. Notwithstanding the effectiveness of neurophysiologic and neuropharmacologic treatment of pain, the multidisciplinary approach is emerging as of equal importance. This approach makes use of physiologic, emotional, cognitive, and social pain relief modalities.[10]

The future is provoked in the statement of the French philosopher Jean-François Lyotard, who describes evaluation and acceptance of postmodernism as related to "metanarratives," in which current ideas lose their power.[11] Among metanarratives he includes Christianity, Marxism, and the organic model of pain. As recently as 1948 an eminent neurologist writing in a text called *Pain* failed to even mention psychosocial aspects.[12]

What is the role of pain in the relationship between disability and impairment? This mundane question has been implied in the cost effectiveness of pain management altering the impairment-causing disability.[13,14] The accepted definition of disability is "lack of ability to perform mental or physical tasks that one can normally do." This contrasts with the definition of impairment as damage, injury, or deterioration.[15] Neither definition has significant objective signs to quantify the documentation. The patient's terms quantify the degree and intensity.

In 1984 an amendment to the Social Security Act (PL 98-460) included the first statutory standard defining how pain should be evaluated in determining eligibility for disability benefits. A committee of the Institute of Medicine clarified some of the confusion.[16]

The Subcommittee on Taxonomy of the International Association for the Study of Pain (IASP 1986) considers pain of 3 months' duration to be chronic pain.[17] Crue considers chronic pain as pain that lasts more than 6 months,[5] Bonica labeled chronic pain as pain that "persists past the usual 'time' for that particular disorder to heal,"[4] and Watson defined chronic pain as "pain that persists one month or past the usual 'time' for that particular disorder to heal."[18] It becomes obvious that these definitions depend on the "expected duration of a specific disease causing pain to abate." "Time" apparently decides when pain goes from acute to chronic and differs with various clinicians.

According to Dwarakanath, "Pain is considered chronic and not related to the significance of tissue injury and thus serves no useful purpose. . . . It is a disorder that can be either somatic or psychological."[19] Acute pain is considered limited and resulting from increased activity of peripheral nociceptors and their afferents. Chronic pain is considered to exist when these afferents continue to discharge after the nociceptive stimuli are no longer active. Mechanoreceptor activity transmitting sensations such as touch and temperature are now considered to be sensitized and capable of initiating pain. Sympathetic mediated pain (SMP) may also be involved,[20] but considering chronic pain to be exclusively mediated via sympathetic nervous pathways is not acceptable.

It has been postulated but not fully accepted that impaired gate control is the neurophysiologic mechanism of chronic pain. Chronic pain is not merely a prolongation of an acute process. It must be viewed as resulting from changes both in the peripheral and the central nervous system.[21]

The terminals of the peripheral nerves at the tissue site of injury undergo chemical and mechanical changes. There are local vasomotor changes with formation of edema that increase the sensitivity of the nerve endings, changing thresholds and allowing them to fire from minimal stimuli. This increased sensitivity allows innocuous stimuli to initiate and prolong the resultant pain.

Chronically and persistently irritated afferent peripheral nerve fibers also lead to hyperexcitability of the spinal cord dorsal horn cells. This has been confirmed experimentally from repeated electrical stimulation, which has demonstrated reformation of the dorsal horn from this bombardment.[22]

Not only have the receptor neurons increased in number and size, but the thresholds of mechanosensitive, nociceptive-specific (NS) neurons, and wide dynamic range (WDR) neurons have been lowered. These findings indicate that the dorsal horn cells are not only more sensitive to peripheral nociceptive impulses but are also more sensitive to mechanical stimuli because of decreased resistance at the synapses.[23,24]

Failure to adequately interrupt bombardment from the peripheral afferents increases the sensitivity of central receptors at the dorsal root ganglia (DRG) and the dorsal horn gray matter.[25]

The reflex myogenic aspect of pain—protective muscle spasm—now becomes an enhancer of nociception as well as a new source of nociception.[26,27] Irritation of a muscle sends afferent impulses through the DRG to the specific area in the dorsal gray column, simultaneously increasing the plasticity of the dorsal ganglion, the neurons in laminae I and II, and the WDR neurons. More input is thus transmitted to the lateral spinothalamic tracts.

Hu identified a similar neuronal composition of the trigeminal nerve (spinal tract nucleus).[28] This peripheral nerve is identical to the dorsal horn cells within the cord.[29,30] Thus there is a similar relationship between the cranial nerves and the more distal cord segmental innervations. Hu also irritated the masseter muscle, a segmentally related muscle, with 5 percent mustard oil injection (Fig. 9–2). This activated small-diameter afferent nerves with a correspondent excitation of the dorsal horn and ventral horn neurons. A similar condition apparently occurs in the cranial nerves as occurs in the spinal cord segments.

Pain can occur in the absence or interruption of peripheral afferent nerves. Afferent impulses originating from destroyed or interrupted axons, termed "deafferentation," may occur from a growth of sprouts at the end of the severed nerve. (Fig. 9–3). These nerve sprouts contain alpha receptors

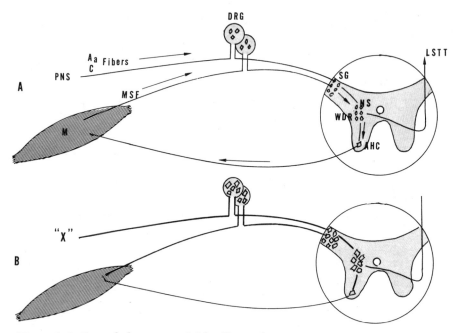

Figure 9–2. Expanded receptive fields of hyperalgesia.

(A), The accepted routes on nociception from the peripheral nociceptive sites (PNS) via the A alpha and C fibers through the dorsal root ganglia (DRG), into the dorsal horn of the cord, into the Rexed layers I and II (substantia gelatinosa [SG]). A response results in the nociceptive specific (NS) neurons with reaction of the wide dynamic range (WDR) neurons. Ultimately, the impulses are transmitted to the limbic system and cortex via the laterospinal thalamic tracts (LSTT) as pain.

Sensory fibers ascending to the DRG are within the muscle sensory fibers (MSF) to the contiguous muscles of the root level. The motor fibers to the muscle descend from the anterior horn cell (AHC), which has internuncial connection to the WDR neurons.

(B), Hyperalgesia occurs from intense, continuous, or repeated nociception in the periphery ("X"). These barrages increase the number and the sensitivity of the nerve cells within the DRG and the SG resulting in increased sensitivity of the entire pathways of pain leading to chronicity.

The increased sensitivity also explains why mechanoreceptors in the periphery entering the WDR may initiate pain although the impulses are not nociceptive. Irritation of the muscle (M) can transmit pain sensation via the MSF to also increase the pain. This theory explains the resultant painful muscle in the region of the nerve root involvement and places muscle as a nociceptive site in chronic pain.

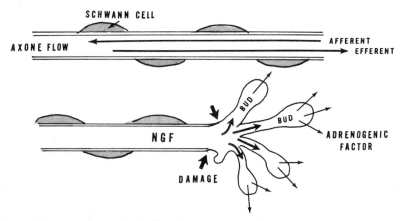

Figure 9–3. Axonal outgrowths forming a neuroma.
After a nerve injury with compression or partial to total severance, the nerve growth factor (NGF) stimulates the nerve to advance distally and form "buds," which create more endings than the normal nerve shown in the upper drawing.
By virtue of the greater secretion of adrenogenic factors from these additional buds, the nerve becomes more sensitive to adrenogenic agonists and transmits more potential pain fiber impulses to the spinal cord.

that are sensitive to adrenaline and become more sensitive to mechanical stimuli (Fig. 9–4). Sensitivity is neither altered nor reversed by local treatment directed to the peripheral tissue site.

Peripheral nociceptor sites considered to be in the arteries postulate a neural pathway in migraine, migraine variants, and facial neuralgia (Fig. 9–5).[31] In addition to the vascular component, a muscular component exists in these head and face pain syndromes.

The increased sensitivity of the DRG from increased peripheral sensitivity is proposed in the "pool" concepts (Fig. 9–6). The proteins and peptides created at the DRG are neurotransmitters that are transported distally to the peripheral terminals and centrally to the Rexed layers of the dorsal columns (Fig. 9–7).

When a peripheral nerve is cut, the chemicals in the spinal cord afferents (layers of Rexed I and II: substantia gelatinosa) are diminished, as are those within the dorsal root of that nerve. Variations of this central sensitivity noted after severance of the peripheral nerve may occur to a degree after mere injury to a peripheral nerve.

There are two postulated mechanisms for denervation hypersensitivity: (1) new acetylcholine chemoreceptors appear in the areas of the innervated membrane, and (2) the membrane, now altered, undergoes changes in its electrical properties and ionic permeability, especially with regard to sodium and potassium ions.[32]

These changes not only increase sensitivity but may permit continued

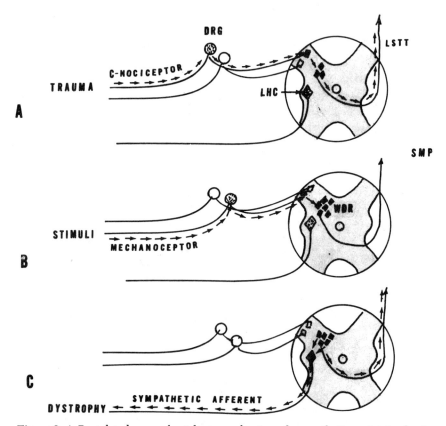

Figure 9–4. Postulated neurophysiologic mechanism of sympathetic-maintained pain (SMP).

The transmission via C-nociceptor fibers *(A)* of impulses from the peripheral tissues that have been traumatized and created peripheral nociceptor chemicals (see details in text). These impulses pass through the dorsal root ganglion (DRG) to activate the gray matter of the cord in the Rexed layers. When sensitized, they are termed wide dynamic range (WDR) neurons. The WDR, becoming very irritated, receive impulses from the periphery via the A-mechanoreceptors fibers *(B)*, which normally transmit sensations of touch, vibration, temperature and so on. When the periphery is stimulated (skin touch, pressure, or joint movement), these impulses enhance and maintain the irritability of the WDR. The impulses from the WDR continue cephalad through the laterospinal thalamic tracts (LSTT) to the thalamic centers with resultant continued pain. The WDR impulses irritate the lateral horn cells (LHC), which generate sympathetic impulses that innervate the peripheral tissues resulting in the symptoms and findings of dystrophy *(C)*.

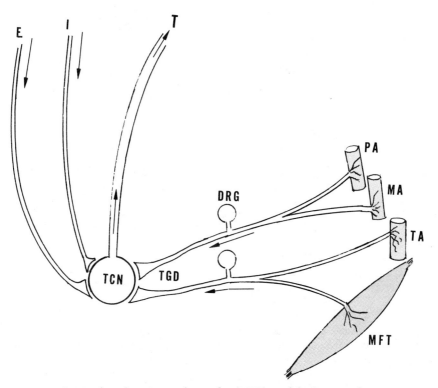

Figure 9–5. Myofascial supraspinal vascular (MSV) model of pain pathways.

The input into the pain neural pathways are depicted in this MSV model. The afferent impulses originating from the pial arteries (PA), meningeal arteries (MA), and the temporal arteries (TA), compete with the nociceptive impulses of the myofascial tissues (MFT).

All impulses converge through their dorsal root ganglia (DRG) to the trigeminal ganglion (1st) division nucleus (TCN). Modulation of these impulses that ultimately enter the thalamus (T) occurs from descending excitatory (E) and inhibitory (I) fibers from cortical levels.

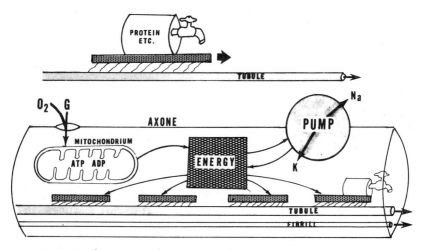

Figure 9–6. Axoplasmic neural transport, a theory.

The flow of protein and other derivatives begins with entry of glucose (G) into the fiber. Glycolysis and phosphorylation occurs (O_2) in the mitochondria through metabolism of adenosine triphosphate (ATP), which creates the energy to the sodium pump. This pump regulates balance of sodium (Na) and potassium (K) and determines nerve activity.

The transport filaments (F) move along the axon by oscillation and carry the nutritive protein elements along the nerve pathway. (*Data from* Ochs: Axoplasmic transport—A basis for neural pathology.)

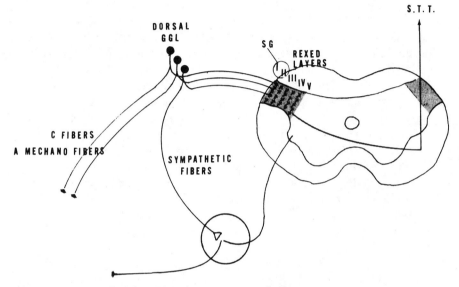

Figure 9–7. Causalgic (autonomic) transmission of pain sensation.
Trauma irritates somatic afferent C-fibers, A-mechanofibers, and sympathetic fibers, whose impulses proceed to the dorsal column of the cord. A cord interneuron connection transmits efferent impulses via the autonomic system to the periphery, which sensitizes the skin to mechanical (light touch) input.

At the cord, the afferent fibers initiate neuronal activity in the Rexed layers of the dorsal column. The Rexed layers I and II are the substantia gelatinosa. (Modified from Roberts, WS: A hypothesis on the physiological basis for causalgia and related pains. Pain 24:297, 1986.)

afferent impulses to be transported via the unmyelinated and A-alpha sparsely myelinated nerves and interfere with the synaptic inhibition at the gate of the dorsal horn. This "dissociation" at the gate may result in chronic pain.

All the above neurophysiologic aspects of chronic pain emphasize the visceral basis; yet current chronic pain concepts appear to have a psychologic basis. Acute pain is made worse by anxiety and anticipation, which is not as apparent in chronic pain. Patients with chronic pain appear more depressed with symptoms of sleep disturbance, reduced energy, difficulty in concentration, irritability, and other similar mood changes.

Chronic pain is considered to be pain behavior with a learned component. The term *psychogenic pain* is no longer accepted as its original description was "symptoms from psychological causes." This led to pain differentiation as "psychogenic versus genuine (organic) pain."[33]

Depression accompanying pain has been viewed as either "the" cause or "a result": the latter is considered to be a reactive depression. Various terms have evolved, such as *learned pain* or *operant pain*.[34] Chronic pain behavior is divided into two variants: respondent behavior or operant behavior. *Respondent behavior* was termed appropriate as a response to a nociceptive stimulus and unrelated to a learned reaction or influenced by the environment. *Operant behavior*, on the other hand, is considered to be related to the patient's past learning and influenced by the current environment. Reward is prominent: the greater the "reward," the greater the reaction.

Both respondent and operant reactions apply in many cases, and patients with significant organic lesions develop secondary emotional changes, justifying treating chronic pain as a somatic illness while addressing the psychologic aspects.[35] There is a need to delineate the illness into subgroups depending on the percentage of organic to psychologic reaction.

Meaningful outcome assessments are desperately needed to clarify this situation. Sternbach claimed that there was no proof that operant programs work any better than other intervention programs, as there are no adequate controlled studies.[36]

A multidisciplinary team can furnish this expertise and determine appropriate psychotherapy, be it analytic, supportive, group, or cognitive.[37–40] The available expertise and prejudices of the pain center often determine the form of psychotherapy that is recommended.

Chronic pain is often treated according to a uniform protocol, whether appropriate or not. Wherein lies the high rate of failure. For example, patients with low back pain routinely undergo exercise and education in body mechanics by the physical therapist and occupational therapist, biofeedback, transcutaneous electrical nerve stimulation (TENS), operant conditioning, nerve blocks, family counseling, assertiveness training, stress management, and systemic medication, usually of antidepression type. Whether these factors are all pertinent appear irrelevant.[41] All patients with this diagnosis are similarly approached and equally treated.

Temporomandibular joint (TMJ) arthralgia has also been categorized as a homogeneous group with all patients undergoing similar treatment.[42] Individual differences of the patients suffering this malady are ignored; thus, the quality of life remains unchanged after therapeutic intervention.[43]

A change in this homogeneous classification was proposed by the Institute of Medicine.[44] Subgroups divided according to diagnostic criteria and definitions have been designed.[45,46] However, similar studies have not yet evolved to ascertain the appropriate treatment and outcomes assessment for each of these classifications.

The diagnostic criteria classify subgroups according to (1) body region, (2) system involved, (3) temporal characteristics, (4) intensity and duration of symptoms, and (5) etiology.[47] Factors such as age, education, personality, psychopathology, socioeconomic status, and response to previous treatment are not included in this subgroup classification.

Recently, the psychologic aspects of pain have been emphasized, studied, and classified, but much remains to be discovered, as the psychosocial aspects—ethnic, racial, religious, and educational—have been only partially explored.[48] The same is true of specific demographics such as disease status, prior treatment, pending litigation, or compensation. It raises the question, Are current studies that classify psychopathology adequate and appropriate?[49]

The Minnesota Multiphasic Personality Inventory (MMPI) test has been used to assess the personality of pain patients,[50] but this test was originally standardized on psychiatric patients, not on general medical patients.[51] The MMPI describes four different subgroups of chronic pain patients: those with hypochondriasis, reactive depression, somatization, and manipulative reaction. The MMPI remains conjectural as to its accuracy, implications, and categorization of chronic-pain patients.[52,53]

Patients with chronic-pain proneness profiles on the MMPI have elevated scores for hypochondriasis and hysteria and lower scores for depression.[54] This configuration has been termed "conversion-V," indicating that the patient being tested uses physical symptoms to cope with psychologic distress that he or she is unable to confront or resolve. This finding has been questioned as there are many variables among subjects and the same profile is found among medically ill patients who feel disabled by their illness.[55,56] Chronic-pain patients produce MMPI profiles similar to patients with chronic hypertension and diabetes.[57]

The Symptom Checklist-90 (SCL-90) has been suggested as a possible test for chronic-pain patients.[58] This test is a 90-item checklist of psychiatric and physical symptoms involving somatization, obsession, interpersonal sensitivity, depression, anxiety, hostility, phobic anxiety, paranoia, and psychotic behavior. All items are graded on a scale from 0 to 5, with 0 being

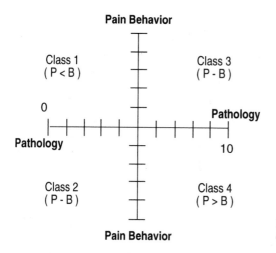

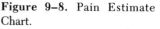

Figure 9–8. Pain Estimate Chart.

"not at all" and 5 being "extremely." The SCL-90 test was also devised for psychiatric patients and faces the same scrutiny as does the MMPI.[59]

Depression is frequently noted in chronic-pain patients, and its relationship to cognitive factors is significant.[60]

The Automatic Thoughts Questionnaire (ATQ), which consists of 30 negative statements, has been used to determine depression in chronic-pain patients.[61] The significance of depression in a chronic-pain patient influences the therapeutic approach.[62] A questionnaire is available to assess depression, but it is time-consuming.[63] It is best utilized by psychologists or psychiatrists, not by family practitioners or primary physicians.

If pain syndromes are not broken down into subgroups with categorized treatment and meaningful outcome assessment, all chronic pain management will remain empirical.

To validate a more precise test than the MMPI in determining pain behavior, Hendler devised the Mensana Clinic Back Pain Test (MCBPT).[64] Whereas the MMPI measures personality traits, the MCBPT measures the impact of pain on the patient's life and is considered a better predictor of the validity of the pain complaint. The Hendler 10-minute screening test for chronic back pain patients is a patient's verbal determination of the pain and has been used primarily to predict the possible success of surgery in relieving pain.[65]

Brena and Koch proposed the pain estimate chart (Fig. 9–8) to qualify and quantify chronic pain.[66] There are numerous factors used to compile this model: (1) a physician-based pathology assessment, (2) a patient-based pain assessment, (3) a physician-based assessment of pathology behavior correlates, and (4) a resultant pain state classification and description.

The physician-based pathology assessment relies on physical examination, neurologic examination, radiology studies, and laboratory studies. None explain the significance of pain other than revealing "organic pathology." The patient-based assessment is a self-determination of pain as depicted by verbalization of the pain quantity, level of patient activity permitted by the pain, drug use, and MMPI, which measures the psychologic adjustment to the pain.

The physician-based assessment of pathologic behavior correlates is divided into classes using terms such as "pain amplifiers," "pain verbalizers," "chronic sufferers," and "pain reducers," indicating the use or overuse of drugs. All these are subjective and are interpreted by the physician, who estimates the value of the complaints and the complainer.

This test, which aims to objectively quantify pain and explain its predominant components, fails to be truly objective and has not been reproducible by varying examiners. The "pathology" ascertained by the physician (or therapist) includes joint range of motion, strength, and endurance, which cannot be standardized.

The classes determining behavior are subjective and cannot be objectively quantified. According to Brena class 4 patients, who have a high score on pathology and a low score on pain behavior, ideally should be able to cope with pain and should not be considered candidates for comprehensive therapy, but merely recipients of the somatic aspects of the programs offered.

The significance of financial gain from pain is being objectively studied, but its value is not yet ascertained.[67]

Of the estimated 450 chronic-pain treatment centers in the United States as of 1989, approximately 20 were truly multidisciplinary.[68] These centers are divided into broad categories: outpatient monomodal clinics, multidisciplinary outpatient, inpatient monomodal clinic, inpatient multidisciplinary clinic, and free-standing multidisciplinary clinic. Being in the medical model, their relationship to hospitals is implied.

In most treatment centers, the treatment goals for a particular patient determine the type of treatment setting and personnel that the physician selects. The desires or needs of the patient depend on the treatment facilities and personnel available.

The goals of current centers are (1) changing patient behavior, which is often accomplished while the patient is in the inpatient service but not always appropriate for the discharge environment, and (2) treating a "specific" disorder when a clear-cut disorder can be diagnosed. This is difficult in most cases of chronic pain. The somatic diagnosis is rarely the specific cause of the pain yet it is predominantly addressed. Drug withdrawal, a basic intent, is not necessarily effective and may be detrimental.

Treatment of depression or anxiety is advocated and acceptable, but as depression and anxiety may be secondary to chronic pain, it often responds to the relief of pain and disability.

Pain therapies such as TENS, biofeedback, acupuncture, physical therapy, psychopharmacologic intervention, hypnosis, and so forth are valuable but are nonspecific and may be used interminably without permanent or significant benefit. Their use, albeit beneficial and desirable, should not constitute the major or only modality; this is the criticism of centers that are predominantly nerve block, acupuncture, or physical therapy centers.

Improved family relations, including marital and sexual problems, must be approached as an aspect of multidiscipline intervention but must not be stated to be the major or only factor in chronic pain.[68]

A major concern is patient selection. A patient suffering chronic cancer pain needs numerous components of the treatment protocols tailored to the disease, its duration, severity, psychologic impairment, and acceptance by the patient.

The pain center clinic personnel remain in the medical model, usually with a physician as director.[69] This raises an important question as to what qualifications and training this physician must have to be the director. The "specialization" of the director usually indicates the model that the center will embody. Currently, there is no regulatory body for licensing and certifying chronic pain centers, nor is the specialty of chronic pain management, the "algologist," as yet a certified or accepted specialty.

Last but not least in evaluating the benefit to the patient undergoing chronic-pain therapy is the compliance of the patient with the program both during care and after discharge.[70] Outcome assessment of any program, any precise diagnosis of a subclass, and any proffered treatment program must address patient compliance.

An acceptable effective model of pain management—and hence the goal of a multidisciplinary center— must address *all* components of pain mentioned heretofore. The West Haven–Yale Multidimensional Pain Inventory has been proposed to assess pain patients.[71,72] This inventory contains (1) a report of pain severity and suffering "as felt and quantified by the patient"; (2) an assessment of how the pain interferes with the patient's life, including professional and social life, family relationships, and sexual functioning; (3) the level of satisfaction or dissatisfaction with the current level of functioning at work, in the family, and in recreational and social areas; (4) an appraisal of any or all support received; (5) assessment of the patient's ability to control his or her life (that is, to cope); (6) the affective distress experienced and attributed to the pain, such as depression, irritability, anxiety, and tension; and (7) patient activity levels, determined both subjectively and objectively.

All these factors can be enhanced by additional tests such as the McGill Pain Questionnaire,[73] the Pain Behavior Checklist,[74] or the Beck Depression Inventory,[75] as well as the other tests mentioned in this text. Reliance on just one of these tests is to be avoided. Only when incorporated in the overall inventory should they be given credence.

Specific subgroups of pain can be determined from careful evaluation of this inventory, and treatment programs can be customized to the needs of the patient.

1. The somatic aspect of the subgroup, such as reflex sympathetic dystrophy, rheumatoid arthritis, or cancer, can be addressed.
2. The resulting dysfunction from the somatic illness can be ascertained and therapeutically approached.
3. The psychologic aspects influencing or enhancing the impairment can be diagnosed and treatment can be directed at the precise diagnosis. Psychopharmacologic therapy can be instituted with or without cognitive-behavioral guidance.
4. Family and/or marital support can be developed or ameliorated if pertinent. Litigation can be addressed, hastened, or terminated.
5. The patient can be completely involved in the program at the level that the patient's education and intellect permit.
6. Ongoing outcome assessment can be structured so that meaningless or ineffectual treatment does not persist.

Diagnostic and therapeutic "homogeneity" of the pain patient must not be accepted. Every aspect of the multidisciplinary group must be mobilized to meet the needs of the patient's specific pain.

REFERENCES

1. Morris, DB: The Culture of Pain. University of California Press, Berkeley, 1991.
2. Brena, SF (ed): Chronic Pain, America's Hidden Epidemic. Atheneum/SMI, New York, 1978.
3. Sternbach, RA: Pain Patients: Traits and Treatment. Academic Press, New York, 1974.
4. Bonica, JJ: The Management of Pain. Lea & Febiger, Philadelphia, 1953.
5. Crue, BL (ed): Pain: Research and Treatment. Academic Press, New York, 1975.
6. Crue BL: The centralist concept of chronic pain. Semin Neurol 3:331, 1983.
7. Cailliet, R: Chronic pain: Is it necessary? Arch Phys Med Rehab 60, 1979.
7a. Crue, BL: The Courage to Risk Being Wrong. Bull LA Neurol Soc 26:5, 1981.
8. Cousins, N: Anatomy of an Illness. New Engl J Med 295(26):1463–1485, 1976.
9. Fry, C: Comedy. In Corrigan, RW (ed): Comedy: Meaning and Form. Chandler Publishing, San Francisco, 1965, p 15.
10. Crue, BL: Pain and Suffering. Charles C Thomas, Springfield, IL, 1970.
11. Lyotard, J-F: The Postmodern Condition: A Report on Knowledge. University of Minnesota Press, Minneapolis, 1984.
12. Wolff, HG and Wolf, S: Pain. Charles C Thomas, Springfield, IL, 1948.
13. Hirsch, T: Work in America. Report of a Special Task Force to the Secretary of Health, Education and Welfare. MIT Press, Cambridge, MA, 1973.
14. Jones, LK (ed): The Encyclopedia of Career Change and Work Issues. Oryx Press, Arizona, 1992.
15. Palmer, G: Compensation for Incapacity. Oxford University Press, Wellington, England, 1979.
16. Osterweis, M, Kleinman, A, Mechanic, D (eds): Pain and Disability. Institute of Medicine, National Academy Press, Washington, DC, 1987.
17. International Association for the Study of Pain, Subcommittee on Taxonomy: Classification of chronic pain. Pain (Suppl) 3:S1–S225, 1986.

262 PAIN: MECHANISMS AND MANAGEMENT

18. Watson, CPN: Chronic pain model. Can Med J 38:1365–1369, 1983.
19. Dwarakanath, GK: Pathophysiology of pain. In Warfield, CA (ed): Manual of Pain Management. JB Lippincott, Philadelphia, 1991, pp 8–9.
20. Wall, PD and Gurnick, M: Ongoing activity in the peripheral nerve: Physiology and pharmacology of impulses originating from a neuroma. Exp Neurol 43:580, 1974.
21. Wall, PD: Introduction. In Wall, PD and Melzack, R (eds): Textbook of Pain. Churchill-Livingstone, New York, 1985, pp 1–16.
22. Dubner, R: Neuronal plasticity and pain following peripheral tissue inflammation or nerve injury. In Bond, MR, Charlton, JE, and Woolf, CF (eds): Proceedings of the VIth World Congress on Pain. Elsevier, Amsterdam, 1991, pp 263–276.
23. Menetry, D and Besson, JM: Electrophysiological characteristics of dorsal horn cells in rats with cutaneous inflammation resulting from chronic arthritis. Pain 13:343–364, 1982.
24. McMahon, SB and Wall, PD: Receptive fields of rat lamina I projection cells move to incorporate a nearby region of injury. Pain 19(3):235–247, 1984.
25. Hylden, JLK, Hahin, RI, Traub, RJ, and Dubner, R: Expansion of receptive fields of spinal lamina I projection neurones in rats with unilateral adjuvant-induced inflammation: The contribution of dorsal horn mechanisms. Pain 37:229–243, 1989.
26. Cailliet, R: Low Back Pain Syndrome, ed 4. FA Davis, Philadelphia, 1988.
27. Cailliet, R: Neck and Arm Pain, ed 3. FA Davis, Philadelphia, 1991.
28. Hu, JW, Sessle, BJ, Raboisson, P, Dallel, R, and Woda, A: Stimulation of craniofacial muscle afferents induces prolonged facilitatory effects in trigeminal nociceptive brain-stem neurones. Pain 48:53–60, 1992.
29. Dubner, R, Sessle, BJ and Storey, AT: The Neural Basis of Oral and Facial Functions. Plenum Press, New York, 1978.
30. Yokota, T: Anatomy and physiology of intra- and extracranial nociceptive afferents and their central projections. In Oleson, J and Edvinsson, L (eds): Basic Mechanisms of Headache, Pain Research and Clinical Management, Vol 2. Elsevier, Amsterdam, 1988, pp 117–128.
31. Olesen, J: Clinical and pathophysiological observations in migraine and tension-type headache explained by integration of vascular, supraspinal and myofascial inputs. Pain 46:125–132, 1991.
32. Thesleff, S: Physiology Rev 40:734–752, 1960.
33. Lewis, A: "Psychogenic": A word and its mutations. Psychol Med 2:209–214, 1972.
34. Fordyce, WE: Behavioral Methods for Chronic Pain and Illness. CV Mosby, St. Louis, 1976.
35. Woodforde, JM and Mersky, H: Personality traits of patients with chronic pain. J Psychosom Res 16:167–172, 1972.
36. Sternbach, RA: Fundamentals of psychological methods in chronic pain. In Bonica, JJ, Lindblom, U, and Iggo, A (eds): Advances in Pain Research and Therapy, Vol 5. Raven Press, New York, 1983.
37. Malan, D: The Frontier of Brief Psychotherapy. Plenum Press, New York, 1976.
38. Pilowsky, I, Bassett, D: Individual dynamic psychotherapy for chronic pain. In Roy, R and Tunks, E (eds): Chronic Pain: Psychosocial Factors in Rehabilitation. Williams & Wilkins, Baltimore and London, 1982.
39. Pinsky, JJ, Griffin, SE, and Agnew, DC: Aspects of long-term evaluation of pain unit treatment program for patients with intractable benign pain syndrome: Treatment outcome. Bull LA Neurol Soc 44:53–59, 1979.
40. Khatami, M and Rush, AJ: A one-year follow-up of multimodal treatment for chronic pain. Pain 14:45–49, 1982.
41. Gallagher, RM, Rauh, V, Haugh, LD, Milhous, R, Callas, PW, Langelier, R, McClallen, JM, and Frymoyer, J: Determinants of return-to-work among low back pain patients. Pain 39:55–67, 1989.
42. Cailliet, R: Head and Face Pain Syndromes, ed 1. FA Davis, Philadelphia, 1992.

43. Tait, RC, Duckro, PN, Margolis, RB, and Wiener, R: Quality of life following treatment: A preliminary study of in- and outpatients with chronic pain. Int J Psychiatry Med 18:271–282, 1988.

44. Osterweis, M, Kleinman, A, and Mechanic, D (eds): Pain and disability: Clinical, behavioral and public policy perspectives. National Academy Press, Washington, DC, 1987.

45. Merskey, H: Classification of chronic pain. Descriptions of chronic pain syndrome and definitions. Pain (Suppl) 3:S1–S225, 1986.

46. Florence, DW: The chronic pain syndrome: A physical and psychological challenge. Postgrad Med 70:218–228, 1981.

47. Olesen, J: Classification and diagnostic criteria for headache disorders, cranial neuralgias and facial pain. Cephalalgia (Suppl) 7:9–96, 1988.

48. Waddell, G, Main, CJ, Morris, EW, Paola, MD, and Gray, ICM: Chronic low-back pain, psychological distress, and illness behavior. Spine 9:209–213, 1984.

49. Maruta, T, Swanson, DW, and Swenson, WM: Chronic pain: Which patients may a pain-management program help? Pain 7:321–329, 1979.

50. Herron, L, Turner, J, and Weiner, P: Does the MMPI predict chemonucleolysis outcome? Spine 13:84–88, 1988.

51. Snyder, DK: Assessing chronic pain with the Minnesota Multiphasic Personality Inventory. In Miller, TW (ed): Chronic Pain. International Universities Press, Madison, 1990, pp 181–214.

52. Watson, D: Neurotic tendencies among chronic pain patients: An MMPI item analysis. Pain 14:365–385, 1982.

53. Smythe, HA: Problems with the MMPI. J Rheumatol 1:417–418, 1984.

54. Fordyce, W, Brena, S, De Lateur, B, Holcombe, S, and Loeser, J: Relationship of patient semantic pain predictors to physician judgment, activity level measures and MMPI. Pain 5:293–303, 1978.

55. Snyder, DK and Power, D: Empirical descriptors of unelevated MMPI profiles among chronic pain patients: A typologic study. J Clin Psychol 37:602–607, 1981.

56. Pincus, T, Callahan, LF, Bradley, LA, Vaughn, WK, and Wolfe, F: Elevated MMPI scores for hypochondriasis, depression, and hysteria in pateints with rheumatoid arthritis reflect disease rather than psychological status. Arthritis Rheum 29:1456–1466, 1986.

57. Naliboff, BD, Cohen, MJ, and Yellin, AN: Does the MMPI differentiate chronic illness from chronic pain? Pain 13:333–341, 1982.

58. Shutty, MS and DeGood, DE: Cluster analysis of responses of low back pain patients to the SCL-90: Comparison of empirical versus rationally derived subscales. Rehab Psychol 32:133–144, 1987.

59. Buckelew, SP, DeGood, DE, Schwartz, DP, and Kerler, RM: Cognitive and somatic item response pattern of pain patients, psychiatric patients, and hospital employees. J Clin Psychol 42:852–860, 1986.

60. Rudy, TE, Kerns, RD, and Tirk, DC: Chronic pain and depression: Toward a cognitive-behavioral mediational model. Pain 35:129–140, 1988.

61. Hollon, SD, and Kendall, PC: Cognitive self-statements in depression: Development of an Automatic Thoughts Questionnaire. Cognitive Therapy Research 4:342–383, 1980.

62. Ingram, RE and Wisnicki, KS: Assessment of positive automatic cognition. J Consult Clin Psychol 56:898–902, 1988.

63. Keefe, FJ, Bradley, LA, and Crisson, JE: Behavioral assessment of low back pain: Identification of pain behavior subgroups. Pain 40:153–160, 1990.

64. Hendler, N, Molett, A, Talo, S, and Levin, S: A comparison between the Minnesota Multiphasic Personality Inventory and the "Mensana Clinic Back Pain Test" for validating the complaint of chronic back pain. J Occup Med 30(2):98–102, 1988.

65. Hendler, N, Viernstein, M, Gucer, P, and Long, D: A preoperative screening test for chronic back pain patients. Psychosomatics 20(12):801–803, 1979.

66. Brena, SF and Koch, DL: A "pain estimate" model for quantification and classification of chronic pain states. Anesthes Rev 2:8–13, 1975.
67. Talo, S, Hendler, N, and Brodie, J: Effects of active and completed litigation on treatment results: Workers Compensation compared with other litigation patients. J Occup Med 31(3):265–269, 1989.
68. Hendler, N and Talo, S: Role of the pain clinic. In Foley, KM and Payne RM (eds): Current Therapy of Pain. BC Decker, Philadelphia, 1989, pp 23–32.
69. Hendler, N: Organization of a chronic pain treatment center. In Diagnosis and Nonsurgical Management of Chronic Pain. Raven Press, New York, 1981, p 163.
70. Turk, DC and Rudy, TE: Neglected topics in the treatment of chronic pain patients—relapse, noncompliance, and adherence enhancement. Pain 44:5–28, 1991.
71. Turk, DC and Rudy, TE: Towards an empirically derived taxonomy of chronic pain patients: Integration of psychological assessment data. J Consult Clin Psychol 56:233–238, 1988.
72. Kerns, RD, Turk, DC, and Rudy, TE: The West Haven–Yale Multidimensional Pain Inventory (WHYMPI). Pain 23:345–356, 1985.
73. Melzack, R: The McGill Pain Questionnaire: Major properties and scoring methods. Pain 1:277–299, 1975.
74. Turk, DC, Wack, JT, and Kerns, RD: An empirical examination of the "pain behavior" construct. J Behav Med 8:119–130, 1985.
75. Beck, AT, Ward, CH, Mendelson, M, Mock, J, and Erbaugh, J: An inventory for measuring depression. Arch Gen Psychiatry 4:561–571, 1961.

CHAPTER 10

Cancer Pain

Pain from cancer is pain associated with a disease that has a poor or questionable prognosis and has the propensity of being chronic, unremitting, and often of increasing severity. Cancer pain should be considered as pain resulting from cancer, its invasion, and/or its treatment. It varies as to site, pathology, clinical manifestations, and response to therapy.[1] Management of the pain from cancer necessitates treatment of the symptoms as well as of the underlying pathology because merely treating the disease may or may not influence the pain, and alleviating the pain may have no influence on the disease.

There are no clinical characteristics of the pain as related to the underlying pathologic lesions. The International Association for the Study of Pain (IASP) taxonomy does not clarify this predicament other than to list the diseases and/or lesions that produce the pain.[2] Bonica laments that pain related to cancer has failed to be statistically classified in cancer studies.[3] Daut concluded that 20 to 50 percent of patients when first diagnosed as having cancer experienced pain, whereas 55 to 95 percent experienced pain in far advanced cases.[4] In most malignancies pain does not act as a warning system but is a sign of advanced disease. Foley found pain to be caused by the tumor in 62 percent of patients, by the therapy in 28 percent, and with no relationship in 10 percent.[5]

The most acceptable mechanism of cancer pain is direct tumor involvement of the peripheral nerves in the region. Pain considered to be neuropathic may not respond to epidural opioid analgesia; cancer pain must be differentiated as somatic, visceral, or neuropathic.[6,7] Other causative mechanisms have been considered to result from cancer treatment, physiologic and biochemical disorders of the cancer, or a combination of both.[8]

In treating pain originating from cancer in which the pain mechanism is considered to be visceral, the organ must be identified. Cancer pain that is neuropathic or the result of deafferentiation presents a therapeutic problem.[9] Deafferentiation pain responds better to opioid and anti-inflammatory treatment, whereas neurogenic pain may not respond to nonsteroidal anti-inflammatory drugs (NSAIDs).[10]

Cancer-pain syndromes often manifest more than one kind of pain.[11] Acute pain can result from certain diagnostic procedures and from certain therapeutic procedures such as bone transplants, chemotherapy, or radiation therapy.[12] Regardless of the mechanism, alleviating the pain allows time to evaluate and treat the organic component.

The nervous system that is in direct proximity or in direct relation to the organ must be considered as the site of pain. Diagnostic and possibly therapeutic intervention of the nerve supply to the organ is afforded by anesthetic nerve blocks. Benefit may also suggest pain of a neurogenic etiology.

Metastasis of systemic cancer may involve the central nervous system as well as the peripheral nervous system. Diffuse head pain is common in metastasis of lung, breast, anal, and testicular malignancies. The mechanism of these head pains is involvement of the meninges, intracranial sinus veins, and meningeal arteries. This pain is ultimately accompanied by signs and symptoms of neurologic deficit: cortical, spinal, plexi, or peripheral nerves.

Obstruction of hollow viscera from cancer with resultant distension may be the mechanism of pain. Distension causes intense contraction of smooth muscles of the viscera, resulting in visceral pain that is usually poorly localized and diffuse but usually referred to the same dermatomal area of the cord segments of the viscera.

Pain from tumor involvement of parenchymal viscera such as the liver, spleen, pancreas, and kidney results from acute distension of the pain-sensitive fascia. They contain many mechanical receptors, and pain results when they are acutely stretched or placed under tension. This pain is poorly defined, dull, and generally located in the dermatomal region of the involved organ.

Cancer of the pancreas, a well-documented painful visceral malignancy, raises the possibility of pain resulting from necrosis from enzymolytic autodigestion. Destruction from the enzyme, combined with tumor invasion and stenosis of the excretory ducts causing visceral distension, enhances the pain mechanism.

Tumor invasion of adjacent blood vessels may also be a mechanism responsible for causing pain. This mechanism is a result of either perivascular lymphangitis causing vasospasm, occlusion with resultant ischemia, venous engorgement, or edema: Any of these can cause severe increasing pain. Management of this pain is obviously to release the entrapment and the resultant distension.

Pain can also result from necrosis of a mucous membrane caused by cancer of the lips, mouth, face, gastrointestinal system, or genitourinary system. The pain in the affected region is the result of inflammation, which lowers the threshold of nociceptors in those tissues.

Pain from cancer therapy must always be considered. Surgical intervention of the cancer can damage adjacent tissues, resulting in pain. Examples of these surgical therapeutic conditions are postthoracotomy, postmastectomy, radical neck dissections, peripheral limb resections resulting in mechanical neurogenic pains, or pain from deafferentiation.

Postchemotherapy pains have been described. Alkaloid medications may cause polyneuritis with resultant painful dysesthesia. Chronic steroid therapy can cause a residual pain state from pseudorheumatism and aseptic bone necrosis. Acute herpes zoster and postherpetic neuralgia occur in a high percentage of patients with cancer or those receiving chemotherapy for cancer. Postradiation plexopathy or myelopathy can also result in pain.

Evaluation and management of cancer pain remains a challenge to the medical team employing all aspects of acute as well as chronic pain management. Volumes of literature are appearing constantly as management of specific malignancies is evolving. Pain related to malignancy is also receiving more attention.

MANAGEMENT OF CANCER PAIN

The presence of pain and a diagnosis of cancer, possibly or probably related, result in severe anxiety. Chronic pain induces physiologic, psychologic, affective, and psychosocial reactions in most patients; this is probably enhanced in patients having pain and cancer. These factors enhance the intensity of the perceived pain and must be addressed in the management of pain from cancer.

Patients with cancer usually have greater sleep problems, loss of appetite, depression, and physical debility than other patients. All these factors, together with anxiety, depression, hypochondriasis, and neuroticism, accentuate the perception of pain.[13]

The reaction to a diagnosis of cancer varies with each individual: some are withdrawn, while others may be combative. The latter attitude actually has been considered to increase longevity.[14] The presence of pain with the cancer causes the patient to be more emotionally disturbed; this probably increases the perception of pain and admits a more ominous interpretation.[15]

Hospitalized patients with cancer and pain have significantly higher levels of depression, anxiety, hostility, and somatization than patients treated at home.[16] This supports the hypothesis that cancer-related pain is a complex multidimensional phenomenon composed of sensory, affective, cognitive, and behavioral components. Pain coexisting with cancer interferes with physiologic functioning and enhances psychologic decompensation. This comprehensive hypothesis is the basis for multidisciplinary treatment of the cancer patient having related pain.[17]

The increasing expense of the treatment, accompanied by loss of time on the job due to illness, adds a psychosocial aspect to the pained cancer patient. New research may increase longevity, but the quality of life for the patient, relatives, and family remains a concern.

The question always arises, Is there a scientific basis for the will to live? Does this will to live influence the rapidity and severity of the malignancy? These questions have been studied intensely.[18,19] Laboratory studies on animals have been carried out to reach a conclusion.[20] The current tendency is to believe that the mind-set influences the outcome; this supports psychotherapeutic intervention.

Angell claimed that the evidence does not support the theory that personality and mental status affect the onset, treatment, or cure but that it is anecdotal and largely folklore.[21] She used this claim to argue that patients should not be held responsible for the outcome of their disease. However, there is enough clinical evidence, albeit anecdotal, to justify patient optimism and cooperation in treatment management.

Numerous measures have been developed to quantify cancer pain and resulting functional impairment; the Minnesota Multiphasic Personality Inventory (MMPI) has received the greatest consideration.[22–24]

In the management of cancer pain the multidisciplinary team approach is the most effective. Primary therapy, including chemotherapy, radiation therapy, hormonal therapy, and/or surgical therapy, must be undertaken and supervised by the primary physician. During this stage there must be communication with the patient and family to initiate coping skills, personal care, and realistic reassurance.

If there is pain associated with the cancer, symptomatic therapy must be instituted; this includes NSAIDs, opioids, regional and local anesthesia, intraspinal narcotics, or whatever modality or medication is needed to diminish or eliminate pain. This should be considered basic to cancer therapy.

If after a thorough trial pain persists, other forms of therapy should be instituted: psychologic therapy, meaningful physical therapy, trigger point injections, acupuncture, and transcutaneous electrical nerve stimulation (TENS). If deemed necessary, neurolytic blocks and intraspinal opioids should be used, and in intractable pain, hypophysectomy, spinal cord stimulation, deep brain stimulation, and cordotomy may be tried. The severity and duration of the pain influence the choice of these more formidable pain intervention techniques.

Studies show that 38 percent of patients in all stages of cancer experience pain, with 40 percent in the intermediate stages and 55 to 85 percent in advanced or terminal stages.[25] In a World Health Organization interview it was reported that less than 10 percent of those suffering severe pain obtained complete relief from their treatment, and 29 percent of patients with moderate pain reported little or no relief.[26] These statistics indicate that pain from cancer is a worldwide problem.

Cancer is characterized by progressive pain.[27] Progressive pain gradually demoralizes the patient, causing mental and physical exhaustion. The fear of addiction must be put into its proper context, and early effective levels of medication should be instituted before any of the sequelae of the cancer and its pain take their toll.

Pain must be addressed while the cause and extent of the cancer undergo evaluation and treatment. Nonopioid medication with or without an adjuvant medication usually constitute initial pain therapy; they both act centrally and peripherally to intercept the receptor site.

Nonopioid drugs include

- Acetylsalicylic acid (aspirin)
- Acetaminophen (Tylenol)
- Indomethacin (Indocin)
- Proprionic acid derivatives (Motrin, Nuprin, and so on)

Adjuvant drugs include

- Corticosteroid (Prednisone)
- Progestin
- Antidepressants (Amitriptyline, Sinequan, Tofranil, and so on)
- Haloperidol (Haldol)
- Carbamazepine (Tegretol)
- Dextroamphetamines (Dexedrine)

The use of opioid analgesics should not be delayed unnecessarily or too long. These include

- Weak opioids: Codeine
- Potent opioids: Morphine, Methadone

Once the decision is made that the pain requires stronger opioids, the dosage and mode of administration must be ascertained to give the patient sufficient amounts to provide satisfactory and sustained pain relief with minimal side effects. This mandates that the effective dose be given at the proper fixed period to assure continuous pain relief. Stronger opioids should be combined with nonopioids and adjuvant drugs to ensure maximum relief.

The concept of "PRN" (necessary for the patient's pain) implies that the patient or the nurse evaluates when and if medication is to administered. Neither have currently been educated in proper interpretation of this term. Both physicians and nurses have been trained to minimize medication for fear of addiction, dependence, and respiratory embarrassment. The patient, who sees administration of medication based on a clock, becomes anxious; this enhances the perception of pain.[29]

A nurse's perception of patient pain is influenced by his or her own beliefs about suffering; this belief system is influenced by cultural factors, religion, and ethnic background.[29,30]

The use of narcotics in treating cancer pain has undergone intensive study because of the claimed unattended complaint of pain in many medical settings. One study showed that 73 percent of hospitalized patients with cancer pain remained in severe pain.[31] The presiding physician rarely prescribed the recommended dose of meperidine, and the nurses administered inadequate PRN medication.

In another study that surveyed the knowledge, attitudes, and experience of medical personnel, half of those surveyed thought that[32]

1. PRN medication caused patients to develop a tolerance to the medication, requiring additional dosage and ultimate addiction.
2. Just enough medication should be used to allow the pain "to be noticed but not distressing."
3. Most patients are overmedicated rather than undermedicated, although pain persisted in the terminally ill.

One survey revealed that intuition rather than a quantitative process was used by nurses in making their decision regarding the quantity and frequency of medication.[33]

Experts managing cancer pain patients have concluded that "inadequate knowledge of the pharmacology of analgesics and the misconceptions and attitudes of those health care professionals who are involved in the care of people who have pain caused by cancer . . . are largely responsible for the failure of analgesics to control pain."[34]

A recommended protocol for using narcotics in malignancy based on the following premises is offered:[35]

1. The intent of drug therapy is to relieve pain at rest, on standing, and during activity.
2. Analgesics should be given around the clock on a regular basis to maintain a therapeutic blood level in order to keep the patient pain-free. The prescription of PRN is to be avoided.
3. When nonnarcotic agents are no longer effective, narcotic drugs, including weak and strong opioids, should be added. The "stepladder" approach of gradual increase in dosage and use of stronger opioids should evolve.

For example, nonnarcotic agents should be followed by weak narcotics, such as codeine 30 to 60 mg every 3 to 4 hours. Gradually the use of stronger narcotics such as morphine, Dilaudid (hydromorphone) and Dolophine (Methadone) can be substituted or added.

The recommended protocol is as follows:

1. Start with a specific analgesic drug that is appropriate for the pain.

2. Know the pharmacokinetic properties of the drug, that is, the duration of action, analgesic doses, methods of administration, and availability of the drug.
3. Adjust the route of administration to the patient's needs:
   a. Oral use if effective and accepted by the patient.
   b. Rectal suppositories if oral route is unacceptable or ineffective.
   c. Sublingual administration if oral is not possible or effective.
4. Change to parenteral use if patient's comfort and convenience demand. Rotate injection sites.
   a. Intravenous as either a bolus or a continuous-drip infusion pump, as decided.
   b. Controlled analgesia by subcutaneous means.
5. Monitor the patient's response to the drug and the duration of the drug's effectiveness.
6. Combine drugs to reduce the side effects such as constipation, drowsiness, nausea, and vomiting.
7. Prevent insomnia by larger bedtime doses. Awaken patient if needed to ensure continuous medication level.
8. Meperidine given repeatedly may cause irritability, shakiness, tremors, twitches, and generalized motor seizures. It must be carefully monitored if used in repeat doses. Painful muscle damage with fibrosis can occur from intramuscular route.
9. Adjuvant medications such as steroids, tranquilizers, antidepressants, and antianxiety agents promote better pain management and, although not analgesic per se, can be combined with any of the above.

Inadequate knowledge of available analgesic medication adversely influences pain management of the cancer patient and especially of the terminally ill. Prevalent misconceptions must be dispelled by proper education of the medical personnel. Concerns about addiction currently result in improper use of opioids in adequately treating pain of the cancer patient.

Longitudinal studies of treatment outcomes in patients with advanced cancer pain have been difficult to assess and have been sparsely reported in the literature.[36] A recent report from a clinic devoted to treating pain of cancer etiology evaluated treatment outcomes and expressed concern about treating pain in a homogeneous context.[37] Cancer pain is a subgroup that must further be subdivided, and all pertinent components of the team must be evaluated.

Conventional analgesic therapy fails to provide pain relief in many cancer patients or at certain phases of the cancer. The multidisciplinary clinic tailors analgesic medication, anesthetic procedures, and psychologic intervention and supportive care. Such a clinic offers care not readily available from a single primary physician, even a trained oncologist.

Gourlay and colleagues[38] reported on individualized treatment made

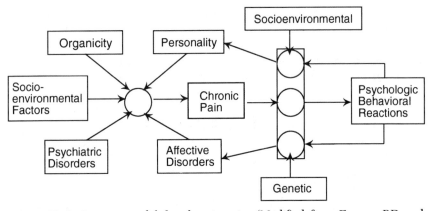

Figure 10–1. Systems model for chronic pain. (Modified from France, RD and Krishnan, KRR: Pharmacological intervention in pain. In Miller, TW [ed]: Chronic Pain, Vol 1. International Universities Press, Madison, CT, 1990, p 185.)

available to patients with pain classified as (1) pain at rest, (2) pain in motion, and (3) pain interrupting sleep. In this longitudinal study many modalities were used, but the initial benefit was derived from appropriate medications. Progressive or nonresponsive patients were treated by neurolytic blocks or neuroablative surgical procedures.

One of the modalities—epidural morphine—was evaluated as to benefit from continuous infusion or intermittent bolus. It was concluded that both were equally effective, an important finding with implications for the out-patient situation.

Ongoing surveillance is possible in a comprehensive multidisciplinary pain clinic. The cancer pain, at each episode and stage, the psychosocial impact of the disease, and the support groups, including family, can be monitored to improve the quality of life.[39]

The systems approach to the assessment and management of chronic pain is shown in Fig. 10–1.

Cancer may not be increasing substantially, but the management of the disease and pain from the disease is making gratifying progress.

REFERENCES

1. Ventafridda, V and Caraceni, A: Cancer pain classification: A controversial issue. Pain 46:1–2, 1991.
2. International Association for the Study of Pain, Subcommittee on Taxonomy; Classification of chronic pain. Pain (Suppl) 3:S1–S225, 1986.
3. Bonica, JJ: Cancer pain. In The Management of Pain, ed 2. Lea & Febiger, Philadelphia, 1990, p 400.

4. Daut, RL and Cleeland, CS: The prevalence and severity of pain in cancer. Cancer 50:1913–1918, 1982.
5. Foley, KM: Pain syndromes in patients with cancer. In Bonica, JJ and Ventafridda, V (eds): Advances in Pain Research and Therapy, Vol 2. Raven Press, New York, 1979, pp 59–78.
6. Arner, S and Arnier, B: Differential effects of epidural morphine in the treatment of cancer-related pain. Acta Anaesthesiol Scand 29:32–36, 1985.
7. Samuelson, H and Hedner, T: Pain characteristics in cancer patients and the analgesic response to epidural morphine. Pain 46:3–8, 1991.
8. Ashbury, AK and Fields, HL: Pain due to peripheral nerve damage: An hypothesis. Neurology 34:1587–1590, 1984.
9. Fields, HL: Can opiates relieve neuropathic pain? Pain 35:365, 1988.
10. Ventafridda, V, Caraceni, A, and Gamba, A: Field testing of the WHO guidelines for cancer pain relief. In Foley, KM, Bonica, JJ, and Ventafridda, V (eds): Advances in Pain Research and Therapy, Vol 16. Raven Press, New York, 1990, pp 451–464.
11. Twycross, RG and Fairfield, S: Pain in far-advanced cancer. Pain 14:303–310, 1982.
12. Chapman, R, Syrjala, KS, and Sargur, M: Pain as a manifestation of cancer treatment. Semin Oncol Nurs 1:100, 1985.
13. Bond, MR: Cancer pain: Psychological substrates and therapy. In Fields, HL, Rubner, R, and Cervero, F (eds): Advances in Pain Research and Therapy, Vol 9. Raven Press, New York, 1985, pp 559–567.
14. Derogatis, LR, Aboloff, MD, and Melisartis, N: Psychological coping mechanisms and survival time in metastatic breast cancer. JAMA 242:1504, 1979.
15. Woodforde, JM and Fielding, JR: Pain and cancer. In Weisenberg, M (ed): Pain: Clinical and Experimental Perspectives. CV Mosby, St. Louis, 1975, pp 326–335.
16. Ahles, TA, Blanchard, EB, and Ruckdeschel, JC: The multidimensional nature of cancer-related pain. Pain 17:227–228, 1983.
17. Ventafridda, V, Tamburini, M, and De Conno, F: Comprehensive treatment in cancer pain. In Fields, HL, Dubner, R, and Cervero, F (eds): Advances in Pain Research and Therapy, Vol 9. Raven Press, New York, 1985, pp 617–628.
18. Simonton, C, Mathews-Simonton, S, and Creighton, J: Getting Well Again. Bantam Books, New York, 1981.
19. Strickland, B: Internal-external expectancies and health-related behaviors. J Consult Clin Psychol 46:1192–1211, 1979.
20. Angell, M: Disease as a reflection of the psyche. New Engl J Med 312:1570–1573, 1985.
21. Richter, C: On the phenomenon of sudden death in animals and men. Psychosom Med 19:191–198, 1957.
22. Ventafridda, V, et al: A new method of pain quantification based on weekly self-descriptive record of the intensity and duration of pain. In Bonica, JJ, Lindblom, U, and Iggo, A (eds): Advances in Pain Research and Therapy, Vol 5. Raven Press, New York, 1983, pp 891–895.
23. Karnofsky, DA and Burchenal, JH (eds): The Clinical Evaluation of Chemical Chemotherapeutic Agents in Cancer. Columbia University Press, New York, 1949.
24. Snyder, DK: Assessing chronic pain with the Minnesota Multiphasic Personality Inventory (MMPI). In Miller, TW (ed): Chronic Pain, Vol 1. International Universities Press, Madison, CT, 1990, pp 215–257.
25. Foley, KM: The Management of Cancer Pain, Vol 1. Hoffman La Roche, Nutley, NJ, 1981.
26. World Health Organization: Cancer Pain Relief. Geneva, 1986.
27. Jacox, A and Stewart, M: Psychosocial Contingencies of Pain Experience. University of Iowa Press, Iowa City, 1973.
28. Shawyer, MM: Pain associated with cancer. In Jacox, AK (ed): Pain: A Source Book for Nurses and Other Health Professionals. Little, Brown, Boston, 1977, pp 373–389.
29. Jacox, A: Assessing pain. Am J Nurs 79(5):895–900, 1979.

30. Davitz, LL and Davitz, JR: Nurses' Responses to Patient's Suffering. Springer, New York, 1980.
31. Marks, RM and Sacher, MD: Undertreatment of medical inpatients with narcotic analgesics. Ann Intern Med 78(2):173–181, 1973.
32. Charap, AD: The knowledge, attitudes, and experience of medical personnel treating pain in the terminally ill. Mt Sinai J Med 45(4):561–580, 1978.
33. Grier, MR, Howard, M, and Cohen, F: Beliefs and values associated with administering narcotic analgesics to terminally ill patients. In Clinical and Scientific Sessions. American Nurses Association, Washington, DC, 1979, pp 211–222.
34. Jacox, A and Rogers, AG: The nursing management of pain. In Marino, LB (ed): Cancer Nursing. CV Mosby, St. Louis, 1981, pp 381–404.
35. Rankin, MA: Using drugs for cancer pain. In Miller, TW (ed): Chronic Pain, Vol 2. International Universities Press, Madison, CT, 1990, pp 667–724.
36. Moulin, DE: Treatment outcome in a multidisciplinary cancer pain clinic by Banning et al. Pain 47:127–128, 1991.
37. Banning, A, Sjogren, P, and Henriksen, H: Treatment outcome in multidisciplinary cancer pain clinic. Pain 47:129–134, 1991.
38. Gourlay, GK, Plummer, JL, Cherry, DA, Onley, MM, Parish, KA, Wood, MM, and Cousins, MJ: Comparison of intermittent bolus with continuous infusion of epidural morphine in the treatment of severe cancer pain. Pain 47:135–140, 1991.
39. Gonzales, GR, Elliot, KJ, Portenoy, RK, and Foley, KM: The impact of a comprehensive evaluation in the management of cancer pain. Pain 47:141–144, 1991.
40. France, RD and Rama Krishnan, KR: The systems approach to the assessment and management of chronic pain. In Miller, TW (ed): Chronic Pain, Vol 1. International Universities Press, Madison, CT, 1990, p 185.

CHAPTER 11
Depression in Patients with Chronic Pain

Admittedly, many patients with chronic pain are depressed, but not all depression is pain-related. The causal relationship of chronic pain and depression remains obscure, and whether depression causes or is the sequela of chronic pain remains unconfirmed.[1]

If chronic pain has resulted in depression, the obvious therapeutic approach is to eliminate or moderate the pain, and the depression will ultimately diminish or subside. Depression also causes pain, or at least aggravates the disabling symptomatology. In this case, moderating or eliminating the depression may need to precede pain relief.

A better understanding of depression is mandated because its role in chronic pain may be overlooked or magnified by the examining physician. The manner in which the diagnosis of depression is ascertained and how it is explained to the patient has often been mismanaged. The physician should fully understand and recognize the symptoms that lead to the diagnosis of depression and identify its specific type.

The symptoms of depression are numerous and vary with the individual. The American Psychiatric Association has documented the criteria for depression (see Table 11–1).[2]

The average physician may not have sufficient knowledge or time to specifically ascertain the degree and type of depression. The need for recognition or its possibility, nevertheless, is obvious so that the condition can be addressed and treated.

As noted in Table 11–1, to be diagnostic, at least five of the symptoms must have been present during the same 2-week period and represent a change from previous functioning. The patient must have exhibited a depressed mood and diminished interest or pleasure in all or almost all activities of

Table 11–1. DIAGNOSTIC CRITERIA FOR MAJOR DEPRESSIVE EPISODES

A. At least five of the following symptoms have been present during the same 2-week period and represent a change from previous functioning, or at least one of the symptoms is either (1) a depressed mood, or (2) loss of interest or pleasure. (Do not include symptoms that are clearly due to a physical condition, mood-incongruent delusions or hallucinations, incoherence, or marked loosening of association.)

(1) Depressed mood (or can be irritable mood in children and adolescents) most of the day, nearly every day, as indicated either by subjective account or observation by others.
(2) Markedly diminished interest or pleasure in all, or almost all, activities most of the day, nearly every day, as indicated either by subjective account or observation by others of apathy most of the time.
(3) Significant weight loss or weight gain when not dieting (e.g., more than 5 percent of body weight in a month) or decrease or increase in appetite nearly every day in children (consider failure to make expected weight gains).
(4) Insomnia or hypersomnia nearly every day.
(5) Psychomotor agitation or retardation nearly every day (observable by others, not merely subjective feelings of restlessness or being slowed down).
(6) Fatigue or loss of energy every day.
(7) Feelings of worthlessness or excessive or inappropriate guilt (which may be delusional) nearly every day (not merely self-reproach or guilt about being sick).
(8) Diminished ability to think or concentrate, or indecisiveness, nearly every day (either subjective account or as observed by others).
(9) Recurrent thoughts of death (not just fear of dying), recurrent suicidal ideation without a specific plan for committing suicide.
B. (1) It cannot be established that an organic factor initiated and maintained the disturbance.
(2) The disturbance is not a normal reaction to the death of a loved one (uncomplicated bereavement). (Morbid preoccupation with worthlessness, suicidal ideation, marked functional impairment or psychomotor retardation of prolonged duration suggest bereavement complicated by major depression.)
C. At no time during the disturbance have there been delusions or hallucinations for as long as 2 weeks in the absence of prominent mood symptoms (i.e., before the mood symptoms developed or after they have remitted).
D. Not superimposed on schizophrenia, schizophreniform disorder, delusional disorder, or psychotic disorder NOS.

Source: American Psychiatric Association. Diagnostic and Statistical Manual of Mental Disorders, ed 3 rev. Washington, DC, 1987.

daily living for those 2 weeks. Often a patient expresses depression, but the examining physician fails to notice. The depression may be denied by the patient, or it may be hidden except for subtle signs and symptoms.

When a patient with chronic pain meets the criteria outlined in Table 11–1, the psychiatric diagnosis is apparent, but it remains obscure when the

Table 11–2. DIAGNOSTIC CRITERIA FOR BIPOLAR MANIC EPISODE

A. A distinct period of abnormally and persistently elevated expansive or irritable mood.
B. During the period of mood disturbance, at least three of the following symptoms have persisted (four if the mood is only irritable) and have been present to a significant degree.
   (1) Inflated self-esteem or grandiosity.
   (2) Decreased need for sleep, e.g., feels rested after only 3 hours of sleep.
   (3) More talkative than usual or pressure to keep talking.
   (4) Flight of ideas or subjective experience that thoughts are racing.
   (5) Distractibility, i.e., attention too easily drawn to unimportant or irrelevant external stimuli.
   (6) Increase in goal-directed activity (either socially, at work or school, or sexually) or psychomotor agitation.
   (7) Excessive involvement in pleasurable activities that have a high potential for painful consequences, e.g., the person engages in unrestrained buying sprees, sexual indiscretions, or foolish business investments.
C. Mood disturbance sufficiently severe to cause marked impairment in occupational functioning or in usual social activities or relationships with others or to necessitate hospitalization to prevent harm to self or others.
D. At no time during the disturbance have there been delusions or hallucinations for as long as 2 weeks in the absence of prominent mood symptoms (i.e., before the mood symptoms developed or after they have remitted).
E. Not superimposed on schizophrenia, schizophreniform disorder, delusional disorder, or psychotic disorder NOS.
F. It cannot be established that an organic factor initiated and maintained the disturbance (somatic antidepressant treatment, e.g., drugs, ECT); that it apparently precipitates a mood disturbance should not be considered an etiological organic factor.

Source: American Psychiatric Association. Diagnostic and Statistical Manual of Mental Disorders, ed 3 rev. Washington, DC, 1987.

criteria are not precisely met. This type of patient taxes the expertise and efficiency of the therapist.

The depressed patient suffering from chronic pain often becomes defensive when questioned about being depressed for fear of being considered crazy or being told that all the symptoms are "mental." Many patients have been inappropriately approached by their physician or have been exposed to inaccurate information from newspapers, magazine articles, television programs, or personal contacts.

A reliable structured-interview technique for diagnosing DSM-III-R disorders has recently been published,[3] but unfortunately it is time-consuming and is usually used only by psychiatrists or psychologists. It appears best, therefore, to make an appropriate referral for further diagnosis in a manner that allies rather than accuses or threatens the patient. The relationship of depression as a contributing or causative factor in chronic pain must also be carefully evaluated.

The distinction between unipolar and bipolar disorders must also be made. The diagnostic criteria for bipolar disorders are listed in Table 11–2. Other categories of diagnostic criteria include melancholic type of depressive episodes, dysthymia, atypical depression, and masked depression. It must also always be remembered that depression may be a sequela of a medical disorder, such as central nervous disease or endocrine disorder, or the residual of drug use and withdrawal.

Depression has been discussed in the preceding sections on sympathetic mediated pain, chronic pain, and cancer pain and in numerous specific anatomic entities. The management of depression has also been discussed. The addition of this chapter was to offer the diagnostic criteria for major depressive disorders so that the term *depression* not be casually bandied about as the cause of chronic pain or an expected sequela.

Chronic pain will almost always have a component of depression. Homogeneity in the diagnosis of depression applies here as it does in other diagnostic and therapeutic criteria. Its recognition, quantification, and management depend on this clarification.

REFERENCES

1. Dworkin, RH and Gitlin, MJ: Clinical aspects of depression in chronic pain patients. Clin J Pain 7:79–94, 1991.
2. American Psychiatric Association. Diagnostic and Statistical Manual of Mental Disorders, ed 3 rev. Washington, DC, 1987.
3. Spitzer, RL, Williams, JBW, Gibbon, M, and First, MB: Users' guide for the structured clinical interview for DSM-III-R. American Psychiatric Association, Washington, DC, 1990.

CHAPTER 12

Pain in Children

It must be assumed that even premature newborns experience pain, although parents and physicians may not realize it. Rather than subjective demonstration by the patient indicating pain, there are behavioral and physiologic responses that occur: crying, stiffening, facial expression, and visible physiologic features such as sweating and tachycardia. Response to acute pain and illness is ultimately associated with fear and anxiety. Children over age 3 can locate the site of pain, the basis of which can then be confirmed.

It is difficult enough to measure pain in adults, and even more so in children as their language is less precise and descriptive. Often it is the parent who realizes that the child is in pain based on the child's reaction and crying. Pain in the neonate is even more difficult to ascertain and is probably more often ignored than adults appreciate.[1]

Postoperative acute pain is frequently noted in children, but unfortunately it is largely ignored because of the myth that children do not experience pain in the same way as adults and need less medication because of their age and size.

Painful orthopedic problems are frequent and, if recognized, can be easily managed with appropriate medication. Oral analgesics are effective in appropriate doses and duration. In painful operative incisions, neural blocks using long-acting analgesic agents are effective. When pain persists or is excessive, caudal analgesic blocks are effective.

Any painful medical or orthopedic condition can respond to the approach taken in adults. The medication, modality, and method of administration are similar. Chronic pain does exist in children. Even though children are unable to clearly verbalize their feelings, realizing that they can experience pain is important in managing their treatment.[2]

Pain is common in children with cancer; it may result from the cancer itself, the anticancer therapy, or the diagnostic and therapeutic measures

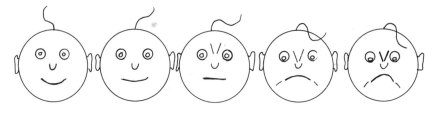

NONE   MILD   MODERATE   SEVERE   VERY SEVERE

Figure 12–1. Picture face scale to evaluate pediatric pain.
This scale allows children with limited vocabulary to identify, by pointing to a picture, the degree of pain they are experiencing. (From Rogers, AG: The assessment of pain and pain relief in children with cancer. Pain 11(Suppl):S11, 1981; with permission.)

used. The following is a partial list of tumor types that can cause pain in children.

- Acute lymphoblastic leukemia
- Chronic myelogenous leukemia
- Hodgkin's disease
- Primary brain tumor
- Rhabdomyosarcoma
- Osteosarcoma
- Ewing's sarcoma
- Wilms' tumor

Whether the site is primary, metastatic, or recurrent must be confirmed. Treatment of the primary disease takes precedence, but the associated pain must also be addressed.

Pain evaluations have been undertaken in specialty medical centers such as pediatric cancer hospitals, but few studies have been undertaken in the general community centers where the primary physician works.[3] Pain in these centers has been largely overlooked and downplayed; medication is often withheld because of a poor understanding of the pain problem and the need for adequate opiate medication.

A child's more limited vocabulary makes verbal grading of the degree of pain in children a difficulty for the pediatrician. A picture face scale (Fig. 12–1), which is graded on a scale of none, mild, moderate, severe, and very severe, may be useful. Such a scale also indicates the severity of the pain from whatever etiology and can then be used periodically to assess the efficacy of the treatment for the pathology and the pain. In using this or any similar scale, the age of the child must be considered; many children below age 3 years cannot be instructed to interpret even these simple drawings.

Pain may result from the treatment or from diagnostic procedures (57 percent) or may occur from other causes of pain unrelated to cancer or its treatment (21 percent).[3] This leaves only 22 percent of cancer patients with pain attributable to the cancer itself.

Of some 5 million patients suffering from cancer, 58 percent complained of intolerable pain.[4] Some figures indicate that 70 percent of patients with advanced cancer have pain as a major symptom.[5]

In adults, pain invokes the feeling of depression, anger, and fear as the pain arises from an "incurable" condition. These feelings may or may not be present in children; it is difficult to be sure in very young children.

Half of patients undergoing anticancer treatment experience pain from the treatment. It is often difficult to differentiate between the disease and the treatment. A proposed management program suggests that the following requirements be met:[4]

1. The patient's pain should be recognized and the patient's assessment of its severity be accepted.
2. The source and mechanism of the pain should be discerned as best as possible.
3. The pharmacology of available analgesics and adjuvants should be fully understood.
4. Analgesic doses and their time factors for administration should be adequate and modified by frequent monitoring.
5. The entire spectrum of available ancillary modalities for addressing pain should be understood.
6. In any management program the low-risk, low-discomfort strategies should be fully explored before resorting to high-risk, complication-prone, invasive and irreversible treatment.

It is thought that chronic pain occurs more frequently in abused and neglected children and in children whose acute pain has been misinterpreted. Medication for acute pain is too often avoided or denied; this allows the pain to persist and compounds the emotional reaction of the abused child. Narcotics in severe pain have been withheld for fear of addiction. The influence on the mother and on the fetus of drug use during pregnancy and breast feeding is being thoroughly studied, but the facts currently remain unclear.

As in adults, pain occurring from cancer may result from tumor invasion (infiltration) of pain-sensitive structures or injury to nerves, bones, and soft tissues as a result of radiotherapy, chemotherapy, or surgery. The three types of pain—somatic, visceral, and deafferentiation—must be ascertained.

Somatic pain occurs from activation of the nociceptors in cutaneous and deeper tissues such as ligaments, bone, and joint tissues. It can usually be localized and will respond to treatment directed at the source and site.

Visceral pain results from infiltration with compression, distension, or stretching of the viscera in the thoracic or abdominal cavity. This pain is poorly localized and is called "deep," "squeezing," or "pressure." Referred pain in a remote area occurs frequently; this may initially confuse the picture. Deafferentiation pain is common. Its mechanism is injury to a peripheral or central nerve component as a consequence of tumor compression, infiltration, or traumatic injury to the nerve resulting from surgery, radiation, chemotherapy, or even the cancer infiltrate. Involvement of these nerves occurs in the periphery, the plexus, or the cord.

Pain in the pediatric population is similar in most respects to pain in adults; only its recognition and acceptance differ. The immediate effects of pain on the infant can be anticipated, but its long-term effects on the psyche remain unclear. Possibly unrecognized and therefore untreated pain in childhood predisposes to ultimate chronic-pain proneness in adulthood. As experience is considered a factor in pain behavior, it seems reasonable to recognize this possibility from underestimating the effects of pain in childhood.

REFERENCES

1. Wilson, PR: Pediatric pain management. Clinical Journal of Pain 7:261, 1991.
2. Anand, KJS, and Hickey, PR: Pain and its effects in the human neonate fetus. N Engl J Med 317:1321, 1987.
3. Elliott, SC, Miser, AW, Dose, AM, Betcher, DL, O'Fallon, JR, Ducos, RS, Shah, NR, Goh, TS, Monzon, CM, and Tschetter, L: Epidemiological features of pain in pediatric cancer patients: A cooperative community-based study. Clinical Journal of Pain 7:263–268, 1991.
4. Abram, SE (ed): Cancer Pain. Kluwer Academic Publishers, Boston, 1989.
5. Foley, KM: The management of pain of malignant origin. In Tyler, HR and Dawson, DM (eds): Current Neurology, Vol 2. Houghton-Mifflin, Boston, pp 279–302.
6. Payne, R: Cancer pain mechanisms and etiology. In Abram, SE (ed): Cancer Pain. Kluwer Academic Publishers, Boston, 1989, pp 1–10.

CHAPTER 13
The Central Pain Syndrome

The concept of central pain expounded by Crue in Chapter 9 is not the same as central pain syndrome, which we address in this chapter. The prevailing definition of central pain syndrome (CPS) is pain arising from disease of the central nervous system: a primary lesion or pathology in the spinal cord, brainstem, or cerebral hemispheres.[1]

Painful lesions that originate in the periphery—with sensitization of the afferents leading to secondary changes in the dorsal root ganglion (DRG), the dorsal horns, and further ascending pathways to the limbic and thalamic system—are not related to CPS. These are secondary changes.

CPS was first identified in the mid-20th century,[3,4] but little additional attention was paid to this syndrome as there were insufficient pathophysiologic information and research until recently.[5]

CLINICAL CHARACTERISTICS OF CENTRAL PAIN SYNDROME

Pain is the most characteristic aspect of CPS. The pain is typically located in the areas of organic sensory loss and is felt deep to the skin surface. This pain is also typically described as aching or burning and is usually described as steady, yet fluctuating in intensity. The pain ranges from moderate to severe. There are often acute brief episodes of intensity described as stabbing pain. Pain is exacerbated by cold temperature, emotions, and even motion.

Stimuli that should not be sensitive can elicit pain in CPS (allodynia) and may be perceived as intense and burning (hyperpathia).

Examination of the CPS patient elicits some neurologic damage or deficit, implying a central neurologic disease. There is often a loss of sensitivity

283

to pinprick and deep stimulation, but tactile, vibratory, and kinesthetic sensation remain intact.[6]

Diagnostic procedures are sparse. Computerized tomographic (CT) and magnetic resonance imaging (MRI) studies may confirm the diagnosis if lesions are found in the area of the central nervous system that is considered the site of organic pathology. Electrically evoked median and tibial somatosensory responses show no significant abnormalities; however, a delay of the potential has been demonstrated.[7]

CPS has been reported in poststroke patients and patients with spinal cord injuries, cord tumors, various thalamic syndromes, and multiple sclerosis.

PATHOMECHANICS OF CENTRAL PAIN SYNDROME

The brain has been considered a passive receptor of afferent information, yet it is constantly modifying experiences even in the absence of normal afferent input. Melzack has demonstrated painful experiences in individuals who have been born without developed limbs. These phantom pains defy explanation by the model of nociceptive afferent impulses and indicate that pain can be experienced without the presence of the limb that would be the site of nociception. Pain can also be experienced by a person with totally interrupted central nervous system pathways such as in paraplegics.[8]

Central nervous system lesions do not merely interrupt afferent impulses to the brain, resulting in the sensation of pain. They possibly disrupt existing neuronal patterns that were there in a dormant or at least inactive status. Melzack postulates that this phenomenon is possible by means of the presence of a substrate of genetically determined body image laid down during maturation. In this concept, the brain is a generator of experiences (sensations) that are modulated by ongoing afferent impulses.

In cat studies, these afferent impulses ascend through spinothalamic tracts and enter the thalamus: 60 percent go to the medial nuclei, 25 percent to the lateral nuclei, and 15 percent to both nuclei.[10] Half of the axons on the neurons in the spinothalamic tracts are found in lamina I of the cord dorsal lamina (Fig. 13–1). The neurons of the dorsal horn respond differently to noxious stimuli and to other forms of stimuli.

The thalamus is located in the very center of the brain; it is enshrouded, except inferiorly, by the cerebrum. It comprises a number of separate discrete nuclei (see Fig. 1–8), which rest directly on top of the midbrain. The thalamus has numerous connections to the cerebral cortex and lies in close apposition to the basal ganglia.

The thalamus is essentially a chief relay station directing sensory and other types of signals from the cord and midbrain into and from the cerebral

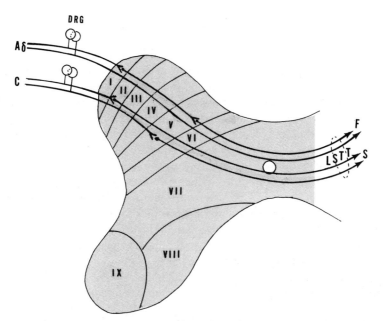

Figure 13–1. Transmission of afferent fibers through the dorsal columns of the cord.
The "acute sharp" signals emit via the A-alpha fibers and the "slow chronic"
signal via the C fibers. On entering the cord they traverse the cord to ascend to the
thalamus via the neospinothalamic tract (fast fibers) and the paleospinothalamic tracts
(slow fibers).
The C fibers synapse within the Rexed layers I and II (SG) and the slow fibers
within the layer V. Some A-alpha fibers initially synapse in layer V.

cortex. It transmits somatesthetic, visual, auditory, and muscle control signals.

As stated in Chapter 1, all pain fiber endings are free nerve endings in
peripheral tissues that use two pathways for transmission: fast-sharp-pain
pathways and slow-chronic-pain pathways. The former are transmitted by
lightly myelinated A-alpha fibers and the latter by unmyelinated C fibers.

Once entering the spinal cord, these fibers synapse within the dorsal
gray matter (Fig. 13–1) into two pathways to the brain. These ascending
tracts are the neospinothalamic and the paleospinothalamic tracts. The former transmit the fast A-alpha impulses and the latter transmit the slower
C-fiber impulses.

Where the C fibers synapse in the dorsal horn, they are believed to
release substance P, a neuropeptide. This peptide builds up slowly at the
synapse, but it is also destroyed slowly, lasting several seconds to several
minutes. This may explain why pain may persist after the painful stimulus
has been removed. The spinothalamic fibers further ascend to terminate at
synapses within the thalamus.

In lower animals the cerebral cortex is not fully developed, whereas the thalamus plays a great role in sensory interpretation. Humans can lose much, if not most, of the cerebral cortex and still retain the ability to perceive pain. This denotes the major role of the thalamus in processing pain sensation.

Without the thalamus, the cortex is essentially useless. The thalamus drives the cortex to activity and relays signals to the cortex from lower spinal and midbrain structures. The thalamus also provides great memory storage, which is constantly available to the cortex for its use.

It has been proposed that neurons in the principal sensory nucleus of the thalamus signal acute pain.[11] When this activity is altered, the activity can generate symptoms of CPS. Increased neuronal activity has been found in these neurons in patients suffering from CPS. This increased activity, termed "bursting," is related to calcium conductance and occurs in specific regions of the nucleus corresponding to the specific part of the body to which the patient relates the pain complaint.

This concept postulates that the thalamus has specific areas related to peripheral regions (Fig. 13–2), and that spontaneous or aberrant activity causes the thalamic nuclei to now generate, as well as transmit, pain impulses. The number and size of cells allegedly increase in the area of the thalamus representing the region of the body. These physiologic activities are influenced by calcium-binding proteins.[12,13]

A lesion of the thalamus causes loss of representation of a part of the body from which there were sensory afferents. Besides being the site of afferent impulses, these groups of cells are also involved in the recovery of these cells lost from the injury.[14]

The ventrobasal complex is topographically organized in what appears to be discriminating sensory function. The medial thalamic nuclei receive a substantial number of neurons from lamina I of the dorsal horn (Fig. 13–1) and may actually encode intensity of the afferent impulses.[15] Direct spinal tract projections to the hypothalamus have been identified in the rat.[16]

Numerous factors influence the excitability of ascending spinothalamic tract neurons. A single lesion in the cord can affect the excitability of the ascending neurons.[17] Descending pathways to the dorsal horn from the periaqueductal gray area may diminish excitability (see Chapter 1). It is well recognized that electrical stimulation of these descending systems produces analgesia. Interruption of these pathways by a cord lesion may alter this phenomenon. Lesions of the medial reticular formation have produced hypoalgesia in cats, but when extended ventrally they produce hyperalgesia, indicating specificity of the function of the thalamic nuclei.

It is accepted that intense or repetitive peripheral nociceptive activity may cause transient or even permanent changes in input: either excitatory or inhibitory. These changes can occur in areas remote from the lesion itself. Nociceptive input can cause central changes in the dorsal horn neurons that

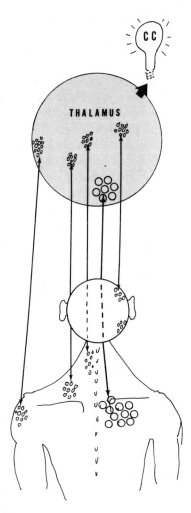

Figure 13–2. Cryptarchitecture of the thalamus.

Cells stimulated in the deep structures such as muscles, joints, and tendons have localization within precise areas of the thalamus (small cells).

With persistent or intense stimulation of these peripheral sites there is an increase in size and number of thalamic cells (large cells).

In cord lesions of the ascending tracts there appears to be an increase in the large active cells that may account for central pain syndrome as these "new" cells generate activity.

make subsequent input more effective or inhibitory mechanisms less effective. This is the plasticity of the central nervous system and also reinforces the concept of Melzack that lesions interfere with the preconceived genetic neural patterns.[8]

These changes can occur in more central regions of the central nervous system than the dorsal horn, including the thalamus. These neurotransmitter changes are of various types of chemical reactions that include calcium calmodulin–dependent protein kinase (gamma-aminobutyric acid [GABA]). Recently, researchers are discovering these various chemicals, and they may ultimately be countered in treatment protocols.

The types of changes in the dorsal horn may also occur at the thalamic level and may include the toxic effect of excitatory amino acids, which cause loss of inhibition by GABA.

The focus of pain perception and modulation is apparently the thalamus, where increased or abnormal activity will result in pain. This conforms to Bonica's classification of reflex sympathetic dystrophy into major and minor components, with the thalamic syndrome being one of the three major reflex sympathetic dystrophy (RSD) (see Chapter 2). CPS has been observed following a thalamic infarct,[18] and CT scans and MRI studies have demonstrated lesions within the central nervous system that relate to the perceived pain.[19] The thalamus remains involved with somatosensory abnormalities in CPS.

The thalamus is an important terminus for spinal pain transmission systems,[20] and transmits pain from the trigeminal system.[21] Electrical stimulation of the thalamus evokes pain. The principal sensory nucleus of the thalamus is the ventralis caudalis and specifically localizes in its structure and function.

CPS apparently disorganizes and reorganizes the somatotropic aspect of the thalamus. Recovery from any of these lesions varies according to time factors as well as to the precise neuronal and pathologic aspects of the lesions.

The ultimate site of pain interpretation, the cerebral cortex, is also being studied molecularly.[22] In 1911, Head and Holmes discovered that destruction of the cortex alone did not disturb the threshold for pain sensation but could actually elevate the pain threshold and markedly diminish the brain's ability to localize the site of noxious stimuli.[23]

It is obvious that in CPS the mechanism of pain originating from the neural structures of the cord, midbrain, thalamus, and cerebral cortex remains obscure.[24] The central nervous system—originally considered inert and insensitive—is now known to be a nociceptive site, with the site being in the cord.

Pain modulation has been well documented. An analgesia system exists in which pain can be modified by ascending and descending pathways. The presence of a pain facilitatory system is now being postulated.[25] Efferent excitation of the dorsal horn pain transmission system is proposed.

These on-cells emit from the rostral ventromedial medulla (RVM) and invoke a reaction in the T cells of the dorsal horn. This seems to be an apparent contradiction to the gate theory of pain, yet it is neurophysiologically also related to this theory. Nociceptive modulation is thus facilitatory and/or inhibitory.[26,27] A feedback loop system may alter negative to positive pain modulation and will, if confirmed, involve the neurophysiologic neurochemical afferent-efferent system from the midbrain periaqueductal and the RVM. What actually triggers incitatory impulses remains obscure.

With further study, neural pathways, both electrical and chemical, will emerge that will probably shed light on peripheral mechanisms, central mechanisms, and neurotransmitter chemicals. Effective treatment could emerge that will benefit both peripheral and central pain mechanisms.

TREATMENT

Treatment of CPS is notoriously difficult depending on the etiologic lesions, the intensity of the pain, its duration, and the toleration and acceptance by the patient. Treatment remains palliative in that most efforts appear to reduce rather than eliminate the pain.

Most clinicians consider opiate medications and serotonin-enhancing drugs ineffective.[28,29] There are treatment centers, however, that have found these drugs to be effective if properly used for sufficient time.

The antidepressant drugs are generally considered to be the most effective. Their value in peripheral neurogenic pains (see Chapter 4) does not necessarily translate to CPS, however. Amitriptyline and carbamazepine have been favorably evaluated against placebos and found effective, with approximately 50 percent of patients experiencing relief for 2 to 24 months.[30]

The mechanism by which antidepressants work is not clearly understood. They may influence serotonergic noradrenergic, cholinergic, or dopamine systems, with inhibition of reuptake of serotonin by the central nervous system as the most probable conclusion. Desipramine, a norepinephrine reuptake blocker, relieves pain, suggesting that this action is a possible mechanism.[31]

Intravenous administration of lidocaine, which has been effective in treating chronic diabetic painful neuropathy, is being studied in treating CPS.[32] If so, oral lidocaine-like medications may be effective.[33]

Anticonvulsive drugs have been effectively used in peripheral neuropathies and probably exert their effect through inactivation of calcium channels,[34] whereas clonazepam and sodium valproate bind to a receptor associated with GABA. Determination of adequate plasma concentration is important in giving effective doses of the above.

Adrenergic drugs have also been effective in neurogenic pain treatment. Clonidine, an alpha$_2$-adrenergic agonist, appears to modulate serotonin and norepinephrine release in the dorsal horn.[35] In multiple sclerosis, which is a source of CPS, clonidine has been effective in relieving painful spasms and symptoms of CPS.[36]

Cholinergic drugs increase pain thresholds by either systemic or spinal administrative routes. These include acetylcholine, physostigmine, and distigmine. Physostigmine given subcutaneously and followed by oral medication has proven effective.[37]

Local anesthetics (lidocaine) and antiarrhythmic drugs related to lidocaine have also been advanced.[38] Intravenous lidocaine used diagnostically and found beneficial is followed by mexiletine administered orally.

Use of physical agents to influence CPS has merit and is being assessed. To be effective they must (1) destroy or diminish spontaneous activity in the cells within the sensory system that is considered to be causative of pain, (2) interrupt the sensory input of the aspects of the sensory system considered

290 PAIN: MECHANISMS AND MANAGEMENT

to be disrupted, (3) normalize these disrupted inhibitory activities, (4) increase the activity of normal inhibitory mechanisms, and/or (5) influence the analysis of sensory information by the cortex.

Transcutaneous electrical nerve stimulation (TENS) has been generally disappointing in treating CPS, but because some patients have received relief for up to 2 years it merits evaluation.[39]

Spinal cord stimulation would appear to be a logical modality in CPS as it allegedly affects the spinal inhibitory mechanisms of the ascending tracts.[40] There are currently few reports of its use in CPS, but those that have been reported have expressed optimism.[41] The fact that spinal cord stimulation destroys ascending mechanoceptive fibers implies a limited benefit for long-term relief.

Deep-brain stimulation with electrode implants in the periaqueductal gray or periventricular gray has been used in chronic pain syndromes since the early 1970s,[42] but significant experience with CPS is not yet ascertained.[43]

Ablative procedures in which a portion of the central nervous system is destroyed are considered a last resort, as some of these procedures have caused rather than relieved pain.[44] These ablative procedures relate to destruction of the spinal cord, brainstem, and brain.

Destructive procedures of the spinal cord affect the dorsal root entry zone and substantia gelatinosa. They are performed by radiofrequency electrode or surgical incision (see Fig. 8–41). Anterolateral cordotomy at the cervical level has been reported as effective up to 1 year.[45]

Spinothalamic tractotomy in the medulla oblongata (brainstem ablation) has been used for chronic intractable pain especially from cancer. As yet, there are few reports of its use in CPS, but in a limited series it has been promising.[46]

Cortectomy (brain ablation) procedures have been successful, but limited in their benefit as to duration.[44] Final beneficial reports of ablative procedures are needed, but most ablative procedures are used in the stage of last resort and only in intractable, severely disabling conditions of CPS when all other treatment modalities have been exhausted.

REFERENCES

1. Mersky, H (ed): Classification of chronic pain. Pain (Suppl) 3:S1–S225, 1986.
2. Dubner, R: Neuronal plasticity in the spinal and medullary dorsal horns: A possible role in central pain mechanisms. In Casey, KL (ed): Pain and Central Nervous System Disease: The Central Pain Syndrome. Raven Press, New York, 1991, pp 143–155.
3. Bonica, JJ: The Management of Pain. Lea & Febiger, Philadelphia, 1953.
4. Cassineri, V and Pagni, CA: Central Pain: A Neurosurgical Survey. Harvard University Press, Cambridge, MA, 1969.
5. Casey, KL (ed): Pain and Central Nervous System Disease. Raven Press, New York, 1991, pp 1–11.

6. Boivie, J and Leijon, G: Clinical findings in patients with central poststroke pain. In Casey, KL (ed): Pain and Central Nervous System Disease. Raven Press, New York, 1991, pp 65–75.

7. Holmgren, H, Leijon, G, Boivie, J, Johansson, I and Ilievska, L: Central post-stroke pain-somatosensory evoked potentials in relation to location of the lesion and sensory signs. Pain 40:43–52, 1990.

8. Melzack, R and Loeser, JD: Phantom body pain in paraplegics: Evidence for central "pattern generating mechanisms" for pain. Pain 4:195–210, 1978.

9. Melzack, R: Central pain syndromes and theories of pain. In Casey, KL (ed): Pain and Central Nervous System Disease. Raven Press, New York, 1991, pp 59–64.

10. Craig, AD Jr, Linington, AJ, and Kniffki, K-D: Cells of origin of spinothalamic tract projection to the medial and lateral thalamus in the cat. J Comp Neurol 2289:558–585, 1989.

11. Lnz, FA: The ventral posterior nucleus of thalamus is involved in the generation of central pain syndromes. APS Journal 1(1):42–51, 1992.

12. Kohr, G, Lambert, CE, and Mody, I: Inactivation of HVA calcium currents in granule cells following kindling-induced epilepsy: The Ca-2 buffering role of calbinding D 28K (CaBP). Soc Neurosci Abstr 16:623, 1990.

13. Sloviter, RS: Calcium-binding protein (calbinding-D28K) paralbumin immunocytochemistry: Localization in the rat hippocampus with special reference to the seizure activity. J Comp Neurol 280:183–196, 1989.

14. Wall, PD and Egger, MD: Formation of new connections in adult rat brains after partial deafferentiation. Nature 232:466–475, 1971.

15. Bushnel, MC and Duncan, GH: Sensory and affective aspects of pain perception: Is [the] medial thalamus restricted to emotional issues? Exp Brain Res 78:415–418, 1989.

16. Burstein, R, Cliffer, KD, and Geisler, JG, Jr: Direct somatosensory projections from the spinal cord to the hypothalamus and teleocephalon. Neuroscience 7:4159–4164, 1987.

17. Zimmermann, M: Central nervous system mechanisms modulating pain-related information: Do they become deficient after lesions of the peripheral or central nervous system disease? In Casey, KL (ed): Pain and Central Nervous System Disease. Raven Press, New York, 1991, pp 183–199.

18. Dejerine, J and Roussay, G: La syndrome thalamique. Rev Neurol (Paris) 14:521–532, 1906.

19. Lewis-Jones, H, Smith, T, Bowsher, D, and Leijon, G: Magnetic resonance imaging in 36 cases of central poststroke pain (CPSP). Pain (Suppl) 5:S278, 1990.

20. Willis, WD: The pain system. Basel: Karger, 1985.

21. Cailliet, R: Head and Face Pain Syndromes, ed 1. FA Davis, Philadelphia, 1992.

22. Black, IB: Information in the Brain: A Molecular Perspective. MIT Press, Cambridge, MA, 1991.

23. Head, H and Holmes, G: Sensory disturbances from cerebral lesions. Brain 34:102–254, 1911.

24. Casey, KL, Huang, GC-H, and Marrow, TJ: The role of cortical, thalamic and subthalamic neurones in pain: Evidence from laser-evoked potentials and sensory testing in patients and normal subjects. Soc Neurosci Abstr 470:15, 1989.

25. Fields, HL: Is there a facilitating component to central pain modulation? APS J 1(2):71–78, 1992.

26. Gebhart, GF: Can endogenous systems produce pain? APS J 1(2):79–84, 1992.

27. LeBars, D, Villanueva, L, and Willert, J-C: Pain modulation: From a negative to a positive feedback loop. APS J 1(2):85–89, 1992.

28. Hammond, DL: Do opioids relieve central pain? In Casey, KL (ed): Pain and Central Nervous System Disease. Raven Press, New York, 1991, pp 233–241.

29. Leijon, G and Boivie, J: Pharmacological treatment of central pain. In Casey, KL (ed): Pain and Central Nervous System Disease. Raven Press, New York, 1991, pp 257–266.
30. Leijon, G and Boivie, J: Central post-stroke pain: A controlled trial of amitryptyline and carbamazepine. Pain 36:27–36, 1989.
31. Kishore-Kumar, R, Max, MB, and Schafter, SC: Desipramine relieves post-herpetic neuralgia. Clin Pharmacol Ther 47:305–312, 1990.
32. Kastrup, J, Petersen, P, Dejgard, A, Angelo, HR, and Milstedt, J: Intravenous lidocaine infusion—a new treatment of chronic painful diabetic neuropathy. Pain 28:69–75, 1987.
33. Loeser, JD: Personal communication, 1992.
34. Swerdlow, M: Anticonvulsants in the therapy of neuralgic pain. Pain Clinic 1:9–19, 1986.
35. Gordt, T: Alpha-2 Adrenoreceptor Agonist Drugs for Spinal Analgesia—From Hypothesis to Clinical Use. Doctoral dissertation, Uppsala University, 1987.
36. Glynn, C, Jamous, MA, Teddy, PJ, Moorea, RA, and Lloyd, JW: Role of spinal noradrenergic system in transmission of pain in patients with spinal cord injury. Lancet 2:1249–1250, 1986.
37. Schott, GD and Loh, L: Anticholinesterase drugs in the treatment of chronic pain. Pain 20:201–206, 1984.
38. Lindstrom, P and Lindstrom, U: The analgesic effect of tocainide in trigeminal neuralgia. Pain 28:45–50, 1987.
39. Sjolund, BH: The role of transcutaneous electrical nerve stimulation, central nervous system stimulation, ablative procedures in central pain syndrome. In Casey, KL (ed): Pain and Central Nervous System Disease. Raven Press, New York, 1991, pp 267–274.
40. Shealy, CN, Mortimer, JT and Resnick, J: Electrical inhibition of pain by stimulation of the dorsal column: Preliminary clinical reports. Anesth Analg 46:489–491, 1967.
41. Richardson, RR, Meyer, PR, and Cerullo, L: Neurostimulation in the modulation of intractable paraplegic and traumatic neuroma pains. Pain 8:75–84, 1980.
42. Richardson, DE and Akil, H: Long-term results of periventricular gray self-stimulation. Neurosurgery 1:199–202, 1977.
43. Tasker, RR: Pain resulting from central nervous system pathology (central pain). In Bonica, JJ (ed): The Management of Pain, ed 2. Lea & Febiger, Philadelphia, 1990, pp 264–286.
44. Cassnari, V and Pagni, CA: Central pain: A neurosurgical survey. Harvard University Press, Cambridge, MA, 1969.
45. Turnbull, F: Chordotomy for thalamic pain: A case report. Yale J Biol Med 11:411–414, 1939.
46. Amano, K, Kawamura, H, Tanikawa, T: Long-term follow-up study of rostral mesencephalic reticulotomy for pain relief: Report of 34 cases. Appl Neurophysiol 49:104–111, 1986.

Index

An "f" following a page number indicates a figure.

293